Conduct Disorders in Children and Adolescents

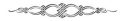

Conduct Disorders in Children and Adolescents

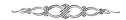

Edited by
G. Pirooz Sholevar, M.D.

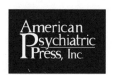

Washington, DC
London, England

Copyright © 1995 American Psychiatric Press, Inc.
ALL RIGHTS RESERVED
Manufactured in the United States of America on acid-free paper
98 97 96 95   4 3 2 1
First Edition

American Psychiatric Press, Inc.
1400 K Street, N.W., Washington, DC 20005

Library of Congress Cataloging-in-Publication Data
Conduct disorders in children and adolescents / edited by G. Pirooz Sholevar.
        p.   cm.
    Includes bibliographical references and index.
    ISBN 0-88048-517-5
    1. Conduct disorders in children. 2. Conduct disorders in adolescence.   I. Sholevar, G. Pirooz.
    [DNLM: 1. Child Behavior Disorders—therapy. 2. Social Behavior Disorders—in adolescence. 3. Child Behavior Disorders—etiology. 4. Child Behavior Disorders—diagnosis.   WS 350.6 C746 1994]
    RJ506.C65C66 1994
    616.92′89—dc20
    DNLM/DLC   94-26150
    for Library of Congress   CIP

British Library Cataloguing in Publication Data
A CIP record is available from the British Library.

This book is
dedicated
to my son,

Darius.

Contents

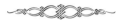

Section I: Overview, Etiology, and Assessment

Contributors

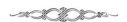

Balkozar Adam, M.D.
Assistant Professor and Medical Director, Arkansas Children's Hospital, Turning Point Child Unit; Division of Child and Adolescent Psychiatry, University of Arkansas for Medical Sciences, Little Rock, Arkansas

Seth Aronson, Psy.D.
Assistant Director, Child and Adolescent Psychiatry, Bronx Municipal Hospital Center, Albert Einstein College of Medicine, Bronx, New York

Efrain Bleiberg, M.D.
Executive Vice President/Chief of Staff, The Menninger Clinic, Topeka, Kansas

David Boulifard, B.A.
Harvard Medical School, Division of Child and Adolescent Psychiatry, The Cambridge Hospital, Boston, Massachusetts

Ana Campo-Bowen, M.D.
Department of Psychiatry, University of Miami School of Medicine, Miami, Florida

Elizabeth L. Hart, Ph.D.
Research Fellow, Yale Child Study Center, Yale University, New Haven, Connecticut

Benjamin B. Lahey, Ph.D.
Visiting Professor, Department of Psychiatry, University of Chicago, Chicago, Illinois

Richard Livingston, M.D.
Professor and Director, Division of Child and Adolescent Psychiatry, Department of Psychiatry, New Jersey Medical School—University of Medicine and Dentistry of New Jersey, Newark, New Jersey

Rolf Loeber, Ph.D.
Professor, Department of Psychiatry, University of Pittsburgh School of Medicine, Western Psychiatric Institute and Clinic, Pittsburgh, Pennsylvania

Karen Longest, M.A.
Psychology intern, Department of Psychiatry, Oklahoma University Health Sciences Center, Oklahoma City, Oklahoma

Keith McBurnett, Ph.D.
Assistant Professor, Department of Pediatrics, University of California Child Development Center, Irvine, California

John Meeks, M.D.
Clinical Professor of Psychiatry, Georgetown University Medical School, Washington, DC

Jeffrey Metzner, M.D.
Associate Clinical Professor of Psychiatry and Director of Young Sex Offenders Treatment Program, University of Colorado Health Sciences Center, Henry Kempe National Center for Prevention and Treatment of Child Abuse and Neglect, Denver, Colorado

Kerim Munir, M.D., Sc.D.
Assistant Professor, Department of Psychiatry, Harvard Medical School; Director, Pediatric Psychopharmacology, Division of Child and Adolescent Psychiatry, The Cambridge Hospital, Cambridge, Massachusetts

Steven I. Pfeiffer, Ph.D.
Director of Clinical Training and Research, Devereux Foundation, Devon, Pennsylvania; Faculty, Temple University, Philadelphia, Pennsylvania

Ronald J. Prinz, Ph.D.
Carolina Research Professor, University of South Carolina, Columbia, South Carolina

Gail D. Ryan, M.A.
Director, Perpetration Prevention Project, Henry Kempe National Center for Prevention and Treatment of Child Abuse and Neglect, Denver, Colorado

Jon A. Shaw, M.D.
Professor and Director, Division of Child and Adolescent, Department
of Psychiatry, University of Miami School of Medicine, Miami, Florida

Saul Scheidlinger, Ph.D.
Emeritus Professor of Psychiatry (Child Psychology), Albert Einstein
College of Medicine, Bronx, New York; Adjunct Professor of Clinical
Psychology in Psychiatry, Cornell University Medical College,
Westchester Division, White Plains, New York

Ellen Harris Sholevar, M.D.
Director, Division of Child and Adolescent Psychiatry, Department of
Psychiatry, Temple University School of Medicine, Philadelphia,
Pennsylvania

G. Pirooz Sholevar, M.D.
Professor and Chair, Department of Psychiatry, Cooper Hospital/
University Medical Center, Robert Wood Johnson Medical School,
University of Medicine and Dentistry of New Jersey, Camden, New
Jersey

E. Eugene Walker, Ph.D.
Professor, Department of Psychiatry and Behavioral Sciences,
Oklahoma University Health Sciences Center, Oklahoma City,
Oklahoma

Karen C. Wells, Ph.D.
Associate Professor of Medical Psychology, Duke University Medical
Center, Durham, North Carolina

Gregory G. Wilkins, Ph.D.
Director of Psychology, Brandywine Center, The Devereux
Foundation, Devon, Pennsylvania

Jacquelyn Miller Zavodnick, M.D.
Clinical Professor of Psychiatry, Robert Wood Johnson Medical
School, University of Medicine and Dentistry of New Jersey, Camden,
New Jersey

Acknowledgment

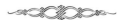

I wish to thank Linda Schwoeri, M.A., M.F.T., for her valuable and sensitive editorial assistance with this manuscript, particularly Chapters 1, 10, and 16.

Introduction

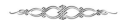

Conduct disorder is the most commonly referred psychological problem to child psychiatric and mental health services. The prevalence of antisocial behavior is estimated to be significantly higher in the general population than in the clinical cases; however, such behaviors remain unreported in many instances and these children do not receive intervention at an early age. The etiology of conduct disorder in children and adolescents is highly complex. Among the more recognized etiological factors are parental skill deficits, social immaturity and narcissistic vulnerability of the child, sociological factors affecting the parental psychosocial and economic status, and school and neighborhood environment. The temperament of the child may also be a significant contributor to the development of the disorder, although the nature of its contribution is poorly understood.

This volume examines the complexities involved in the etiology, diagnosis, and treatment of conduct disorder in children and adolescents. The book is divided into two sections.

In Section I, the phenomenology, etiology, and diagnosis of conduct disorder are examined. Chapter 1 presents an overview of conduct disorders as a group of serious and chronic psychiatric disorders. Prevalence, symptomatology, longitudinal course, and duration, as well as subtypes distinguished in the DSM-III-R (American Psychiatric Association 1987), are discussed. Chapter 2, on the psychobiology of conduct disorder, explores the possible role of biological factors in various subgroups of conduct disorder. In addition to Gray's theory of dysfunction in reward and inhibition systems, the new investigations with serotonin may shed light on some of the biological characteristics and vulnerabilities of children with conduct disorder, particularly in the area of irritability. Chapter 3 examines the stability of aggression as a developmental and personality characteristic and its relationship to conduct disorder. The significant issue of comorbidity of conduct disorder with other childhood disorders, such as attention-deficit hyperactivity disorder (ADHD) and depression, is discussed in Chapter 4. A review of the use of multiple rating scales with youths with conduct disorder is provided in Chapter 5. In addition to serving as diagnostic tools, rating scales may be helpful in demonstrating the level of improvement in conduct disorder with intervention. Chapters 6 and 7 examine the overlap between conduct disorder and criminal behavior with serious consequences—specifically, murderous actions and sexual offenses.

In Section II, therapeutic and preventive interventions are highlighted. Multiple chapters address the application of different treatment and preventive modalities with children and adolescents with conduct disorder. Chapter 8 describes the use of individual psychotherapy with youths with conduct disorder and its application to their narcissistic vulnerability. Chapter 9 summarizes the work of Paulina Kernberg and Saralea Chazan in providing a manual-based intervention for children with conduct disorder, both individually and in a group, as well as interventions with their parents. Various approaches to family intervention with children with conduct disorder, including the schools of functional family therapy, structural family therapy, and psychodynamic family therapy, are reviewed in Chapter 10; the interfaces among family intervention, hospitalization, and residential treatment are considered as well. In Chapter 11, two parent management training programs—those of Hanf-Forehand and of Patterson and Reid—are described. A review of the empirical basis and outcome studies for these programs is included. Chapters 12 and 13 outline the rationale and methodology of group therapy and behavior therapy, respectively, with youths with conduct disorder. The various psychopharmacological agents used in the treatment of children with conduct disorder are examined in Chapter 14. In Chapter 15, an overview of the multiple functions of hospitalization for children with conduct disorder is presented, followed by a discussion of the use of hospitalization as a crucial element in the range of psychotherapeutic modalities necessary for treatment of this disorder. Chapter 16 describes the role of residential treatment centers—a modality that is being increasingly applied in interventions with children with conduct disorder. The significant issue of preventive intervention and multiple preventive models with children with conduct disorder is considered in Chapter 17. Finally, Chapter 18 contemplates new directions in research findings with conduct disorder.

G. Pirooz Sholevar, M.D.

Section I

Overview, Etiology, and Assessment

Chapter 1

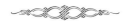

Overview

G. *Pirooz Sholevar, M.D.*
Ellen Harris Sholevar, M.D.

Conduct disorder comprises a pervasive group of serious and chronic psychiatric disorders in children and adolescents. These disorders are characterized by persistent aggression, theft, vandalism, fire setting, running away, truancy, defying authority, and other behaviors referred to as "antisocial." Such behaviors violate the basic rights of others and deviate from age-appropriate societal norms and rules. A variety of terms have been applied to this group of behaviors, including *delinquency, antisocial behavior, externalizing behavior,* and *conduct disorder.* Although seemingly diverse, these behaviors usually cluster together; violate legal, familial, or academic codes as well as major societal rules and expectations; and constitute transgressions against persons and property. They represent "recurrent violations of socially prescribed patterns of behavior" (Loeber and Schmaling 1985b, p. 338; Simcha-Fagan et al. 1975).

Antisocial behavior is a term that broadly refers to any behavior that violates social rules or represents an action against others. Such behavior includes fighting, lying, and stealing. The term *conduct disorder* (CD) refers to patterns of antisocial behavior exhibited by children or adolescents coupled with significant impairment in everyday functioning at home or school to the degree that the behavior is considered unmanageable by significant others. The term is reserved for antisocial behavior that is clinically significant and clearly beyond the range of normal functioning and that brings the youth into contact with various social agencies, including mental health services and the

The authors wish to thank Ben Lahey, Ph.D., for his valuable contribution to this chapter. Dr. Lahey's work is mainly reflected in the section on subgrouping of conduct disorders.

juvenile justice system. Such behavior frequently requires assignment to special educational settings or programs within the school system. Therefore, CD refers to a severe level of antisocial behavior in which the everyday functioning of the individual is impaired, as defined by parents, teachers, and significant others.

CD is one of the most common and serious psychiatric disorders affecting children and adolescents. It disrupts the developmental course during childhood and adolescence and creates impairment and suffering both for the child and for those who most interact with him or her. CD is of major concern to child and adolescent psychiatrists because it constitutes the most common reason for referral to child and adolescent clinical services. Many additional cases of CD exist that are never referred for treatment; the total number of such untreated cases remains uncertain (Robins et al. 1991). Unfortunately, this disorder has proven highly resistant to psychosocial interventions (Kazdin et al. 1987). Therefore, it can serve as a forerunner to adult antisocial personality disorder, substance abuse, and other serious social problems in adulthood. When grown up, youths with CD are likely to exhibit significant social maladjustment or criminal behavior and to pass along antisocial behaviors to their children, who continue the cycle. The prognosis for children with CD is poor: about half of the children referred to clinics will exhibit antisocial behavior in adulthood (Robins 1966, 1978).

In DSM-III-R (American Psychiatric Association 1987), CD is grouped with attention-deficit hyperactivity disorder (ADHD) and oppositional defiant disorder (ODD) under the category of disruptive disorders. Both ADHD and ODD are possible precursors to some forms of CD, and their presence with CD usually denotes a poorer prognosis than for CD that appears first in adolescence. In DSM-IV (American Psychiatric Association 1994), ODD and CD are grouped into one category in recognition of their frequent co-occurrence.

Both undersocialized and socialized patterns of CD have been firmly and empirically established. The undersocialized aggressive pattern of CD is particularly ubiquitous and well defined empirically. Hyperactivity, as a behavioral characteristic, is frequently found to be associated with the undersocialized type of CD. One study identified a subgroup of children with CD who are developmentally overactive as well as aggressive (Stewart and Behar 1983; Stewart et al. 1981). Stewart and Behar (1983) suggested that individuals with CD who also exhibit hyperactivity and attentional problems are more likely to show cognitive, linguistic, and academic deficits.

Sociocultural and family aggression has shown a marked association with CD. More recently, biological vulnerability has been suspected in CD, especially CD accompanied by aggression.

Individuals with CD may be identified by other categories and "labels" by non–child psychiatrists. They may be defined as "aggressive" by school psychologists, as "learning disabled" or "hyperactive" by pediatricians and educators, and as "delinquent" by criminologists. Many of the behaviors of delinquent youths and youths with CD overlap and are conventionally viewed as antisocial behavior. Although there are considerable similarities between CD and delinquency, there are also many differences. Youths with CD may not necessarily engage in behaviors that are defined as delinquent or have any contact with police and courts.

Prevalence

It is difficult to measure the prevalence of CD because of a variety of factors, including differences in the criteria used for definition and variations in the rate of conduct problems in children of different ages, sexes, socioeconomic classes, and geographical locales. Estimates of the rate of CD among children have ranged from approximately 4% to 10% (Rutter et al. 1970, 1975). Epidemiological studies have provided varying estimates of the frequency of CD in children of different ages in the general population; these estimates range from 3.2% for 10-year-olds in Isle of Wight, United Kingdom (Rutter et al. 1970), to 5.5% of 4- to 16-year-olds in Ontario, Canada (Offord et al. 1987), to 6.7% of 10-year-olds in Queensland, Australia (Connell et al. 1982), to 6.9% of 7-year-olds in Dunedin, New Zealand (McGee et al. 1984).

The prevalence of CD tends to be reported as much greater when nonclinical populations are assessed by an anonymous survey. Large-scale evaluations conducted among nonclinical children and adolescents who were asked to report on their delinquent and antisocial behaviors have revealed much higher prevalence rates of antisocial and delinquent behavior than usually shown in official records (Elliott et al. 1981; Farrington 1978; Johnston et al. 1982). These studies have provided important information about antisocial youths and their families.

Evaluations of the prevalence rate of CD should consider the age of the children. In the large-scale study of Werry and Quay (1971), children of both sexes exhibited a high prevalence of disruptive, disobedient, fighting, hyperactive, restless, boisterous, and attention-seeking behavior. In another large-scale, anonymous survey of a midwestern high school, Cernkovich and Giordano (1979; cited in Achenbach 1982 and in King and Noshpitz 1991) reported rates of the following behaviors for boys and girls, respectively: burglary of occupied residences—10% and 2%; burglary of unoccupied residences—17% and 4%; theft—13%–34% and 5%–26%; early sexual intercourse—78% and 62%; sex for money—5% and 1%; carrying a weapon—34% and 17%; running away from home—16% for both sexes; using hard drugs—15% and 19%; selling marijuana—35% and 20%; and school probation/suspension/expulsion—32% and 27%.

In a questionnaire study of a nonclinical population of high school students, Offer et al. (1987) reported a prevalence rate for CD of 11% for boys and 8.4% for girls. Among youths 13 to 18 years of age, more than 50% admitted to theft, 35% to assault, 45% to property destruction, and 60% to engaging in more than one type of antisocial behavior.

In terms of *geographical distribution and settings,* Rutter et al. (1975) reported a prevalence rate of approximately 4% for CD in a rural context. Graham (1979) reported a prevalence rate of 8% within an urban setting in a population of boys and girls. The prevalence of CD was found to be 1.5% in 4- to 16-year-olds in Puerto Rico (Bird et al. 1988); 3.2% in 10-year-olds in the Isle of Wight, United Kingdom (Rutter et al. 1970); 3.4% in 11-year-olds (Anderson 1987) and 6.9% in 7-year-olds in Dunedin, New Zealand (McGee et al. 1984); and 5.5% in 6- to 13-year-olds in Ontario, Canada (Boyle et al. 1987). These epidemiological studies report a preponderance of the disorder in boys (Anderson 1987; McGee et al. 1984; Offord et al. 1987). In the Isle of Wight cohort, for example, the high male preponderance of CD was responsible for the overall elevated rate of psychopathology in males (Rutter et al. 1970). The total population prevalence varies depending on the characteristics of the sample (e.g., age of subject), the setting (e.g., urban or rural), and the sampling method and classification instrument used to measure disorders (Costello 1989).

The *precise sex ratio* of CD is hard to specify because of different methodologies used by different investigators. However, it seems that antisocial behavior is at least three times more common among boys than among girls (Graham 1979). Sex differences are also apparent in the age at onset of the disorder. Robins (1966) has reported that the median age at onset of the disorder for children referred for conduct problems is in the 8- to 10-year age range. Most boys had an onset before the age of 10 (median = 7 years old). For girls, onset was in the 14- to 16-year-old range (median = 13 years old). For boys, aggression and/or theft was the most likely presenting problem, whereas for girls it was sexual misconduct.

The diagnosis of CD in children is seldom made before school age (Robins 1978; Robins and Price 1991). In clinical populations, 50% of children with CD are believed to continue to exhibit antisocial behaviors into adulthood. Early-onset CD (prior to the advent of puberty) is believed to have a more persistent course compared with later-onset forms (Robins 1966, 1978; Robins and Price 1991).

CD and antisocial behavior are the major reasons for referral to outpatient and inpatient psychiatric services. It is estimated that between one-third and one-half of all children and adolescents referred to outpatient services have a diagnosis of CD or antisocial behavior (Gilbert 1957; Herbert 1978; Robins 1981). Costello and Angold (1988) have reported that 2.6% of 7- to 11-year-olds in pediatric primary care populations in the United States are referred for CD and antisocial behavior.

— — — — — — — — — — — —

Longitudinal Course

CD is relatively stable over time, a characteristic that sets it apart from many other disorders of childhood. It is unlikely that a child with consistent antisocial behavior will "grow out of it." Because of the stability of the condition and its resistance to conventional treatment, the long-term prognosis for CD is relatively poor. CD in childhood continues into adulthood and manifests itself in a range of disturbances that include criminal behavior, alcoholism, antisocial personality, and other diagnosable psychiatric disorders. Adults who as children had CD tend to have poor marital and occupational adjustment (Robins 1966; Wolfgang et al. 1972).

The limited information on population studies points to the stability of CD and oppositional defiant symptoms throughout the course of development. Early-onset aggressive behaviors are believed to persist (Loeber 1982). Antisocial behaviors are also believed to be stable, as noted in the Dunedin Longitudinal Study of children from birth to 15 years of age (White et al. 1991). The Dunedin study showed that 84% of children who were found to be uncontrollable at age 11 years met criteria for stable and pervasive antisocial disorders when reassessed at age 13 years.

Antisocial behavior at age 13 was predicted by "externalizing behavior" at age 3 and behavior problems at age 5 (White et al. 1991). The same study suggested that, compared with early-onset CD, antisocial behavior that appears for the first time at around 13 years of age tends to have a benign course, particularly in girls (Moffitt 1990; Robins 1980). Such behavior is usually related to problems surrounding puberty and could be considered "normative adolescent delinquency."

Robins and Wish (1977) have described a possible course for CD. Shortly after first entering school, the child is repeatedly truant. Academic difficulties follow, often culminating in school failure. Alcohol abuse appears, accompanied or followed by sexual misconduct—typically in the form of promiscuity—and progressing to school dropout, drug abuse, and delinquency.

A study of the early infancy of children who subsequently developed CD identified a high incidence of early object loss, particularly between 6 and 12 months of age (King and Noshpitz 1991). The behavioral problems of hyperactivity, invasiveness, destructiveness, persistent biting, running away, and power struggles surfaced in the second year of life. Cruelty to pets and aggressive behavior toward peers and siblings were common, as were enuresis, learning difficulties, and frequent problems with truancy.

Although systematic, prospective studies—beginning in infancy—of children who subsequently develop CD are lacking, parents of children with CD often recall early irritability and uncooperativeness dating back to their offsprings' infancy. The New York Longitudinal Study, which followed children from infancy and early childhood (cited in Achenbach and Edelbrock 1981), presented some evidence that the "quiet" child may be more likely to develop this disorder. A systematic study of 2,600 children between the ages of 4 and 16 (Achenbach and Edelbrock 1983) identified argumentativeness, stubbornness, and tantrums as the early signs of subsequent CD. Those behaviors are followed by oppositional behavior, fire setting, and stealing. The last behaviors to appear are truancy, vandalism, and substance abuse. Achenbach and Edelbrock (1981) conclude that tantrums and fighting decline with age, lying appears at all ages, stealing increases until age 10 and then declines, and truancy and substance abuse increase throughout the age span. Loeber (1982) suggests that those arrested early are more likely to be recidivist and to have subsequent arrests.

Aggressive behavior in childhood is the most stable of early detectable personality characteristics. Olweus (1979) reviewed 18 follow-up studies that estimated a 0.63 correlation between early and subsequent aggression—a stability exceeded only by that of IQ.

Grown-Up Children With CD

Longitudinal studies of children with CD have consistently shown that clinically referred youths continue to exhibit social dysfunction, problematic behavior, and poor school adjustment as they age (Bachman et al. 1978; Glueck and Glueck 1950; Huesmann et al. 1984; Robins 1966, 1978). As adults, these individuals display a high level of criminal behavior, symptomatology, and dysfunction. Compared with control subjects, adults who as children had CD exhibit greater psychiatric impairment, including antisocial personality, anxiety, and somatization symptoms; drug and alcohol abuse; and high rates of psychiatric hospitalization. They likewise show higher rates of arrest, conviction, and imprisonment for relatively serious criminal acts. Occupationally, these adults have high rates of unemployment, employment of short duration and in lower status jobs, frequent job changes, and dependence on financial assistance from welfare. Compared with control subjects, youths with CD have higher rates of school dropout and—for those who remain in school—lower educational attainment. When grown, individuals who had childhood CD have higher rates of divorce, remarriage, and separation; less contact with relatives, friends, and neighbors; and little participation in organizations such as churches. Mortality rates and rates of hospitalization for physical and psychiatric problems are also disproportionately high (Kazdin et al. 1987).

Robins (1966) evaluated the status of aggressive children with CD in a 30-year follow-up study. She concluded that childhood antisocial behavior predicted multiple problems in adulthood. Compared with a matched clinical and nonclinical population, adults who as children had CD exhibited greater psychiatric symptomatology and dysfunction such as criminal behavior, physical health problems, and social maladjustment. However, less than 50% of the children with CD grew up to become antisocial adults. Factors contributing to a poor outcome included parental antisocial behavior, alcoholism, poor parental supervision, harsh or inconsistent disciplinary practices, parental and marital discord, large family size, and older siblings who were antisocial. The most significant predictors of long-term outcome were characteristics of the child's antisocial behavior. Early onset of antisocial behaviors, antisocial acts evident across multiple settings (e.g., home and school), and the presence of diverse antisocial behaviors (e.g., several overt and covert antisocial behaviors) were predictive of a poor long-term prognosis (Loeber and Dishion 1983; Rutter and Giller 1983).

The Epidemiological Catchment Area (ECA) project (Robins et al. 1991) has clearly correlated CD in childhood with a variety of psychiatric problems in adult life, including antisocial behavior, substance abuse, general health problems, mania, schizophrenia, and obsessive-compulsive disorder. Using the National Institute of Mental Health ECA project data, Robins and Price (1991) examined the effects of childhood CD problems on 10 DSM-III (American Psychiatric Association 1980) psychiatric disorders, including somatization disorder, phobia, obsessive-compulsive disorder, depression, mania, alcohol and drug use disorders, schizophrenia, and antisocial personality. They found that conduct problems had equal predictive power for males and females and noted that an increased number of conduct problems correlated with an increase in prevalence of these internalized disorders. Robins and Price further suggested that the increasing rate of CD in younger cohorts may be adding to the rising rates of other disorders.

The findings of the ECA project may be summarized as follows:

1. The study of the relationship between age at onset and extent of symptomatology presented the following conclusions about the consequences of CD: The incidence of subsequent antisocial behavior is the highest for those with a *high level* of conduct symptomatology (eight or more symptoms), particularly when the symptoms appear before the age of 6.
2. The rate of subsequent antisocial personality for the children with eight or more CD symptoms was 71% if symptoms appeared before the age of 6, 53% if they appeared between the ages of 6 and 12, and 48% if they appeared after age 12.
3. For those with *moderate* CD (five to seven symptoms), the rate of antisocial personality development was 24% if symptoms appeared before the age of 6, 16% if they appeared between the ages of 6 and 12, and 10% if they appeared after age 12.
4. For those with *minimal* CD symptoms (three or four), the rate of adult antisocial personality was 3.2% if symptoms appeared before the age of 6,

1.9% if they appeared between the ages of 6 and 12, and 0.9% if they appeared after age 12 (Robins and Price 1991).

In summary, one-quarter of the children who reported at least three CD symptoms prior to age 15 went on to develop antisocial personality in adulthood.

There is also a powerful association between childhood CD and later substance abuse; this association has been established in a large number of studies (Hesselbrock 1986; Robins 1978).

In addition to the consequences of adult antisocial personality and substance abuse, adults who had CD in childhood have a high incidence of elevated scores on general health questionnaires, indicating depression and anxiety, psychiatric disability, or psychiatric illnesses. There is a wide-ranging poor prognosis in multiple areas of adult functioning:

1. The rate of marital breakup is high.
2. There is a high mortality rate due to violent death (Rydelius 1988).
3. There are high rates of school failure, joblessness, financial dependency, and poor interpersonal relationships, particularly marital conflict and marital breakups. The excessive days missed in elementary school have been correlated with subsequent truancy in the offspring of adult patients who had CD when they were children (Robins et al. 1979).

Defining and Identifying Antisocial Behavior

Defining and identifying CD and antisocial behavior is difficult because of the high frequency of many antisocial behaviors in the course of normal development. Longitudinal studies by MacFarlane et al. (1954) have shown that many antisocial behaviors—for example, lying, disobedience, and destruction of property—are quite common among children ages 4 to 6, particularly in boys. However, the frequency of such behaviors decreases significantly as children become older. The children who tend to continue their antisocial behavior exhibit a variety of characteristics, such as frequent and intense antisocial actions, and their behavior tends to be more repetitive and chronic. The antisocial behavior of children with CD also manifests in a range of settings, which makes them unmanageable and prompts clinical referral. At times children can be referred for treatment for behaviors of low frequency but high intensity, such as injuring a sibling, threatening a parent with a weapon, setting a fire, or killing a pet.

Many of the behaviors of delinquent youths and youths with CD overlap. *Delinquency* is a legal designation referring to official contact with courts. Such contact includes legal encounters for offenses that are criminal if committed by an adult (e.g., robbery) or behaviors that are illegal because of the age of the offender. These activities are referred to as *status offenses.*

Large-scale self-report studies conducted among "normal" children and adolescents have shown much higher prevalence rates of antisocial and delinquent behavior than official records usually reveal (Elliot et al. 1981; Farrington 1978; Johnston et al. 1982).

The antisocial behaviors in CD form a syndrome or constellation of symptoms that are unlike the antisocial behavior exhibited during the course of normal development, which tends to occur as isolated and infrequent individual symptoms. CD, as a syndrome, includes several core features such as fighting, throwing temper tantrums, stealing, being truant, destroying property, defying or threatening others, and running away (Quay and Werry 1979).

The destructive consequences associated with antisocial behavior in childhood and adolescence do not disappear as adulthood is reached. A large number of such patients remain impaired as adults and transfer the same types of behavior to their offspring, thereby sustaining the cycle (Huesmann et al. 1984). The behavior of antisocial youths—because of vandalism, fire setting, and theft—tends to be very costly to the community in monetary terms. In addition, the victims of those antisocial actions suffer a very high and unjustified cost. The problem is made worse by the absence of a clear and effective treatment method for such youth.

Diagnostic Approaches

A number of alternative approaches to diagnosing conduct and antisocial behavior disorders have been proposed (Achenbach and Edelbrock 1984; Kazdin et al. 1990; Quay and Werry 1979). These include:

— Clinically derived diagnosis (categorical or typological)
— Multivariate approaches (dimensional)
— Salient symptom approach
— Overt/covert types of antisocial behavior

These approaches are described in detail in the following sections.

Clinically Derived Diagnosis

Clinically derived diagnoses rely on clinical observations and abstractions from these observations to identify a discrete constellation of behavior or symptoms. The diagnostic systems here are categorical or typological. The two major categorical diagnostic systems are those of the World Health

Organization (*International Statistical Classification of Diseases and Related Heath Problems* [ICD]) and the American Psychiatric Association (*Diagnostic and Statistical Manual of Mental Disorders* [DSM]). The revised third edition of the DSM (DSM-III-R) defines the essential feature of CD as "a persistent pattern of conduct in which the basic rights of others or major age-appropriate societal norms or rules are violated" (American Psychiatric Association 1987, p. 53). The problematic behavior must have a duration of at least 6 months for the diagnosis to be made. The CD diagnosis depends on the presence of at least 3 of 13 symptoms.

Multivariate Approaches

Multivariate approaches to diagnosis are fundamentally dimensional rather than categorical. Unlike clinically derived diagnoses, these approaches do not lead to the statement that a person has a particular disorder; rather, they describe the degree to which one or many characteristics are evident. Multivariate approaches depend on determining the correlations among several specific characteristics (e.g., symptoms or problems) and then summarizing them with quantitative techniques. Individuals' responses to a large number of items are subjected to factor analysis that correlates them. Rating scales yield multiple factors; an individual child has a score on each of the different factors or dimensions. In factor analytic studies, the most common characteristics associated with CD are fighting, disobedience, temper tantrums, destructiveness, impertinence, and uncooperativeness (Quay 1986).

Salient Symptom Approach

The salient symptom approach identifies prominent symptoms and determines how family characteristics, associated features, response to treatment, and prognosis vary among individuals with these symptoms. Two symptoms in CD yield reliable and clinically meaningful ways of segregating different types of antisocial behavior (Patterson 1982): aggression and stealing. Accordingly, two categories of children with CD have been designated: aggressors and stealers. Aggressors have a history of fighting and engaging in assaultive behavior. Stealers have a history of repeated theft and contact with the courts. Although these characteristics often go together, subpopulations of "pure" aggressors and stealers can be readily identified.

Compared with children who steal, aggressive children engage in significantly more aversive and coercive behaviors in their interactions in the home and are less compliant with their parents' requests. Parents of stealers show greater emotional distance from their children than do parents of aggressors.

Parent management training has been more effective with children in the aggressive category, and the parents of these children have been found to be more likely to continue what they have learned in treatment at home (see Chapter 11 for a description of parent management training). The coercive child-parent interactions do not appear to be a central characteristic of family life among stealers, and the parents of such children tend to cease applying what they have learned in treatment over time. Children with "mixed" symptoms of aggression and stealing are especially at risk for child abuse (Patterson 1982).

Overt/Covert Types of Antisocial Behavior

Loeber and Schmaling (1985a, 1985b) distinguished two types of CD behavior: overt and covert. Overt behavior consists of confrontative actions such as biting, arguing, and temper tantrums; covert behavior includes stealing, truancy, lying, and fire setting.

Some children exhibit both overt and covert types of behavior. Compared with children who exhibit only one or the other type, those who exhibit both types of CD behavior have more severe family dysfunction and a poorer long-term prognosis, resulting in subsequent contact with police.

There are commonalities among clinically derived, multivariate, and other approaches to diagnosis. Each approach recognizes a constellation of antisocial behavior among children and adolescents. Some consistencies also exist in the subtyping of antisocial behavior, such as aggressive type (fighting) and covert delinquent type (running away, lying). Different types of antisocial behavior may be associated with different characteristics, prognoses, and developmental sequences.

Symptomatology

In DSM-III-R, 13 symptoms for CD are listed in descending order of discriminating power (these symptoms are based on data from a national field trial of the DSM-III-R criteria for disruptive behavior disorders):

1. Has stolen without confrontation of a victim on more than one occasion (including forgery)
2. Has run away from home overnight at least twice while living in parental or parental surrogate home (or once without returning)
3. Often lies (other than to avoid physical or sexual abuse)
4. Has deliberately engaged in fire setting
5. Is often truant from school (for older person, absent from work)
6. Has broken into someone else's house, building, or car

7. Has deliberately destroyed others' property (other than by fire setting)
8. Has been physically cruel to animals
9. Has forced someone into sexual activity with him or her
10. Has used a weapon in more than one fight
11. Often initiates physical fights
12. Has stolen with confrontation of a victim (e.g., mugging, purse snatching, extortion, armed robbery)
13. Has been physically cruel to people

Nine of the these symptoms characterize the *aggressive* type of symptomatology in CD; four of them (running away, lying, truancy, and fire setting) distinguish the *nonaggressive* type.

DSM-III-R also establishes criteria for the severity of conduct disorder. In mild cases, there are few symptoms in excess of the three required to make the diagnosis, and the conduct problems cause only minor harm to others. In moderate cases of CD, the number of conduct problems and their effects on others are intermediate between "mild" and "severe." In severe cases, many problems are present in excess of those required for the diagnosis, and the conduct problems cause considerable harm to others (e.g., serious physical injury to victims, extensive vandalism or theft, prolonged absences from home).

DSM-III-R proposes three subtypes of CD, which largely correspond to categories derived from empirical studies: *group type, solitary aggressive type,* and *undifferentiated type.* In group type (1312.20) CD, the essential feature is that the conduct problems occur mainly as a group activity with peers. Aggressive physical behavior may or may not be present. In solitary aggressive type (1312.00), the central feature is aggressive physical behavior, usually directed toward both adults and peers, that is initiated by the person (not as a group activity). In undifferentiated type (1312.90), a mixture of clinical features is present that cannot be classified as either solitary aggressive type or group type.

In the earlier diagnostic and classification systems of DSM-III and ICD-9 (World Health Organization 1977), a distinction was made between "socialized" and "unsocialized" subtypes of CD. Socialized CD was characterized by the presence of enduring friendships, altruistic behavior, feelings of guilt or remorse, refraining from blaming others, and feelings of concern for others; the socialized subtype required the presence of two or more of these five indicators. Both DSM-III-R and ICD-10 (World Health Organization 1992) deemphasize the socialized/unsocialized distinction, indicating a move away from the view that disorders explained by genetic and parenting defects can be clearly distinguished from disorders explained primarily by subcultural variation. Research support for this distinction has been uneven (Robins and Price 1991).

Subtypes

It is clear that CD is a heterogeneous diagnostic category (Farrington 1978; Kazdin et al. 1990; Lahey and Loeber 1991). Subtypes of CD have been proposed, therefore, in an effort to capture differences in behavior, development, and assumed etiology. Moreover, strong evidence already exists that CD is not homogeneous in terms of biological correlates, and that this biological heterogeneity may be associated with behavioral subtypes of CD (Rogeness et al. 1990). We will look briefly, therefore, at subtypes of CD that have been suggested on the basis of the individual's capacity for maintaining social relationships, the presence or absence of aggression, the age at onset, and the presence or absence of comorbid diagnoses.

Subtypes based on "socialization."   A distinction is made in DSM-III-R between group and solitary types of CD. In DSM-III, essentially the same subtypes were referred to as socialized and undersocialized, respectively. The distinction is made between those youths with CD who are capable of maintaining social relationships and who primarily commit antisocial behavior with other deviant peers (socialized or group type) and those youths with CD who are not capable of maintaining social relationships and who primarily commit antisocial acts alone (undersocialized or solitary type).

The distinction between socialized and undersocialized CD was originally derived from a number of consistently replicated multivariate studies of psychiatric outpatients and incarcerated juvenile delinquents (Jenkins and Hewitt 1944; Quay et al. 1987). These studies suggest that, compared with youths with socialized CD, those with undersocialized CD are more aggressive, adjust less well to juvenile detention facilities, are less successful in work-release programs, and are more likely to violate probation and to be rearrested after release. The biological evidence reviewed in Chapter 2 is consistent with the hypothesis of Quay et al. (1987) that socialized and undersocialized subtypes of CD differ in biological substrates. However, the "capacity for maintaining social relationships" is a vague concept that needs to be operationalized.

Subtypes based on aggression.   The socialized and undersocialized subtypes of CD distinguished in DSM-III were each subdivided into aggressive and nonaggressive subtypes. Because of the social importance of aggression and its stability over time, there is strong reason to believe that youths with CD who are physically aggressive should be distinguished from those who are not. Stattin and Magnusson (1989) found that troubled youths rated as physically aggressive were significantly more likely to commit violent acts, including assault, murder, and rape, as adults.

The symmetrical subtyping of CD in DSM-III, together with the socialized/undersocialized and aggressive/nonaggressive dimensions, was dropped in DSM-III-R in favor of two subtypes that captured some aspects of these distinctions. A solitary aggressive type was distinguished, but no solitary nonaggressive subtype was provided on the assumption that few such cases of CD would be identified. The group type can include both aggressive and nonaggressive youths, but no distinction was made on the basis of aggression in this subtype.

A study by Rogeness et al. (1990) is consistent with the DSM-III-R approach to subtypes of CD. Among 345 children and adolescents who were inpatients in a psychiatric hospital and who were given a DSM-III diagnosis of CD:

— 46% were given the diagnosis of socialized aggressive CD.
— 38% were given the diagnosis of undersocialized aggressive CD.
— 14% received a diagnosis of socialized nonaggressive CD.
— 2% received a diagnosis of undersocialized nonaggressive CD.

Thus, consistent with the DSM-III-R, some youths with socialized CD were found to be aggressive and some were found to be nonaggressive, but virtually all undersocialized youths were found to be aggressive. Note that 84% of the youths with CD exhibited significant aggression, but Rogeness et al. (1990) appropriately warned that selection factors may have been biased in favor of the admission of youths with aggressive CD to their psychiatric hospital.

Subtypes based on age at onset.   Criminologists have long distinguished between early and late onset of juvenile delinquency (Farrington 1978). Late-onset delinquents tend to be less severe in their offending, to be rarely aggressive, and to have a better prognosis for desistance in offending (Loeber 1982). Consistent with this distinction, Robins (1966) found that youths with CD onset before 11 years of age were twice as likely to receive a diagnosis of antisocial personality disorder (sociopathy) in adulthood as those with an onset after age 11.

Moffitt (1990) and McGee et al. (1992) examined the question of late-onset antisocial behavior using data from the Dunedin Longitudinal Study. They identified a large group of male and female youths in a longitudinal sample who exhibited antisocial behavior for the first time after the age of 11. Compared with a group of youths who had shown persistent antisocial behavior since age 5, the late-onset antisocial youths were more likely to be female, to exhibit higher verbal ability and reading scores, to have less family adversity, and to be of higher socioeconomic status. Furthermore, the late-onset group displayed markedly less antisocial behavior and physical aggression and were much less inattentive, impulsive, and hyperactive throughout childhood than the early-onset group. Thus, Moffitt (1990) and McGee et al.

(1992) appear to have identified a group of youths who developed antisocial behavior for the first time around the time of puberty in the absence of a history of oppositional and hyperactive behavior. Gittelman and Mannuzza (1985) also found some evidence of a late-onset type of CD, but more investigation of this issue is clearly needed in prospective studies specifically designed to examine both early- and late-onset CD.

In accord with the findings of Moffitt (1990) and McGee et al. (1992), youths whose delinquent behavior emerges for the first time during adolescence consistently display nonaggressive, covert antisocial behaviors, such as substance use, theft, and truancy, and are infrequently aggressive.

Because, in most cases, late-onset CD is less severe and persistent than early-onset CD, and because it does not show the extended developmental progression (i.e., beginning with ODD during the preschool years) shown by early-onset CD, it seems plausible to assume that the biological correlates of late-onset CD may be different from those of early-onset CD. Indeed, it seems reasonable to speculate that if biological factors do, in fact, play a role in the etiology of CD, they play that role in the early-onset and not the late-onset group.

Subtypes based on comorbid conditions.   ICD-10 distinguishes subtypes of CD based on comorbidity with ADHD and with emotional disorders. The course of CD may be influenced in positive or negative directions by the presence of certain comorbid psychiatric disorders. There is evidence suggesting that youths with CD and comorbid ADHD exhibit a more severe and persistent disorder than youths with CD alone (Offord et al. 1979; Schachar et al. 1981; Walker et al. 1987), but more research is needed to understand the nature of this difference. Recent evidence from the dexamethasone suppression test (DST) also suggests that, compared with youths with CD alone, those with CD and comorbid anxiety disorder exhibit less-severe impairment but higher cortisol levels (McBurnett et al. 1991). On the other hand, a long-term follow-up study of clinic-referred youths in London (Harrington et al. 1990) showed that youths with CD were equally likely to meet criteria for antisocial personality disorder in adulthood regardless of whether a comorbid depression was present (61%) or absent (53%) during childhood. Much remains to be learned about the comorbidity of CD and emotional disorders. Comorbidity with anxiety disorders appears to be extremely important to the understanding of the biological correlates of CD.

___ ___ ___ ___ ___ ___ ___ ___ ___ ___ ___

Associated Features

In addition to the syndrome of CD, which includes fighting, stealing, and other symptoms described in DSM-III-R, associated symptoms are frequently present in CD. Symptoms related to hyperactivity include excess motor activity, restlessness, impulsiveness, inattentiveness, and overactivity in general. The frequent co-occurrence of hyperactivity and CD has given rise to considerable debate about these syndromes' common origins.

Other associated features include boisterousness, showing off, blaming others, academic deficiencies, poor interpersonal relations, rejection by peers, and poor social skills (Quay and Werry 1979). Frequently noted in children with CD are certain cognitive and attributional deficiencies or qualities that give rise to poor problem-solving skills (Dodge 1985; Kendall and Braswell 1985). Cognitive difficulties make children with CD prone to interpreting gestures of others as hostile, which in turn interferes with problem solving. Other common cognitive qualities are resentment, suspiciousness, and irritability in relation to others (Kazdin et al. 1987).

A variety of dysfunctional family characteristics have also been frequently reported in youths with CD.

Psychiatric and Neurological Vulnerabilities

D. O. Lewis and her colleagues have emphasized the high levels of psychiatric symptomatology and neurological vulnerabilities in the histories of patients with CD. Studies of incarcerated delinquents and juveniles condemned to death have found a high level of previously overlooked psychotic symptomatology, such as paranoid ideation and occasional auditory or visual hallucinations (D. O. Lewis and Shanok 1979; D. O. Lewis et al. 1988a, 1988b). The misperception of being insulted or looked at in a threatening way was a common reason for aggressive attacks. Approximately 6% of the incarcerated adolescent boys had been in psychiatric hospitals or residential centers at some time during their childhoods (D. O. Lewis and Shanok 1980), a finding that underlines the chronicity and severity of these individuals' disorders. Suicidal ideation and suicidal attempts were frequent in patients with CD, although these characteristics were not necessarily related to depression.

Drug and alcohol abuse have been commonly reported among children and adolescents with CD. The substance abuse at times dates back to age 11 or 12 years. Possible contextual and individual reasons for substance abuse are many, including attempts to self-medicate for anxiety and depression.

Patients with CD often have histories of injuries, accidents, and illnesses that affect central nervous system (CNS) functioning. However, these disturbances are seldom localized to particular portions of the brain (M. Lewis 1991). A typical finding is a history of symptoms such as frequent and severe headaches, episodes of dizziness, and blackouts. A few patients with severe CD may suffer from epilepsy. A much larger number present with equivocal or diffusely abnormal electroencephalograms (EEGs) because of adverse perinatal histories, accidents, and injuries. Psychomotor seizures are observed on rare occasions, but they are more common in very violent delinquents than in the general population (D. O. Lewis et al. 1982). Psychomotor symptoms such as metamorphopsias (visual distortions) and impaired memory for behaviors are also observed. These symptoms may represent abnormal electrical activity in the CNS that can contribute to behavior problems.

Hyperactivity and attention problems, poor fine motor coordination, inability to skip, and impaired short-term memory are common. Learning disabilities, impaired abstract reasoning, and poor judgment are frequent manifestations of cognitive dysfunction and vulnerability in children with CD.

Assessment

Alternative methods have been used to diagnose and classify CD. These methods, which frequently rely on some form of measurement that may extend beyond diagnosis, are used for a variety of goals (e.g., correlating specific symptoms with other dysfunctional characteristics of the child or the family). Modalities of assessment include the following:

— **Self-report measures** are more likely to be useful with adolescents than with children because of children's limited capacity to identify themselves as having problems. As an auxiliary method of assessment, self-report measures can yield important information on symptoms as well as identify specific problems that may not be readily evident to the parents (Herjanic and Reich 1982).

— **Reports of significant others,** such as parents, teachers, or therapists, are the most widely used and reliable sources of information. Many rating scales can be easily completed by parents and significant others.

— **Peer evaluations** involve different ways of soliciting peer nomination of persons who exhibit particular characteristics, such as aggressiveness. The consensus of the peer group is likely to reflect consistencies in performance and stable characteristics (Huesmann et al. 1984).

— **Direct observation** at home, at school, or in the community is a useful assessment method that provides samples of the actual frequency or occurrence of particular antisocial or prosocial behaviors. The use of home observation of families has been extensively investigated by Patterson (1982). The Family Interaction Coding System (FICS; Patterson 1982) provides particularly useful and reliable information about children's interactions with their parents and siblings at home.

— **Diagnostic interview** yields valuable information by assessing the overall level of the child's ego development, the extent and complexity of behavioral repertoire and social skills, and capacity for relatedness, which are important dimensions of the level of ego development. The capacity for self-observation, for self-reflection, and for relating to the evaluator are other important sources of information during the interview. In addition to its correlation with impulse control and social adjustment, the level of ego development can reveal the child's degree of completion of the separation-individuation process and distortions in selfobject definitions.

A careful and complete medical history should be obtained to unearth adverse medical histories commonly found in many children with CD. Trauma of one sort or another to the CNS is extremely common among especially aggressive offenders, juvenile as well as adults. Compared with white nondelinquents, white delinquent children with CD have far less favorable medical histories.

The nature of the child's symptomatic behaviors should be explored in detail, including the circumstances in which they occur, the precipitants, and the amount of self-control the child seems to have. Sensitivity to seemingly provocative behavior by others, frequently as a result of misperceptions, should be established.

Many youngsters with CD have scars on their faces and bodies that can facilitate the investigation of past traumas. A neurological examination is usually helpful in verifying the existence of nonspecific signs of CNS dysfunction. The EEG may confirm the suspicion of a seizure disorder, although a normal EEG does not rule it out. The diagnosis of complex partial seizure disorder rests on the overall clinical picture. Neuropsychological testing is often very valuable in identifying the kind of CNS dysfunction that may be contributing to a child's adaptational problems. A detailed psychoeducational evaluation can establish the presence of remediable learning problems that can contribute to behavior problems, including school truancy.

Risk Factors

The causes of CD are poorly understood. Deficiencies in parent-child relationships and the impact of social and socioeconomic environments have been extensively investigated and implicated as contributing factors in the genesis of CD. More recently, the role of psychobiological factors and multiple neuroendocrine systems have been the focus of investigation.

Risk factors for CD include the following:

— **Child's temperament**—Children who are difficult and who show oppositional patterns in their emotional responsiveness, level of activity, quality of mood, and social adaptability are more likely to be referred for treatment for aggressive behavior and tantrums than are children with other temperamental characteristics (Thomas and Chess 1977). Other observations have suggested that the "quiet" child may be at especially high risk for CD.

— **Parental factors**—Parental factors include psychopathology and criminal behavior in parents as well as ineffective and confusing parent-child interactions. Separation from one's parents during early childhood and marital discord between one's parents are commonly observed.

— **Birth order and family size**—CD is more prevalent among middle children than among only, firstborn, or youngest children (Glueck and Glueck 1968; McCord et al. 1959; Nye 1958). Family size has frequently been shown to correlate with CD, with more children in the family being associated with higher rates of delinquency (Glueck and Glueck 1968; Nye 1958; West 1982).

— **Social class**—CD occurs at a higher rate in children of families with lower socioeconomic status (West 1982).

— **School-related factors**—Several school-related factors are correlated with a high rate of CD. Poor physical condition of the building, low teacher-student ratio, insufficient emphasis on academics, low teacher time spent on lessons and preparation, and ineffective and punitive methods of teaching contribute to the development of CD.

— **Gender**—The high rate of CD in boys as compared with girls is a common observation reported by all investigators, although the biological or cultural nature of this fact has not been determined.

— **Sustained pattern of aggressive behavior in early childhood**—Next to intelligence, aggression is the most stable characteristic throughout childhood (0.70 for intelligence in comparison with 0.63 for aggression [Olweus 1979]).

— **Other factors**—Other risk factors for CD include parental marriage at a young age, lack of parental interest in the child's school performance, mental retardation in parents, lack of participation by the family in religious or recreational activities, and exposure of the child to violence and aggression on television.

References

Achenbach TM: Developmental Psychology, 2nd Edition. New York, Wiley, 1982

Achenbach TM, Edelbrock CS: Behavioral problems and competencies reported by parents of normal and disturbed children aged four through sixteen. Monogr Soc Res Child Dev 46 (Serial No. 188), 1981

Achenbach TM, Edelbrock CS: Manual for the Child Behavior Checklist and Revised Child Behavior Profile. Burlington, VT, University of Vermont, Department of Psychiatry, 1983

Achenbach TM, Edelbrock CS: Psychopharmacology of childhood. Annu Rev Psychol 35:227–256, 1984

American Psychiatric Association: Diagnostic and Statistical Manual of Mental Disorders, 3rd Edition. Washington, DC, American Psychiatric Association, 1980

American Psychiatric Association: Diagnostic and Statistical Manual of Mental Disorders, 3rd Edition, Revised. Washington, DC, American Psychiatric Association, 1987

American Psychiatric Association: Diagnostic and Statistical Manual of Mental Disorders, 4th Edition. Washington, DC, American Psychiatric Association, 1994

Anderson T: The reflecting team. Fam Process 26:415–428, 1987

Bachman JG, Johnston LD, O'Malley PN: Delinquent behavior linked to educational attainment and post–high school experiences, in Colloquium on the Correlates of Crime and the Determinants of Criminal Behavior. Edited by Otten L. Arlington, VA, The MITRE Corp, 1978, pp 1–42

Bird HR, Canino G, Rubio-Stipec M, et al: Estimates of the prevalence of childhood maladjustment in a community survey in Puerto Rico. Arch Gen Psychiatry 45:1120–1126, 1988

Boyle MH, Offord DR, Hofmann H, et al: Ontario Child Health Study, I: methodology. Arch Gen Psychiatry 44:826–831, 1987

Cernkovich SA, Giordano PC: A comparative analysis of male and female delinquency. Sociological Quarterly 20:131–145, 1979

Connell HM, Irvine L, Rodney J: Psychiatric disorder in Queensland primary school children. Australian Pediatric Journal 18:171–188, 1982

Costello EJ: Developments in child psychiatric epidemiology. J Am Acad Child Adolesc Psychiatry 28:836–841, 1989

Costello EJ, Angold A: Scales to assess child and adolescent depression: checklists, screen, and nets. J Am Acad Child Adolesc Psychiatry 27:726–737, 1988

Dodge KA: Attributional bias in aggressive children, in Advances in Cognitive-behavioral Research and Therapy, Vol 4. Edited by Kendall PC. Orlando, FL, Academic Press, 1985, pp 73–110

Elliott DS, Knowles BA, Canter RJ: The epidemiology of delinquent behavior and drug use among American adolescents, 1976–1978: progress report to NIMH. Boulder, CO, Behavior Research Institute, 1981

Farrington DP: The family backgrounds of aggressive youths, in Aggressive and Antisocial Behavior in Childhood and Adolescence. Edited by Hersov LA, Berger M, Shaffer D. Oxford, UK, Pergamon, 1978, pp 73–93

Gilbert GM: A survey of "referral problems" in metropolitan child guidance centers. J Clin Psychol 13:37–42, 1957

Gittelman R, Mannuzza S: Diagnosing ADD-H in adolescents. Psychopharmacol Bull 21:237–242, 1985

Glueck S, Glueck E: Unravelling Juvenile Delinquency. Cambridge, MA, Harvard University Press, 1950

Glueck S, Glueck E: Delinquents and Nondelinquents in Perspective. Cambridge, MA, Harvard University Press, 1968

Graham PJ: Epidemiologic studies, in Psychopathological Disorders of Childhood. Edited by Quay HC, Werry JS. New York, Wiley, 1979, pp 185–209

Harrington R, Rutter MP, Pickles A, et al: Adult outcomes of childhood and adolescent depression. Arch Gen Psychiatry 47:465–473, 1990

Herbert M: Conduct Disorders of Childhood and Adolescence: A Behavioral Approach to Assessment and Treatment. Chichester, UK, Wiley, 1978

Herjanic B, Reich W: Development of a structured psychiatric interview for children: agreement between child and parent on individual symptoms. J Abnorm Child Psychol 10:307–324, 1982

Hesselbrock N: Childhood behavior problems and adult antisocial disorder in alcoholism, in Psychopathology and Addictive Disorders. Edited by Meyer RE. New York, Guilford, 1986

Huesmann LR, Eron LD, Lefkowitz MM, et al: Stability of aggression over time and generations. Developmental Psychology 20:1120–1134, 1984

Jenkins RL, Hewitt L: Types of personality structure encountered in child guidance clinics. Am J Orthopsychiatry 14:84–94, 1944

Johnston LD, Bachman JG, O'Malley PM: Student Drug Use, Attitudes and Beliefs: National Trends. Washington, DC, National Institute on Drug Abuse, 1982

Kazdin AE, Rodger A, Colbus D, et al: Children's Hostility Inventory: measurement of aggression and hostility in psychiatric inpatient children. J Clin Child Psychol 16:320–328, 1987

Kazdin AE, Bass D, Ayers W, et al: Empirical and clinical focus of child and adolescent psychotherapy research. J Consult Clin Psychol 58:729–740, 1990

Kendall PC, Braswell L: Cognitive-behavioral therapy for impulsive children. New York, Guilford, 1985

King RA, Noshpitz J: Pathways to Growth: Essentials of Child Psychiatry, Vol 2: Psychopathology. New York, Wiley, 1991

Lahey BB, Loeber R: A preliminary psychobiological model of conduct disorder. Presentation to the annual meeting of the Society for Research in Child and Adolescent Psychopathology, Amsterdam, The Netherlands, June 1991

Lewis DO, Shanok SS: A comparison of the medical histories of incarcerated delinquent children and a matched sample of nondelinquent children. Child Psychiatry Hum Dev 9:210–214, 1979

Lewis DO, Shanok SS: The use of a correctional setting for follow-up care of psychiatrically disturbed adolescents. Am J Psychiatry 137:953–955, 1980

Lewis DO, Pincus JH, Shanok SS, et al: Psychomotor epilepsy and violence in an incarcerated adolescent population. Am J Psychiatry 139:882–887, 1982

Lewis DO, Lovely R, Yeager C, et al: Intrinsic and environmental characteristics of juvenile murderers. J Am Acad Child Adolesc Psychiatry 27:582–587, 1988a

Lewis DO, Pincus JH, Bard B, et al: Neuropsychiatric, psychoeducational and family characteristics of 14 juveniles condemned to death in the United States. Am J Psychiatry 145:584–589, 1988b

Lewis M (ed): Child and Adolescent Psychiatry: A Comprehensive Textbook. Baltimore, MD, Williams & Wilkins, 1991

Loeber R: The stability of antisocial and delinquent child behavior: a review. Child Dev 53:1431–1446, 1982

Loeber R, Dishion TJ: Early predictors of male delinquency: a review. Psychol Bull 94:68–99, 1983

Loeber R, Schmaling KB: Empirical evidence for overt and covert patterns of antisocial conduct problems: a meta-analysis. J Abnorm Child Psychol 13:337–352, 1985a

Loeber R, Schmaling KB: The utility of differentiating between mixed and pure forms of antisocial child behavior. J Abnorm Psychol 13:315–355, 1985b

MacFarlane JW, Allen L, Honzik MP: A Developmental Study of the Behavior Problems of Normal Children Between 21 Months and 14 Years. Berkeley, University of California Press, 1954

McBurnett K, Lahey BB, Tuch PF, et al: Anxiety, inhibition, and conduct disorder in children, II: relation to salivary cortisol. J Am Acad Child Adolesc Psychiatry 30:192–196, 1991

McCord W, McCord J, Zola IK: Origins of Crime. New York, Columbia University Press, 1959

McGee R, Williams S, Silva PA: Behavioral and developmental characteristics of aggressive, hyperactive, and aggressive-hyperactive boys. Journal of the American Academy of Child Psychiatry 23:270–279, 1984

McGee R, Feehan M, Williams S, et al: DSM-III disorders from age 11 to age 15 years. J Am Acad Child Adolesc Psychiatry 31:50–59, 1992

Moffitt TE: Juvenile delinquency and attention deficit disorder: boys' developmental trajectories from age 3 to age 15. Child Dev 61:893–910, 1990

Nye FI: Family Relationships and Delinquent Behavior. New York, Wiley, 1958

Offer D, Ostrov E, Howard KI: Epidemiology of mental health and mental illness among adolescents, in Basic Handbook of Child Psychiatry, Vol 5. Edited by Noshpitz JD. New York, Basic Books, 1987, pp 82–88

Offord DR, Sullivan K, Allen N, et al: Delinquency and hyperactivity. J Nerv Ment Dis 167:734–741, 1979

Offord DR, Boyle MH, Szatmari P, et al: Ontario Child Health Study, II: six-month prevalence of disorder and rates of service utilization. Arch Gen Psychiatry 44:832–836, 1987

Olweus D: Stability of aggressive reaction patterns in males: a review. Psychol Bull 86:852–875, 1979

Patterson GR: Coercive Family Processes, Vol 3: A Social Learning Approach. Eugene, OR, Castalia, 1982

Quay HC: A critical analysis of DSM-III as a taxonomy of psychopathology in childhood and adolescence, in Contemporary Directions in Psychopathology: Toward the DSM-IV. Edited by Millon T, Klerman GL. New York, Guilford, 1986, pp 151–165

Quay HC, Werry JS (eds): Psychopathological Disorders of Childhood. New York, Wiley, 1979

Quay HC, Rauth DK, Shapiro SK: Psychopathology of childhood from description to validation. Annu Rev Psychol 38:491–532, 1987

Robins LN: Deviant Children Grown Up: A Sociological and Psychiatric Study of Sociopathic Personality. Baltimore, MD, Williams & Wilkins, 1966

Robins LN: Sturdy childhood predictors of adult outcomes: replications from longitudinal studies. Psychol Med 8:611–622, 1978

Robins LN: Epidemiology of adolescent drug use and abuse, in Psychopathology of Children and Youth: A Cross-Cultural Perspective. Edited by Purcell EF. New York, Josiah Macy Jr. Foundation, 1980

Robins LN: Epidemiological approaches to natural history research: antisocial disorders in children. Journal of the American Academy of Child Psychiatry 20:566–580, 1981

Robins LN, Price R: Conduct problems and adult psychiatric disorders. Psychiatry 54:116–132, 1991

Robins LN, Wish E: Childhood deviance as a developmental process. Social Forces 56:448–471, 1977

Robins LN, Ratcliff KS, West PA: School achievement in two generations: a study of 88 urban black families, in New Directions in Children's Mental Health. Edited by Shamsie SJ. New York, Spectrum, 1979

Robins LN, Tipp J, McEvoy L: Antisocial personality, in Psychiatric Disorders in America. Edited by Robins LN, Regier D. New York, Free Press, 1991

Rogeness GA, Javors MA, Maas JW, et al: Catecholamine and diagnoses in children. J Am Acad Child Adolesc Psychiatry 29:234–241, 1990

Rutter MP, Giller H: Juvenile Delinquency: Trends and Perspectives. New York, Penguin, 1983

Rutter MP, Tizzard J, Whitmore K (eds): Education, Health and Behavior. London, Longman, 1970

Rutter MP, Cox A, Tupling C, et al: Attainment and adjustment in two geographical areas, I: the prevalence of psychiatric disorder. Br J Psychiatry 126:493–509, 1975

Rydelius PA: The development of antisocial behavior and sudden violent death. Acta Psychiatr Scand 77:398–403, 1988

Schachar R, Rutter MP, Smith A: The characteristics of situationally and pervasively hyperactive children: implications of syndrome definition. J Child Psychol Psychiatry 23:375–392, 1981

Simcha-Fagan O, Langner TS, Gersten JC, et al: Violent and antisocial behavior: a longitudinal study of urban youth. Unpublished report of the Agency of Child Development (OCD-CB-480, p 7), 1975

Stattin H, Magnusson D: The role of early aggressive behavior in the frequency, seriousness and types of later crime. J Consult Clin Psychol 57:710–718, 1989

Stewart MA, Behar D: Subtypes of aggressive conduct disorders. Acta Psychiatr Scand 68:178–185, 1983

Stewart MA, Cummings C, Singer S, et al: The overlap between hyperactive and unsocialized aggressive children. J Child Psychol Psychiatry 22:35–45, 1981

Thomas A, Chess S: Temperament and Development. New York, Brunner/Mazel, 1977

Walker JL, Lahey BB, Hynd GW, et al: Comparison of specific patterns of antisocial behavior in children with conduct disorder with or without co-existing hyperactivity. J Consult Clin Psychol 55:910–913, 1987

Werry JS, Quay HC: The prevalence of behavior symptoms in younger elementary school children. Am J Orthopsychiatry 41:136–143, 1971

West DJ: Delinquency: Its Roots, Careers and Prospects. Cambridge, MA, Harvard University Press, 1982

White J, Moffit TE, Earls F, et al: Preschool predictors of conduct disorder. Criminology 28:507–533, 1991

Wolfgang ME, Figlio RM, Sellin T: Delinquency in a Birth Cohort, Chicago, IL, University of Chicago Press, 1972

World Health Organization: Manual of the International Statistical Classification of
    Diseases, Injuries, and Causes of Death, 9th Revision (ICD-9). Geneva, World
    Health Organization, 1977
World Health Organization: International Statistical Classification of Diseases and
    Related Heath Problems, 10th Revision (ICD-10). Geneva, World Health Orga-
    nization, 1992

Chapter 2

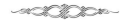

Psychobiology

Benjamin B. Lahey, Ph.D.
Keith McBurnett, Ph.D.
Rolf Loeber, Ph.D.
Elizabeth L. Hart, Ph.D

onduct disorder (CD) has been the subject of a considerable research effort in recent years, perhaps both because of its seriousness and because of the difficulties involved in its treatment. One line of investigation has focused on the biological correlates of CD, including measures of skin conductance, cardiac functioning, monoamine neurotransmitters and their associated metabolites and enzymes in blood and urine, endocrine hormones in saliva, and electroencephalographic (EEG) evoked potentials. There are at least three important reasons for such lines of scientific inquiry.

First, CD is highly familial. The parents of youths with CD frequently exhibit antisocial personality, substance abuse, and criminality (Lahey et al. 1987). Although evidence on the mechanism(s) of this pattern of cross-generational transmission is currently weak, there is some evidence suggesting that heredity may play a role (Raine and Venables 1992). Because the heritability of some of the biological correlates of CD—particularly some of the enzymes involved in monoamine synthesis—are already understood or are under study, knowledge of the biological correlates of CD may facilitate genetic studies by giving researchers reliably measured neurochemical dependent variables in addition to diagnoses of CD. In addition, if CD is partly heritable, knowledge of its biological correlates will provide an important starting place for understanding what is inherited.

The second reason for studying the biological correlates of CD is quite different. In this context, it is worth restating the truism that all patterns of behavior, normal and abnormal, are mediated by biological mechanisms,

27

whether the origins are environmental or endogenous biological processes. If, for example, one were to reinforce a laboratory rat with food pellets for pressing a lever, the resulting change in behavior would be accompanied by changes in the biological systems that provide the substrate for operant learning.

When the etiology of a pattern of behavior is unknown, as is the case for CD, knowledge of the biological correlates of the disorder may lead to hypotheses concerning both the underlying neurobiological mechanisms and the etiology of the disorder. For example, this chapter's literature review will show that serum and urinary catecholamine levels are often abnormal in a subgroup of youths with CD. Previous research has shown that abnormal infant-caretaker interactions are associated with similar catecholamine abnormalities in the developing infant (Reite and Field 1985). If supported by other findings, this may suggest that early experience should be a focus of research on the etiology of CD. In the future, greater knowledge of the neurochemical correlates of CD can be expected to give rise to a variety of leads concerning both environmental and biological variables of potential etiological significance.

The third goal of biological studies of CD is to develop hypotheses regarding treatment. These hypotheses may involve pharmacological interventions to directly manipulate the suspected biological substrate of CD or may consist of prevention strategies based on suspected environmental causes of the biological abnormalities (e.g., preventing certain forms of atypical infant-mother interaction). In addition, knowledge of the biological correlates of CD could lead to hypotheses that facilitate psychotherapy. For example, this chapter will suggest that a subgroup of youths with CD shows dampened sympathetic responsiveness, whereas another subgroup shows heightened sympathetic responsiveness. If confirmed, such findings may lead to hypotheses concerning the role of anxiety and inhibition in CD that may facilitate psychotherapy by focusing the therapist on inhibitory processes in subgroups of youths with CD.

Biological Correlates of CD

A small body of research now exists on the biological correlates of CD. Although fraught with methodological shortcomings, these studies are consistent enough to support some reasonable hypotheses to guide future research on biologically homogeneous subtypes of CD. To date, most studies have focused on peripheral measures linked to sympathetic and parasympathetic activity and peripheral measures of catecholamines, but several studies have examined other biological correlates of CD.

As will be discussed in detail later in this chapter, few biological measures have been found to distinguish individuals with CD, as a group, from control subjects. Most findings suggest that two subgroups of youths with CD differ from control subjects in *opposite* ways. These subgroups are characterized in different ways in different studies, but it appears that youths with CD who are considered to be undersocialized, aggressive, and low in anxiety can be distinguished on a variety of biological measures both from control subjects and from other youths with CD.

CD and Skin Conductance

Because sweating is largely under the control of the autonomic nervous system, measures of skin conductance are often used as an index of sympathetic outflow. Based on early work with adults with antisocial personality disorder, a number of studies of skin conductance have been performed comparing subgroups of youths with CD with a variety of control subjects. Four studies that used a paradigm of habituation to pure tones (Borkovec 1970; Delamater and Lahey 1983; Schmidt et al. 1985; Siddle et al. 1973) found consistently lower skin conductance in CD groups characterized as undersocialized, aggressive, psychopathic, or nonemotional, especially on the first trial. Differences in skin conductance amplitudes per se did not reach customary levels of statistical significance in another study (Raine and Venables 1984), but youths with undersocialized CD exhibited significantly fewer responses that exceeded a preset minimum amplitude. In a mixed sample of referred and nonreferred boys, McBurnett et al. (1991b) found lower skin conductance levels during the administration of a neuropsychological test in boys rated high in oppositional and aggressive behavior.

In contrast, comparisons of CD and non-CD groups using resting skin conductance levels and number of spontaneous fluctuations have sometimes found lower resting levels for youths with CD (Borkovec 1970; Fox and Lippert 1963), but more often have not (Delamater and Lahey 1983; McBurnett et al. 1991b; Schmidt et al. 1985; Siddle et al. 1973). However, the importance of all measures of skin conductance is magnified considerably by two recent studies. The number of skin conductance responses to tones, the resting levels, and the number of nonspecific fluctuations measured at age 15 in a group of nonreferred boys were all found to predict criminal behavior at age 24 (Raine et al. 1990a, 1990b). In addition, Raine et al. (1991) reported that these measures of skin conductance correlated .44–.60 with estimates of prefrontal cortex area in a magnetic resonance imaging (MRI) study of nonreferred subjects. These studies suggest that atypical skin conductance may be related to the most severe and persistent forms of aggressive CD and that atypical skin conductance may be associated with anatomical differences in prefrontal structures that are thought to play an important role in impulse control.

CD and Cardiovascular Measures

Heart rate and blood pressure have been a focus of biological studies of CD because, like skin conductance, these measures are partially influenced by sympathetic arousal. A subgroup of undersocialized, aggressive, and/or non-emotional youths with CD consistently exhibit lower resting heart rate than control subjects (Delamater and Lahey 1983; Raine and Jones 1987; Raine and Venables 1984; Wadsworth 1976). More importantly, three prospective longitudinal studies (Davies and Maliphant 1971; Raine et al. 1990b; West and Farrington 1977) found that lower resting heart rate predicted serious criminal behavior in adolescence or young adulthood, particularly aggressive crime. Thus, resting heart rate appears to be a robust and important biological correlate of aggressive CD and later criminal aggression. In addition, one study found that youths with undersocialized CD had lower systolic blood pressure than control youths without CD (Rogeness et al. 1990b).

CD and Catecholamines

Several studies have examined the association of the catecholamines norepinephrine and epinephrine with CD. These substances serve as neurotransmitters in the hypothalamus and limbic system and are released into the bloodstream as a result of sympathetic arousal (Cooper et al. 1986). Norepinephrine is released principally from sympathetic synapses, whereas epinephrine is released by the adrenal medulla when stimulated by sympathetic neurons.

Dopamine-beta-hydroxylase (DBH), the enzyme that converts dopamine into norepinephrine, is released into serum with norepinephrine from sympathetic synapses. Because levels of DBH are under genetic control and are stable from the age of 6 years (Ciaranello and Boehme 1981; Weinshilboum 1983), DBH is an interesting candidate as a potential marker of biologically homogeneous subtypes of CD. In a series of reports on a single sample that has grown to 559 child and adolescent psychiatric inpatients in the latest report, Rogeness et al. consistently reported lower levels of DBH in boys classified as having undersocialized aggressive CD compared with other CD groups and clinical control subjects (Rogeness et al. 1984, 1990a, 1991). Although this finding was replicated with a separate clinic-referred sample (Bowden et al. 1988), it was not replicated in either an outpatient sample (Pliszka et al. 1988a) or a juvenile detention sample (Pliszka et al. 1988b).

Rogeness and colleagues (Rogeness et al. 1988, 1990a) have suggested that serum levels of DBH reflect the activity of neurons in the central nervous system (CNS) that release the neurotransmitter norepinephrine (noradrenergic neurons). Boys with low levels of serum DBH were found to have a higher ratio of two metabolites of norepinephrine, the ratio of 3-methoxy-

4-hydroxyphenylglycol (MHPG) to vanillylmandelic acid (VMA) in serum, than were boys with higher levels of serum DBH (Rogeness et al. 1988, 1990a). Maas et al. (1987) have hypothesized that the ratio of these metabolites of norepinephrine is an index of noradrenergic neuronal functioning. Higher ratios of MHPG, which is the primary product of metabolism of norepinephrine within the neuron, to VMA, which primarily results from extraneuronal metabolism of norepinephrine, are posited to reflect lower levels of norepinephrine release from neurons. Thus, low levels of DBH in boys with undersocialized aggressive CD may reflect low levels of noradrenergic neuronal activity. However, because the largest pool of DBH in blood originates in peripheral sympathetic neurons that release norepinephrine, it is not clear that levels of serum DBH reflect the activity of CNS noradrenergic neurons.

Similarly, boys with undersocialized CD were found to have lower 24-hour levels of urinary norepinephrine than were boys with socialized CD, but the levels of the undersocialized group did not differ from those of inpatient boys without CD (Rogeness et al. 1989). This finding raises the possibility that the socialized CD group showed abnormally high levels of urinary epinephrine, whereas the norepinephrine levels of the undersocialized group were normal. Unfortunately, however, a nonreferred control group was not included in the study. Interestingly, increased levels of urinary excretion of norepinephrine and its metabolites have been found in inhibited children who are at risk for childhood anxiety disorders (Biederman et al. 1990; Kagan et al. 1987). This finding suggests that the urinary norepinephrine levels of the socialized CD group may be elevated like those of shy and anxious children.

Research with adult offenders has shown that incarcerated adults with high levels of aggression and psychopathic features excrete lower levels of urinary epinephrine than do other offenders and nonoffenders, especially under stressful conditions (Lidberg et al. 1978; Woodman and Hinton 1978). Olweus et al. (1988) found significant negative correlations between average urinary epinephrine excretion levels taken under nonstressful conditions and peer ratings of unprovoked aggression ($r = -.44$) in a small school-based Swedish sample. Urinary epinephrine was also found to be negatively correlated with a self-report measure of extroversion ($r = -.48$) and positively correlated with a self-report measure of anxiety ($r = .42$). In a much larger Swedish school sample ($n = 538$), Magnusson (1988) found significant negative correlations between urinary epinephrine level and ratings of aggressiveness ($r = -.34$) and motor restlessness ($r = -.34$) among 13-year-old boys and girls on the day of a school test. More impressively, urinary epinephrine levels taken under both stressful and nonstressful conditions predicted registered criminality between the ages of 18–26 years.

Other studies have examined monoamine oxidase (MAO) and catechol-o-methyltransferase (COMT), the enzymes that catabolize norepinephrine,

epinephrine, and dopamine. Using a sample of children referred to two attention-deficit disorder specialty clinics, Bowden et al. (1988) found boys with undersocialized CD to have lower levels of platelet MAO than either clinic-referred or nonreferred control subjects. Pliszka et al. (1988a) found no relationship between DSM-III (American Psychiatric Association 1980) clinical diagnoses of CD and either plasma MHPG or platelet MAO in a sample of boys referred to an outpatient mental health center, but both MHPG and MAO were positively correlated ($r = .42$ and $r = .38$, respectively) with two independent ratings of anxiety. In addition, youths rated by parents as high in CD and low in anxiety had significantly lower levels of MHPG than youths rated as low in CD and high in anxiety.

Rogeness et al. (1982) found no differences in platelet MAO, but noted that children with undersocialized CD exhibited lower levels of red blood cell COMT than children with socialized CD. However, as was the case for urinary norepinephrine (Rogeness et al. 1989), the undersocialized CD group did not differ significantly in COMT levels from the inpatient control group, whereas the socialized CD group showed significantly higher levels. Moreover, in a much larger extended sample from the same hospital, Rogeness et al. (1991) failed to find an association between either platelet MAO or red blood cell COMT and either subgroup of CD.

CD and Serotonin

Serotonin (5-HT) also serves as a neurotransmitter in key limbic and hypothalamic brain structures (Cooper et al. 1986). It has been a focus of biological research on CD because of strong evidence from several laboratories that low levels of cerebrospinal fluid (CSF) serotonergic activity are associated with psychopathy, aggressive behavior, and suicide, whereas high levels are associated with anxiety (Gray 1982, 1987; Linnoila et al. 1983; Schalling 1986). Pliszka et al. (1988b) found lower levels of whole blood 5-HT in anxious or depressed male adolescents without CD than in juvenile offenders with CD, especially violent offenders. Youths with CD and comorbid depression or anxiety did not show the low levels of whole blood 5-HT shown by the depressed-anxious control group; rather, they resembled the other youths with CD in showing higher levels of whole blood 5-HT. In addition, Pliszka et al. (1988b) found whole blood 5-HT to be positively correlated with clinician ratings of defiance and aggression and negatively correlated with ratings of anxiety.

The meaning of measures of 5-HT in blood is not clear, as the origin of the great majority of 5-HT in blood is the digestive system and not the brain. Nevertheless, the direction of the relationship between 5-HT in blood and aggression and anxiety reported by Pliszka et al. (1988b) is consistent with one report (McBride 1987) that suggests that levels of whole blood 5-HT are negatively correlated with levels of CNS serotonergic activity. However, although Rogeness et al. (1982, 1991) did not find an association between whole blood 5-HT and CD, they did find significantly lower levels in youths with depression. These findings are consistent with studies suggesting that whole blood 5-HT is reduced in adults with major depression (Coppen et al. 1976; LeQuan-Bui et al. 1985). Interestingly, lower levels of whole blood 5-HT were found only in depressed youths who did not also exhibit CD, suggesting a possible interaction in the relationship of these two diagnoses to 5-HT (Rogeness et al. 1985, 1991).

Moreover, the findings of a study using a more direct measure of CNS serotonergic activity were consistent with the hypothesis that low levels of 5-HT activity in the CNS are associated with aggression. 5-Hydroxyindoleacetic acid (5-HIAA), the primary metabolite of 5-HT, is used as a measure of 5-HT metabolism in the CNS. This metabolite can be measured reliably in CSF obtained by lumbar puncture. Kruesi et al. (1990a) reported the results of an important preliminary study of 5-HT in the CSF of 29 children and adolescents who had at least one DSM-III disruptive behavior disorder (DBD) diagnosis (16 with CD). Compared with an age-, sex-, and race-matched comparison group of youths with obsessive-compulsive disorder, the youths with DBD diagnoses had significantly lower concentrations of CSF 5-HIAA. Perhaps more importantly for the thesis of this chapter, there was a significant negative association between the number of symptoms of aggression reported in a structured diagnostic interview and CSF 5-HIAA ($r = -.65$) in youths in the DBD group. The coefficient of correlation fell to $r = -.40$ when the age of the subjects was controlled using partial correlation; however, this may not have been a necessary correction because the decline in 5-HIAA in this age range may be part of the mechanism underlying the increases in the severity of aggression that occur in youths with CD during this period of development (Loeber 1988). In the full sample, CSF 5-HIAA concentrations were positively correlated with parent ratings of social competence ($r = .39$), suggesting that central serotonergic activity may be negatively correlated with aggression and positively correlated with the capacity for social relationships.

Kruesi et al. (1990b) also examined CSF somatostatin in 10 youths with DBDs and 10 age- and sex-matched comparison subjects with obsessive-compulsive disorder. Somatostatin was studied because of earlier evidence that it stimulates the release of 5-HT in the cortex, hypothalamus, and hippocampus. Consistent with predictions, the DBD youths exhibited lower concentrations of CSF somatostatin when pubertal stage was controlled, and the age-corrected correlation between somatostatin and CSF 5-HIAA ($r = .56$) was statistically significant.

Two other studies designed to shed light on serotonergic functioning in CD have measured platelet imipramine binding sites based on 1) evidence that imipramine binding is associated with 5-HT binding in platelets, and

2) the hypothesis that both may be reflective of CNS neuronal binding of 5-HT. Stoff et al. (1987) found that maximum platelet imipramine binding correlated negatively with parent ratings of aggression in a sample of 10 youths (ages 12–17 years) with aggressive CD and 10 nonreferred control subjects. Birmaher et al. (1990) replicated this study in a sample of inpatient and day patient youths (ages 10–16 years) who met criteria for both CD and attention-deficit hyperactivity disorder (ADHD), excluding youths who were depressed or suicidal to avoid possible confounds. These authors reported significant negative correlations of maximum platelet imipramine binding and parent ratings of hostility ($r = -.53$) and aggression ($r = -.50$).

CD and Neurohormones

McBurnett et al. (1991a) examined cortisol as an index of hypothalamic-pituitary-adrenal (HPA) axis activity in a sample of clinic-referred boys ages 7–12 years. They found that although salivary cortisol concentration was not associated with CD per se, there was a significant interaction between CD and the presence of a comorbid anxiety disorder. Boys with CD in the absence of anxiety disorder showed significantly lower concentrations of cortisol than did boys with CD and comorbid anxiety disorder. Clinical control groups of anxious and nonanxious boys had intermediate values that did not differ from those of either CD group.

In additional analyses of data from the McBurnett et al. (1991a) study, Lahey and Loeber (1991) found cortisol concentrations to be negatively correlated with the number of symptoms of aggression ($r = -.41$, $P < .001$), with the number of peer nominations of the child who is the "meanest" in the class ($r = -.39$, $P < .005$), and with the number of peer nominations of the child who "fights most" ($r = -.40$, $P < .001$). However, the number of nonaggressive symptoms of CD was not correlated with cortisol ($r = -.08$). These findings suggest that the negative correlation with HPA axis activity is specific to aggression. Interestingly, the number of symptoms of anxiety was not correlated with cortisol in the full sample ($r = .14$), but was positively correlated with cortisol among youths with CD ($r = .46$, $P = .05$). This finding suggests an interactive relationship of anxiety and CD to HPA axis functioning.

Urinary free cortisol has similarly been reported to be negatively related to appropriate classroom behavior in nonreferred school children (Tennes et al. 1986) and, more impressively, to be low in habitually violent incarcerated offenders (Virkkunen 1985). However, Kruesi et al. (1989) compared 19 boys with DBDs, mostly CD, with matched nonreferred control subjects and found no differences in 24-hour urinary cortisol output. A positive correlation between salivary cortisol and inhibited social behavior was also shown in Kagan et al.'s (1988) study of inhibited children at high risk for anxiety disorders.

Because extensive research has linked testosterone with social dominance and aggression in both primates and human males, several studies of the association of testosterone to aggression in youths have been conducted. Olweus et al. (1988) found significant correlations between serum testosterone and self-report measures of verbal aggression ($r = .38$) and physical aggression ($r = .36$) in his school-based Swedish sample. Similarly, Mattson et al. (1980) found that recidivist juvenile delinquents had significantly higher levels of serum testosterone than nonreferred control youths when pubertal stage was controlled. Because testosterone is closely linked to HPA axis activity, these differences may be related in some way to the neurohormonal differences described above.

CD and Event-Related Potentials

Event-related EEG potentials (ERPs) are used to assess brain activity associated with information processing. Raine and Venables have published a series of reports on parameters of ERPs based on a sample of 101 nonreferred English boys who were reassessed for antisocial behavior at age 24. At age 15, the boys with the highest scores on a composite of conduct problems and "undersocialized-psychopathic personality" had significantly higher P300 amplitudes to warning signals than did the remainder of the subjects (Raine and Venables 1987). These findings confirmed an earlier finding of a nonsignificant trend toward greater P300 amplitude in sociopathic delinquents (Syndulko et al. 1975), and were, in turn, confirmed in a later study of adult prisoners rated as psychopathic using Hare's (1980) psychopathy checklist (Raine and Venables 1988).

In a follow-up study of the same sample, Raine and Venables found that early adult criminal offending could be predicted by several EEG measures. Boys who had at least one registered criminal offense by age 24 had greater amounts of slow-frequency activity (Raine et al. 1990b) and shorter P300 latencies at age 15 (Raine et al. 1990a). Although the measures that predicted later criminal offending were different from the ones that differentiated the undersocialized-psychopathic group at age 15, these results clearly suggest the need for further studies of ERPs in youths with CD.

Critique of Biological Studies of CD

These studies are important in suggesting that subgroups of youths with CD can be distinguished both from one another and from control subjects on a broad range of physiological measures, including skin conductance, heart rate, cortisol, and several indices of catecholaminergic activity. Several cautionary comments on this literature are important, however.

First, the studies reviewed above were based either on all-male samples or on samples in which the great majority of subjects were male. When females were included in the samples, they were present in insufficient numbers to allow meaningful comparisons of the biological correlates of males and females. Although this is an understandable consequence of the markedly higher prevalence of CD among male children and adolescents, the result is that there is no evidence available concerning possible—or even likely—sex differences in the biological correlates of CD, and nothing is known about the biological characteristics of females with CD. In addition, because sex ratios may not be identical among the various subgroups of CD, it is possible that some findings of differences among subgroups could be artifacts of greater numbers of males in one or more CD subgroup.

Second, although the existing biological studies of CD are rather consistent for the psychophysiological measures of skin conductance and heart rate, they are less consistent for neurochemical variables. Although this lack of consistency is not surprising at the present early stage of biological research on CD, it must be addressed in future studies. The studies reviewed above are marked by lack of standardization in collection of specimens in terms of time of day and other variables, lack of control for drug and nutritional intake, and possible biases in subject referral and recruitment. In addition, many of the existing studies are based on numbers of subjects that are insufficient to provide adequate statistical power.

Third, it is important to keep in mind several concerns about diagnostic classification of CD in the studies reviewed here. Many studies were reviewed that grouped subjects according to parent and teacher behavior rating scales or on the basis of adjudication for delinquent acts, rather than by diagnoses of CD. It is likely that many of these youths would meet current diagnostic criteria for CD, but the proportion cannot be estimated accurately. When diagnostic classification of CD was made, it was usually on the basis of subjective clinical impressions rather than structured diagnostic interviews and protocols, and DSM-III criteria rather than DSM-III-R (American Psychiatric Association 1987) criteria were used in most studies. Thus, although some findings concerning the biological correlates of CD are apparently robust enough to emerge in studies using a variety of weak measures of CD, findings using more stringent DSM-III-R diagnoses based on reliable diagnostic protocols might yield more consistently replicable results. Studies using these improved measures may identify additional—or even different—correlates of CD.

Fourth, future studies of the association of biological variables to subgroups of CD must take both motor hyperactivity and "bizarre" behavior into consideration. In two separate samples, low DBH was found to be associated with those boys with CD who exhibited bizarre/psychotic or behavior or who had diagnoses of borderline personality disorder (Pliszka et al. 1988a; Rogeness et al. 1991). Similarly, studies of adults have reported negative correlations of serum DBH with scores on the Psychopathic Deviance and Schizophrenia scales of the Minnesota Multiphasic Personality Inventory (MMPI; Hathaway and McKinley 1970), suggesting that low DBH may characterize a subgroup of CD antisocial individuals with bizarre behavior (Rogeness et al. 1982). Furthermore, Raine and Venables (1984) have reported that the youths with conduct problems who showed the fewest skin conductance responses to tones were those with schizoid characteristics.

In addition, Klinteberg and Magnusson (1989) have found evidence that the association of urinary epinephrine with aggression may be explained by the association of aggression with motor hyperactivity. In the same sample in which urinary epinephrine was significantly correlated (both concurrently and predictively) with aggression, the correlation of urinary epinephrine with ratings of hyperactivity was significant when aggression levels were controlled; however, the opposite was not true. If confirmed in future studies, such associations between biological measures and bizarre/psychotic behavior and motor hyperactivity may clarify the association of biological variables with a subgroup of CD. For example, previous studies have shown that boys with CD who are hyperactive are more likely to be aggressive than are nonhyperactive boys with CD (Walker et al. 1987). It may well be, then, that an adequate model of the biological correlates will involve complex relationships among aggression, motor hyperactivity, bizarre/psychotic behavior, and other comorbidities such as anxiety and depression.

Finally, although most studies with negative findings were included in this review, some less important, inconsistent results were not summarized. For example, a study of nonreferred school children by Tennes and Kreye (1985) that did not confirm several findings regarding epinephrine, norepinephrine, and cortisol was omitted because it did not include strong measures of CD behaviors. In this sense, then, our review should be considered to be somewhat selective. Moreover, there is an obvious bias toward the reporting of positive findings in the literature. Therefore, one should not conclude that the consistency of findings reported in this chapter reflects the consistency with which such findings could be replicated.

Integrative Hypotheses Regarding Biological Measures

Keeping in mind the criticisms noted above, some tentative integrative hypotheses may be in order for the biological variables reviewed in this chapter. It is possible that most of the biological characteristics described thus far reflect a small number of neurobiological processes. The primary sources of DBH, norepinephrine, and metabolites of norepinephrine in serum are sympathetic synapses, and a major source of epinephrine in urine is the adrenal medulla, which is stimulated by sympathetic fibers. Thus, these variables may all primarily reflect sympathetic activity. Similarly, skin conductance rather directly reflects sympathetic discharge, and heart rate and blood pressure are importantly influenced both by the balance of sympathetic and parasympathetic activity and by circulating epinephrine and norepinephrine. Thus, group differences in skin conductance and heart rate may also reflect differences in sympathetic activity.

Although cortisol secretion by the adrenal cortex is not under direct autonomic control, the same noradrenergic, serotonergic, and other neural tracts that affect sympathetic outflow also influence the hypothalamic centers that modulate the HPA axis. In addition, the HPA axis and the autonomic nervous system interact reciprocally in a number of ways. For example, corticotropin-releasing hormone (CRH)—the hypothalamic neuropeptide that initiates the HPA axis hormonal chain that governs the secretion of cortisol—also affects key limbic structures (e.g., the locus coeruleus and the dorsal vagal complex) that control the autonomic nervous system (Nemeroff 1991). Thus, a wide range of biological correlates of CD could be explained by a small set of CNS mechanisms that affect HPA axis and autonomic functioning. The present findings do not allow strong inferences concerning the nature of that putative CNS pathophysiology, but the very fact that a few common pathways can be hypothesized for the diversity of findings in the present literature gives strength to the hypothesis that one or more subgroup of CD is associated with atypical neurobiologic functioning.

Although much more speculative at this point, some evidence suggests that at least two specific CNS neural systems that influence the sympathetic nervous system and the HPA axis may be linked to aggressive CD. The finding of a significant association between aggression and several measures of serotonergic activity (Birmaher et al. 1990; Kruesi et al. 1990a; Pliszka et al. 1988b; Stoff et al. 1987) suggests that CNS serotonergic neurons may be one of the central systems associated with aggressive CD. This possibility is strengthened by the fact that the P300 component of ERP is both predictive of persistent antisocial behavior and correlated with CSF 5-HIAA.

Similarly, Quay (1988) and Rogeness et al. (1984, 1991) have suggested, based on limited evidence, that CNS noradrenergic systems may play a role in the mediation of CD. This hypothesis is based on three key findings: First, serum DBH has sometimes been found to be low in youths with undersocialized aggressive CD. Second, previous studies have reported positive correlations between serum DBH and CSF DBH and norepinephrine (Lerner et al. 1978; Zuckerman et al. 1983) and among norepinephrine and its metabolites in urine, serum, and CSF (Roy et al. 1988). Third, in the Rogeness studies, boys with low DBH were found to have higher ratios of MHPG to VMA, and Maas et al. (1987) have hypothesized that the ratio of these metabolites of norepinephrine reflects CNS noradrenergic functioning. Although quite speculative at this point, the hypotheses that youths with undersocialized CD exhibit deficits in CNS serotonergic and noradrenergic functioning should receive careful experimental evaluation in the future.

Summary

It seems likely that CD is a heterogeneous disorder in terms of patterns of antisocial behavior, developmental course, and outcome. Too little is known at present to attempt to characterize those youths who initially develop CD around puberty. The developmental histories of these youths, their pattern of nonaggressive antisocial acts, their tendency to commit delinquent acts with peers, and the relative transience of their antisocial behavior suggest that they may not share the same biological characteristics with those with more persistent CD who are younger at onset.

Various diagnostic nomenclatures have attempted to capture the heterogeneity of CD by using a variety of subtyping dimensions that appear to overlap considerably. It may be useful for heuristic purposes to assume that a group of youths with persistent early-onset CD can be identified reliably who can be said to have poor social relatedness, high levels of aggression, and other "psychopathic" characteristics. This group may be quite different from youths with CD who have adequate social relatedness and low levels of aggression.

If one assumes that two such groups of early-onset CD can be distinguished, the literature on the biological correlates of CD is rather consistent in suggesting that the "psychopathic-undersocialized-aggressive" and the "neurotic-socialized-nonaggressive" subgroups are quite distinct. The former is characterized by a variety of measures that appear to reflect lower levels of sympathetic and HPA axis activity. These measures include skin conductance, heart rate, and products reflective of release of norepinephrine by the sympathetic synapses, release of epinephrine by the adrenal medulla, and cortisol. The latter subgroup of CD is characterized by the opposite pattern of the same measures, perhaps reflecting abnormally high levels of sympathetic and HPA axis activity. Hence, these two subgroups of CD appear to have essentially *opposite* biological correlates.

The finding that cortisol levels parallel measures that are reflective of sympathetic arousal suggests that hypothalamic centers that influence both sympathetic outflow and activation of the HPA axis are influenced by the CNS systems that constitute the pathophysiology or pathophysiologies underlying the two putative biologically homogeneous subtypes of CD. Studies of serotonergic and noradrenergic functioning have provided the basis for tentative hypotheses that these CNS systems may be involved in the mechanisms that underlie CD.

It is particularly interesting that the biological variables that predict adult criminal behavior (lower heart rate, less phasic skin conductance to tones, lower urinary epinephrine, and increased P300 latency) are characteristic of those youths with CD who are identified as aggressive, undersocialized, and psychopathic. Because those same behavioral characteristics predict long-term persistence and worsening of antisocial behavior in youths with CD, it appears that this set of biological characteristics identifies the most severe group of CD, both concurrently and predictively.

References

American Psychiatric Association: Diagnostic and Statistical Manual of Mental Disorders, 3rd Edition. Washington, DC, American Psychiatric Association, 1980

American Psychiatric Association: Diagnostic and Statistical Manual of Mental Disorders, 3rd Edition, Revised. Washington, DC, American Psychiatric Association, 1987

Biederman J, Rosenbaum JF, Hirshfeld DR, et al: Psychiatric correlates of behavioral inhibition in young children with and without psychiatric disorders. Arch Gen Psychiatry 47:21–26, 1990

Birmaher B, Stanley M, Greenhill L, et al: Platelet imipramine binding in children and adolescents with impulsive behavior. J Am Acad Child Adolesc Psychiatry 29:914–918, 1990

Borkovec TO: Autonomic reactivity to sensory stimulation in psychopathic, neurotic, and normal delinquents. J Consult Clin Psychol 35:217–222, 1970

Bowden CL, Deutsch CK, Swanson JM: Plasma dopamine-b-hydroxylase and platelet monoamine oxidase in attention deficit disorder and conduct disorder. J Am Acad Child Adolesc Psychiatry 27:171–174, 1988

Ciaranello RD, Boehme RE: Biochemical genetics of neurotransmitter enzymes and receptors: relationships to schizophrenia and other major psychiatric disorders. Clin Genet 19:358–372, 1981

Cooper JR, Bloom FE, Roth RH: The Biochemical Basis of Neuropharmacology. New York, Oxford University Press, 1986

Coppen A, Rowsell AR, Turner P, et al: 5-hydroxytryptamine (5-HT) in the whole blood of patients with depressive illness. Postgrad Med J 52:156–158, 1976

Davies JGV, Maliphant R: Autonomic responses of male adolescents exhibiting refractory behavior in school. J Child Psychol Psychiatry 12:115–127, 1971

Delamater AM, Lahey BB: Physiological correlates of conduct problems in hyperactive and learning disabled children. J Abnorm Child Psychol 11:85–100, 1983

Fox R, Lippert W: Spontaneous GSR and anxiety level in sociopathic delinquents. Journal of Consulting Psychology 27:368–370, 1963

Gray J: The Neuropsychology of Anxiety: An Enquiry Into the Functions of the Septo-Hippocampal System. Oxford, UK, Oxford University Press, 1982

Gray J: The Psychology of Fear and Stress, 2nd Edition. Cambridge, UK, Cambridge University Press, 1987

Hare RD: A research scale for the assessment of psychopathy in criminal populations. Personality and Individual Differences 1:111–120, 1980

Hathaway SR, McKinley JC: Minnesota Multiphasic Personality Inventory, Revised. Minneapolis, University of Minnesota, 1970

Kagan J, Resnick JS, Snidman N: The physiology and psychology of behavioral inhibition in young children. Child Dev 58:1459–1473, 1987

Kagan J, Resnick JS, Snidman N: Biological bases of childhood shyness. Science 240:167–171, 1988

Klinteberg BAF, Magnusson D: Aggressiveness and hyperactive behavior as related to adrenaline excretion. European Journal of Personality 3:81–93, 1989

Kruesi MJP, Schmidt ME, Donnelly M, et al: Urinary free cortisol output and disruptive behavior in children. J Am Acad Child Adolesc Psychiatry 28:441–443, 1989

Kruesi MJP, Rapoport JL, Hamburger S, et al: Cerebrospinal fluid monamine metabolites, aggression, and impulsivity in disruptive behavior disorders of children and adolescents. Arch Gen Psychiatry 47:419–426, 1990a

Kruesi MJP, Swedo S, Leonard H, et al: CSF somatostatin in childhood psychiatric disorders: a preliminary investigation. Psychiatry Res 33:277–284, 1990b

Lahey BB, Loeber R: A preliminary psychobiological model of conduct disorder. Paper presented at the annual meeting of the Society for Research in Child and Adolescent Psychopathology, Amsterdam, The Netherlands, June 1991

Lahey BB, Piacentini JC, McBurnett K, et al: Psychopathology in the parents of children with conduct disorder and hyperactivity. J Am Acad Child Adolesc Psychiatry 27:163–170, 1987

LeQuan-Bui KH, Plaisant O, Leboyer M, et al: Reduced platelet serotonin in depression. Psychiatry Res 13:129–139, 1985

Lerner P, Goodwin FK, van Kammen, et al: DBH in the CSF of psychiatric patients. Biol Psychiatry 13:685–694, 1978

Lidberg L, Levander SE, Schalling D, et al: Urinary catecholamines, stress, and psychopathy: a study of arrested men awaiting trial. Psychosom Med 40:116–125, 1978

Linnoila M, Virkkunen M, Scheinin M, et al: Low cerebrospinal fluid 5-hydroxyindoleacetic acid concentration differentiates impulsive from nonimpulsive violent behavior. Life Sci 33:2609–2614, 1983

Loeber R: Natural history of juvenile conduct problems, delinquency, and associated substance abuse: evidence for developmental progressions, in Advances in Clinical Child Psychology, Vol 11. Edited by Lahey BB, Kazdin AE. New York, Plenum, 1988, pp 73–124

Maas JW, Koslow SH, Davis J, et al: Catecholamine metabolism and disposition in healthy and depressed subjects. Arch Gen Psychiatry 44:337–344, 1987

Magnusson D: Aggressiveness, hyperactivity, and autonomic activity/reactivity in the development of social maladjustment, in Individual Development From an Interactional Perspective: A Longitudinal Study. Edited by Magnusson D. Hillsdale, NJ, Lawrence Erlbaum, 1988, pp 1533–172

Mattson A, Schalling D, Olweus D, et al: Plasma testosterone, aggressive behavior, and personality dimensions in young male delinquents. J Am Acad Child Adolesc Psychiatry 19:476–490, 1980

McBride A: Serotonin in major psychiatric disorders. Paper presented at the annual meeting of the American Psychiatric Association, Chicago, IL, May 1987

McBurnett K, Lahey BB, Tuch PF, et al: Anxiety, inhibition, and conduct disorder in children, II: relation to salivary cortisol. J Am Acad Child Adolesc Psychiatry 30:192–196, 1991a

McBurnett K, Swanson JM, Pfiffner LJ, et al: The Relationship of Prefrontal Test Performance and Autonomic Arousal to Symptoms of Inattention/Overactivity and Aggression/Defiance. Paper presented at the annual meeting of the Society for Research on Psychopathology, Amsterdam, The Netherlands, June 1991b

Nemeroff CB: Corticotropin-releasing factor, in Neuropeptides and Psychiatric Disorders. Edited by Nemeroff CB. Washington, DC, American Psychiatric Press, 1991, pp 75–91

Olweus D, Mattson A, Schalling D, et al: Circulating testosterone levels in adolescent males: a causal analysis. Psychosom Med 50:261–272, 1988

Pliszka SR, Rogeness GA, Medrano MA: DBH, MHPG, and MAO in children with depressive, anxiety, and conduct disorders: relationship to diagnosis and symptom ratings. Psychiatry Res 24:35–44, 1988a

Pliszka SR, Rogeness GA, Renner P, et al: Plasma neurochemistry in juvenile offenders. J Am Acad Child Adolesc Psychiatry 27:588–594, 1988b

Quay HC: The behavioral reward and inhibition system in childhood behavior disorders, in Attention Deficit Disorder, Vol 3. Edited by Bloomingdale LM. New York, Pergamon, 1988, pp 176–186

Raine A, Jones F: Attention, autonomic arousal, and personality in behaviorally disordered children. J Abnorm Child Psychol 15:583–599, 1987

Raine A, Venables PH: Electrodermal responding, antisocial behavior, and schizoid tendencies in adolescents. Psychophysiology 21:424–433, 1984

Raine A, Venables PH: Contingent negative variation, P3 evoked potentials, and antisocial behavior. Psychophysiology 24:191–199, 1987

Raine A, Venables PH: Enhanced P3 evoked potentials and longer P3 recovery times in psychopaths. Psychophysiology 25:30–38, 1988

Raine A, Venables PH: Antisocial behavior: evolution, genetics, neuropsychology, and psychophysiology, in Handbook of Individual Differences. Edited by Gale A, Eysenck M. Chichester, UK, Wiley, 1992

Raine A, Venables PH, Williams M: Autonomic orienting responses in 15-year-old male subjects and criminal behavior at age 24. Am J Psychiatry 147:933–937, 1990a

Raine A, Venables PH, Williams M: Relationships between central and autonomic measures of arousal at age 15 years and criminality at age 24 years. Arch Gen Psychiatry 47:1003–1007, 1990b

Raine A, Reynolds GP, Sheard C: Neuroanatomical mediators of electrodermal activity in normal human subjects: a magnetic resonance imaging study. Psychophysiology 28:548–558, 1991

Reite M, Field T: The Psychobiology of Attachment and Separation. Orlando, FL, Academic Press, 1985

Rogeness GA, Hernandez JM, Macedo CA: Biochemical differences in children with conduct disorder socialized and undersocialized. Am J Psychiatry 139:307–311, 1982

Rogeness GA, Hernandez JM, Macedo MD, et al: Clinical characteristics of emotionally disturbed boys with very low activities of dopamine-b-hydroxylase. Journal of the American Academy of Child Psychiatry 23:203–208, 1984

Rogeness GA, Mitchell EL, Custer GJ, et al: Comparison of whole blood serotonin and platelet MAO in children with schizophrenia and major depressive disorder. Biol Psychiatry 20:270–275, 1985

Rogeness GA, Maas JW, Javors MA, et al: Diagnoses, catecholamine metabolism, and plasma dopamine-B-hydroxylase. J Am Acad Child Adolesc Psychiatry 27:121–125, 1988

Rogeness GA, Maas JW, Javors MA, et al: Attention deficit disorder symptoms and urine. Psychiatry Res 27:241–251, 1989

Rogeness GA, Javors MA, Maas JW, et al: Catecholamine and diagnoses in children. J Am Acad Child Adolesc Psychiatry 29:234–241, 1990a

Rogeness GA, Cepeda C, Macedo CA, et al: Differences in heart rate and blood pressure in children with conduct disorder, major depression, and separation anxiety. Psychiatry Res 33:199–206, 1990b

Rogeness GA, Macedo CA, Fischer C, et al: Biochemical and clinical differences among DSM-III subtypes of conduct disorder. University of Texas Health Science Center at San Antonio, December 1991

Roy A, Pickar D, De Jong J, et al: Norepinephrine and its metabolites in cerebrospinal fluid, plasma, and urine: relation to hypothalamic-pituitary-adrenal axis function in depression. Arch Gen Psychiatry 45:849–857, 1988

Schalling D: The involvement of serotonergic mechanisms in anxiety and impulsivity in humans. Behavioral and Brain Sciences 9:343–344, 1986

Schmidt K, Solanto MV, Bridger WH: Electrodermal activity of undersocialized aggressive children. J Child Psychol Psychiatry 26:653–660, 1985

Siddle OAT, Nicol AR, Foggitt RH: Habituation and over extinction of the GSR component of the orienting response in antisocial adolescents. British Journal of Social and Clinical Psychology 12:303–308, 1973

Stoff DM, Pollack L, Vitiello B, et al: Reduction of 3-H-imipramine binding sites on platelets of conduct-disordered children. Neuropsychophysiology 3:155–162, 1987

Syndulko K, Parker OA, Jens R, et al: Psychophysiology of psychopathy: electrocortical measures. Biol Psychiatry 10:185–200, 1975

Tennes K, Kreye M: Children's adrenocortical responses to clas sroom activities and tests in elementary school. Psychosom Med 47:451–460, 1985

Tennes K, Kreye M, Avitable N, et al: Behavioral correlates of excreted catecholamines and cortisol in second-grade children. J Am Acad Child Adolesc Psychiatry 25:764–770, 1986

Virkkunen M: Urinary free cortisol excretion in habitually violent offenders. Acta Psychiatr Scand 72:40–42, 1985

Wadsworth MEJ: Delinquency, pulse rates and early emotional deprivation. British Journal of Criminology 16:245–256, 1976

Walker JL, Lahey BB, Hynd GW, et al: Comparison of specific patterns of antisocial behavior in children with conduct disorder with or without coexisting hyperactivity. J Consult Clin Psychol 55:910–913, 1987

West DJ, Farrington DP: The Delinquent Way of Life. London, Heinemann, 1977

Weinshilboum RM: Biochemical genetics of catecholamines in man. Mayo Clin Proc 58:319–330, 1983

Woodman DO, Hinton J: Catecholamine balance during stress anticipation: an abnormality in maximum security hospital patients. J Psychosom Res 22:477–483, 1978

Zuckerman M, Ballenger JC, Jimeson OC, et al: A correlational test in humans of the biological models of sensation seeking, impulsivity, and anxiety, in Biological Bases of Sensation Seeking, Impulsivity and Anxiety. Edited by Zuckerman M. Hillsdale, NJ, Lawrence Erlbaum, 1983, pp 229–248

Chapter 3

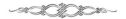

Aggression

Jon A. Shaw, M.D.
Ana Campo-Bowen, M.D.

Anumber of observers have commented on the presence of aggression as a ubiquitous phenomenon in nature and in mankind. As Sigmund Freud (1930/1953) noted, "Men are not gentle creatures who want to be loved, and who at the most defend themselves if they are attacked; they are, on the contrary, creatures among whose instinctual endowment is to be reckoned a powerful share of aggressiveness" (p. 111). Thomas Hobbes (1651/1961), reflecting upon the nature of man in *Leviathan,* observed that "if any two men desire the same thing which nevertheless they cannot both enjoy, they become enemies and in the way to their end, endeavor to destroy or subdue one another" (p. 99). Aggression has been demonstrated in one form or another in virtually every society around the globe.

Much of the confusion in any discussion of aggression is the problem of definition. Joseph (1973) has observed that the term *aggression* is derived from the Latin "to go forward" or "to approach" and has generally been associated with the meaning "to go forward with the intent of inflicting harm" (p. 198). E. O. Wilson, the sociobiologist, has defined aggression as "the abridgement of the rights of others, forcing [them] to surrender something [they] own or might otherwise have attained, either by a physical act or by the threat of action" (Wilson 1975, p. 242). *Webster's New 20th Century Dictionary* (1980) defines aggression as "an unprovoked attack or act of hostility."

The scientific literature has frequently failed to distinguish between aggressive antisocial behavior and conduct-related problems. Loeber (1982) has defined antisocial behavior as "acts that maximize a person's immediate personal gain through inflicting pain or loss upon others" (p. 1432).

It is difficult to talk about antisocial behavior in children without discussing the problem of aggression. One-third to one-half of all child and adolescent clinic referrals are for aggressiveness, conduct problems, and antisocial behaviors (Robins 1981). Aggression in child and adolescent psychiatric disorders is most commonly thought to occur within the diagnosis of conduct disorder. Eight of the 13 DSM-III-R (American Psychiatric Association 1987) criteria used for the diagnosis of conduct disorder specifically probe for symptoms of aggression. Antisocial behavior includes a broad range of actions that violate major age-appropriate societal norms and rules; these actions include stealing, fighting, destroying property, forcing another person into sexual activity, being cruel to animals, and setting fires.

There is increasing recognition that aggressivity is the significant variable determining severity of antisocial behavior. Kupersmidt and Coie (1990) noted that aggression toward peers was a better predictor of adolescent delinquency than either peer rejection or school performance. Rogeness and colleagues (1990), in a study of 345 children and adolescents with conduct disorder using DSM-III-R criteria, found that 84% were ranked as either socialized or undersocialized aggressive, whereas only 16% were in the nonaggressive categories. Aggressive acts are the preferred means by which the rights of others are violated.

Ethological Perspectives

The emergence of ethology as a scientific discipline has contributed to our understanding of aggression. Lorenz (1966) noted that aggressive tendencies are one of the legacies of the evolutionary past and suggested that such tendencies are necessary for the continuing successful existence of various animal groups. In particular, he stressed the importance of ranking order, territoriality, displacement activity, and the various dimensions of animal group behavior in which aggressive tendencies have been inhibited and/or ritualized to sustain the survival of the group.

Lorenz (1966) also observed that ranking order is a principle of organization without which a more advanced social life cannot develop in higher vertebrates. Under this order, every animal in a group knows which members are stronger and which are weaker than itself so that each group member can retreat from the stronger and expect submission from the weaker if they should get in each other's way.

David Hamburg (1973) has noted that ranking order leads to the protection of the weaker members of the group, not to their exploitation. In the rank order, the authority and responsibility for detecting and responding to hostile elements are entrusted to the higher ranking members, and the traits that brought them to power are the ones most likely to have survival value for the group. In this instance, the aim of aggression is not the extermination of fellow members of the species. The establishment of a hierarchy benefits many animal groups. Wild geese are assured that on their long flights the strong will fly first, breaking the force of the wind, and the ranks of the V formation will remain intact. The older and more experienced leaders of a troop of baboons will defend and seemingly sacrifice their lives to defend the troop against a leopard.

With reference to territoriality, it has been noted that the aggressive defense of territory between conspecifics serves the function of putting distance between them, an obvious advantage in the struggle of the species to survive. Territorial boundaries are labeled and demarcated in many ways. Dogs urinate on various trees, male birds sing their arias, while the grizzly bear stands fully erect, rubbing the bark of trees with its back and snout to signal other bears to avoid this district where a bear of such dimensions defends his territory. The largest part of aggressive behaviors among members of a species involves either sexual competition or resource competition. Wynne-Edwards (1962) has postulated that all higher animals have evolved societies in which some form of conventional competition has been substituted for the direct struggle for food.

Wasman and Flynn (1962) distinguished between two subtypes of aggressive behavior: affective aggressive and predatory aggressive. Affective aggressive behavior is characterized by autonomic arousal, threatening or defensive postures and vocalizations, and, often, frenzied attacks. Affective aggression may be reactive, situational, or intraspecific and is not always goal directed. Predatory aggressive behavior, on the other hand, entails less autonomic activation associated with stalking behavior, little posturing and vocalization, appetitive motivation, and lethally directed attacks on interspecific prey.

There is disagreement among ethologists and social scientists as to the existence of an aggressive instinct. Scott (1975) concluded that "there is no such thing as a simple instinct for fighting, in the sense of an internal driving force which has to be satisfied. There is, however, an internal physiological mechanism which has only to be stimulated to produce fighting" (p. 62). Berkowitz (1962) observed that "since spontaneous animal aggression is a relatively rare occurrence in nature, . . . many ethologists and experimental biologists rule out the possibility of a self-stimulating aggressive system in animals" (p. 46). Tinbergen (1953) indicated that no evidence exists of a general aggressive instinct among animals. The fighting that occurs between conspecifics consists mainly of threatening behavior (i.e., bluff) or a reaction to sexual rivalry. Lorenz (1966) appears to be unique in his unquestioning acceptance of aggression as an instinct.

It is apparent that aggression in animal groups may be manifested in several different recognized forms and that it may serve multiple purposes. Wilson (1975) has described eight different kinds of aggression present in vertebrates:

— Territorial
— Dominance
— Sexual
— Parental disciplinary
— Weaning
— Moralistic
— Predatory
— Antipredatory

It would thus seem that aggression is not a unitary concept, but rather refers to a heterogeneous grouping of phenomena.

Genetic and Family Influences

Family, twin, and adoptee studies provide evidence of considerable genetic influence in aggressive behavior tendencies. Hutchings and Mednick (1975) observed that adopted-away offspring of criminal fathers were twice as likely as those of noncriminal fathers to be antisocial. There was likewise an interaction effect between genetic and family environment factors. The highest criminality rate was found among those adoptees who had both a biological and an adopting father with a police record. Studies of Swedish adoptees have confirmed the increased rates of criminality in the biological parents of petty criminals (Bohman et al. 1982). O'Connor et al. (1980) demonstrated a higher concordance for behaviors such as bullying, restlessness, and school problems in identical twins than in fraternal twins. Christiansen (1976) reported on the criminality of 3,586 male twin pairs in Denmark and noted that the concordance for criminality between monozygotic twins was 51% compared with 22% for dizygotic twins. Offord (1989) has suggested, however, that whereas the evidence for genetic influences in a subgroup of adult criminals has been demonstrated, there is little proof that genetic factors play an important etiological role in conduct disorder in children.

The best predictor of aggressive behavior in human relationships is the XY chromosome dyad. Compared with females, males are universally more aggressive, more prone to establish dominance hierarchies, and less empathic and nurturing toward their young.

The role of psychosocial, family, and parental factors in determining aggressive/antisocial behavior is well known (McCord 1988; Patterson et al. 1989; Richman et al. 1982). There is evidence that aggressiveness and antisocial behavior in parents influence the behavior of their offspring. Imitation, social learning, modeling, and identification with the aggressor vis-à-vis aggressive, physically abusing, antisocial, and criminal parents have variously been cited (Fry 1988; Hall and Cairns 1984; West and Farrington 1977) as the mechanism of such influence. Patterson et al. (1989) demonstrated that harsh and inconsistent discipline, lack of positive parenting experiences, and poor parental monitoring result in children who are prone to antisocial behavior and for whom aggression is a legitimate means for resolving conflict. The children of aggressive parents have a greater proclivity to perceive the actions of others as hostile and more readily respond with aggression to such perceived threats (Dodge and Somberg 1987). A factor that may contribute to increased aggressivity in children who have been victimized by aggression is their apparent reduced responsiveness to pain, which may be related to an increase of endogenous opiates (van der Kolk 1989). A lack of responsiveness to pain may contribute to antisocial behavior because anticipatory inhibitions are reduced. Quay (1965) suggested that reduced arousal may also account for sensation seeking. Raine et al. (1990) have demonstrated that underarousal measures (electrodermal, cardiovascular, and cortical) at adolescence predict criminality in young adulthood. McCord (1988) reported that the offspring of aggressive, punitive parents are more prone to be aggressive, to identify situations as justifying annoyance, and to display more egocentricity. West and Farrington (1977) noted a cluster of traits characteristic of delinquents: irregular work habits, immoderation in the pursuit of immediate pleasure, lack of conventional social restraints, and aggressiveness.

Developmental Perspectives on Aggressive/Antisocial Behavior

Anna Freud (1953) observed that "there seems to be universal recognition of the fact that normal and abnormal psychological development cannot be understood without an adequate explanation of the role of aggression played by the aggressive and destructive tendencies and attitudes" (p. 216).

Aggressive, disruptive behavior appears to be a developmental trait that begins in early life and frequently continues into adolescence and adulthood. In an often-cited report, Olweus (1979) reviewed 16 studies on the stability of aggressive reaction patterns from early childhood to early adulthood. He concluded that the degree of stability of aggression is substantial, approaching that found in the domain of intelligence. Marked individual differences in habitual aggression levels were evident during the developmental period and clearly differentiated between individuals by 3 years of age. Olweus suggested that the stability of aggression over time reflects an enduring individual reaction tendency or trait position. Aggression at 8–9 years of age correlated with aggression observed 10–14 years later. Aggressive behavior persists from the preschool into the school years and is the most important variable predicting later aggression and antisocial behavior.

Reid (1986) has suggested that there is nothing that children with conduct disorder do that all children don't do at some time or another. It is just that they tend to do a lot more of these things in specialized ways, and such actions become an enduring pattern of behavior. *Conduct disorder* refers to a persistent pattern of antisocial behavior that is clinically significant and meets syndromal criteria. When specific behaviors are examined and youths are asked to self-report on their activities, the prevalence rates for antisocial behavior are quite high. In a national survey of 3,000 adolescents by the Michigan Institute for Social Research (Bachman et al. 1986) quoted by Siegel and Senna in *Juvenile Delinquency* (1988), 12% reported hurting someone so badly that he or she needed medical attention, 32% admitted to stealing something valued at less than $50, 28% acknowledged shoplifting, and 14% reported having damaged school property.

A number of longitudinal studies have investigated the relationship between early childhood aggression and antisocial behavior and subsequent aggressive, antisocial, and delinquent behavior.

Preschool Children

Henri Parens (1979, 1989), from his observational work with infants, has taken the position that aggression is present at birth and that hostile, destructive aggression is initially evident in the rage reactions of infants who are hungry, frightened, or in pain. The basic aim of such aggression is to act upon one's environment and to assert oneself; it emerges as the result of excessive unpleasure and provocation. It is Parens's belief that around the first year of life, this form of aggression may change from nondirective expressions of rage into increasingly directed aggressive behavior in which the aim is to hurt and humiliate another. However, by 30 months of age, most children will begin to substitute verbal aggression for biting, pushing, hair pulling, throwing objects, and hitting others (Hartup 1974).

Although it has been observed that the frequency and duration of aggressive pushing and hitting decreases between 2 and 5 years of age, the disposition to be physically aggressive remains highly stable in boys. More modest correlations are found among girls. Dimensions of physical aggression at age 2, as manifested by bodily and object-directed aggression, predicted dimensions of physical aggression at 5 years of age (Cummings et al. 1989).

Richman et al. (1982) evaluated every fourth child in a borough outside of London at 3, 4, and 8 years of age using a behavior screening questionnaire that provided a measure of impulsivity, activity level, aggressivity, and discipline problems. Sixty-two percent of those children with disruptive behavior problems at 3 years of age continued to have adjustment problems at age 8. There was evidence of a severity effect: approximately three-fourths of those rated moderate/severe at age 3 continued to have conduct-related behavior at age 8. Antisocial behavior in boys at age 8 years was found to be related to excessive activity level, difficult-to-control behavior, and poor peer relationships at 3 years of age. Girls with conduct-related problems at age 8 often had had difficult sibling relationships and undue fears when they were younger.

Campbell et al. (1986; Campbell and Ewing 1990), in an ongoing longitudinal study of externalizing behaviors first inventoried in children at 3 years of age, observed that half of these children continued to have significant difficulties at school entry and 67% continued to have problems with behavior control at age 9. The severity of hyperactivity and aggression at 3 years of age predicted conduct problems at age 9.

Fischer et al. (1984) reported that discipline problems and aggression in day care predicted ongoing adjustment problems 5–7 years later. Early behaviors such as temper tantrums and grade school troublesomeness were found to significantly predict adolescent and adult offenses (Patterson et al. 1989).

A number of factors—family stress, marital discord, quality of parent-child relationship, maternal depression, low IQ, specific and general developmental delays, and severity of disruptive behavior—have been discovered to contribute to the stability of disruptive/antisocial behavior developmentally in the early childhood years (Campbell and Ewing 1990; Richman et al. 1982).

School-Age Children and Adolescents

First-grade ratings of aggressive behavior in males portend delinquent behavior in adolescence, whereas shy behavior in the first grade appears to be a protective factor against delinquent behavior (Ensminger et al. 1983). When reassessed after 5 years, aggressive/antisocial behaviors—i.e., conflicts with parents, delinquency, and fighting—observed in children and adolescents between 6 and 18 years of age either increased in a pathological direction or remained at a relatively constant level, whereas nonaggressive behaviors declined with advancing age (Gersten et al. 1976). Havighurst et al. (1962) observed that teacher- and peer-related aggressive maladjustment at the sixth-grade level predicted poor adult adjustment at 20 years of age.

Dodge et al. (1990) have described the predictability with which instrumental and reactive aggression in a boy's behavior may rapidly determine his peer status and thus sustain his maladaptive social behaviors. This finding suggests that aggressivity has enduring effects on social valence. The boys in this study were characterized as likely both to interpret ambiguously provocative incidents as intentionally caused by peers and to display aggressive behavior toward their peers.

Kupersmidt and Coie (1990), in a study of 112 fifth graders in a rural elementary school, observed that preadolescent aggression toward peers was predictive of subsequent police or juvenile contacts. Halikas et al. (1990), noting the relationship between attention-deficit hyperactivity disorder

(ADHD) and substance abuse, determined that it is the aggressivity and not the attention-deficit disorder that is predictive of subsequent substance abuse.

Blumstein et al. (1985) found that seven variables predicted chronic offending: conviction for crime prior to age 13; low family income; troublesome rating in school by ages 8–10; poor public school performance by age 10; psychomotor clumsiness; low nonverbal IQ; and having a brother or sister convicted of a crime. Farrington (1983) followed children from 8 to 22 years of age, measuring aggression approximately every 2 years, and substantiated the persistence of aggression as a stable feature in the lives of these children. Half of the violent delinquents had been rated aggressive at ages 8–10 years.

A number of studies suggest that childhood antisocial/aggressive behavior predicts adult antisocial behavior and that criminal behavior in late childhood or early adolescence predicts chronic offenders (Farrington 1983; Glueck and Glueck 1959; Loeber 1982; Robins 1979). Glueck and Glueck (1959) noted that 80% of 500 boys defined as delinquent between 9 and 17 years of age were arrested again within the subsequent 8-year period. Robins (1979) concluded that adults with antisocial behavior had almost always been antisocial children and that the number and diversity of childhood antisocial behaviors were the best predictors of adult antisocial behavior. Loeber (1982) observed that chronically delinquent young adults were more likely than nondelinquent control subjects to have, as children, manifested early onset of antisocial behaviors across more than one setting and to have displayed a wider variety of such behaviors. Although less than half of antisocial youth become antisocial adults and a general decline of overt antisocial acts occurs during the adolescent years, there is evidence that the more extreme the antisocial behavior, the greater its stability over time (Farrington 1983).

Wolfgang et al. (1972) not only demonstrated the ubiquitousness of antisocial behavior in adolescence and early adulthood but, more importantly, described the phenomenon of the chronic delinquent offender. Six percent of their original cohort were responsible for 51.9% of the 10,214 offenses perpetrated.

Henn et al. (1979) studied a group of delinquent adolescents and observed that behavior evaluated as undersocialized aggressive was predictably related to adult arrests, convictions, and imprisonments for violent crimes. Loeber (1991) has suggested that disruptive/antisocial behavior stabilizes before midadolescence and that malleability decreases subsequently; thus, intervention programs should be directed toward the younger age groups.

Robins (1966) has demonstrated that, compared with control subjects, children who were initially referred for antisocial behavior were, at a 30-year follow-up, more likely to have been arrested for nontraffic crimes, to be imprisoned, to be divorced, to be heavy drinkers, and to be physically aggressive. All the rapes and murders that had been committed in the adult sample had been perpetrated by those who had been antisocial youths.

Adults with antisocial behavior were almost always antisocial children, and it is extremely rare for antisocial behavior to arise de novo in adult life. Although antisocial behavior remains relatively stable throughout childhood, more than half of these children do not grow up to be antisocial adults. Nevertheless, there is agreement that the child's behavior is a better predictor of adult antisocial behavior than family characteristics or social dimensions. The longitudinal research evidence suggests that antisocial behavior in childhood, particularly when some estimate of severity is taken into account, is the single most powerful predictor of later adjustment problems (Kolhberg et al. 1984).

There is general agreement that antisocial behavior that is characterized by early onset, frequency, and diversity and that occurs across different social situations increases the risk of adult antisocial behavior.

Although frequent and relatively severe childhood antisocial behavior is a necessary condition for predicting adult antisocial behavior, it is also clear that antisocial behavior declines with age, particularly in the period between 25 and 40 years of age (Kohlberg et al. 1984). It is known that whereas 15- to 18-year-old adolescents represent only 6% of the population, they commit 25% of index crimes, while those over 45 years of age, who constitute 30% of the population, commit only 6% of index crimes (Uniform Crime Report 1985 [1986]). A sample of more than 2,300 former child guidance clinic patients who were judged initially to have manifested excessive aggressive behavior were found at 30-year follow-up to have significantly higher mortality rates. Eighty-two percent of the total deaths were related to suicide, accidents, or abuse of alcohol and drugs (de Chateau 1990). Similarly, Robins (1970) observed that 17% of antisocial boys died before their mid-40s, compared with 10% of control subjects.

Summary

Aggressive behavior is a measurable behavior trait that—although determined and influenced by the exigencies of biological, developmental, and social-familial processes throughout the life cycle—is remarkably stable, particularly when severity is taken into account as a measure. Individual differences in aggressive reaction levels are evident by 3 years of age and predict subsequent aggressive behavior. Aggressive behavior stabilizes in the early preschool years and predicts disruptive behaviors in elementary school. Antisocial/aggressive behavior not infrequently emerges as a developmental trait in childhood, continues throughout adolescence, and may persist into adult life. Antisocial behavior stabilizes during middle childhood and maintains a high degree of stability over time. The prevalence of conduct disorder increases throughout adolescence and gradually remits, with only about 50% of youths going on to exhibit adult antisocial personality. *Early onset* of antisocial behavior expressed in a *variety* of different ways with *high frequency across different social situations* is the most powerful predictor of adult antisocial behavior. Although antisocial and aggressive behavior declines in frequency and duration from 25 to 40 years of age, the individual disposition to physical aggression seems to be individually determined and remains characterologically true throughout the life cycle.

References

American Psychiatric Association: Diagnostic and Statistical Manual of Mental Disorders, 3rd Edition, Revised. Washington, DC, American Psychiatric Association, 1987

Bachman JG, Johnston LD, O'Malley PM: Monitoring the Future: Questionnaire Responses from the Nation High School Seniors, 1986. Ann Arbor, MI, Institute for Social Research, 1986

Berkowitz L: Aggression: A Social Psychological Analysis. New York, McGraw-Hill, 1962

Blumstein A, Farrington D, Moitra S: Delinquency careers: innocents, desisters, and persisters, in Crime and Justice: An Annual Review, Vol 6. Edited by Tonlry M, Morris N. Chicago, IL, University of Chicago Press, 1985, pp 187–220

Bohman M, Cloninger CR, Sigvardsson S, et al: Predisposition to petty criminality in Swedish adoptees. Arch Gen Psychiatry 39:1233–1241, 1982

Campbell SB, Ewing LJ: Follow-up of hard-to-manage preschooler: adjustment at age 9 and predictors of continuing symptoms. J Child Psychol Psychiatry 31:871–889, 1990

Campbell SB, Ewing LJ, Breaux AM, et al: Parent-referred problem three-year-olds: follow-up at school entry. J Child Psychol Psychiatry 27:473–488, 1986

Christiansen KO: The genesis of aggressive criminality: implications of a study of crime in a Danish twin study, in Determinants and Origins of Aggressive Behavior. Edited by Wit DDfe, Hastings W. The Hague, The Netherlands, Mouton, 1976

Cummings EM, Iannotti RJ, Zahn-Waxler C: Aggression between peers in early childhood: individual continuity and developmental change. Child Dev 60:887–895, 1989

de Chateau P: Mortality and aggressiveness in a 30-year follow-up study in child guidance clinics in Stockholm. Acta Psychiatr Scand 81:472–476, 1990

Dodge KA, Somberg DR: Hostile attributional biases among aggressive boys are exacerbated under conditions of threats to the self. Child Dev 58:213–224, 1987

Dodge KA, Coie JD, Pettit GS: Peer status and aggression in boys' groups: developmental and contextual analyses. Child Dev 61:1289–1309, 1990

Ensminger M, Kellam E, Rubin B: School and family origins of delinquency: comparisons by sex, in Prospective Studies of Crime and Delinquency. Edited by Van Dusen KT, Mednick SA. Boston, MA, Kluwer-Nijhoff, 1983, pp 73–98

Fischer M, Rolf JE, Hasazi JE, et al: Follow-up of a preschool epidemiological sample: cross-age continuities and predictions of later adjustment with internalizing and externalizing dimensions of behavior. Child Dev 55:137–150, 1984

Farrington DP: Offending from 10 to 25 years of age, in Prospective Studies of Crime and Delinquency. Edited by Van Dusen KT, Mednick SA. Boston, MA, Kluwer-Nijhoff, 1983, pp 17–37

Freud A: The bearing of the psychoanalytic theory of the instinctual drives on certain aspects of human behavior, in Drives, Affects, Behaviors, Vol 1. Edited by Lowenstein R. New York, International Universities Press, 1953, pp 259–277

Freud S: Civilization and its discontents (1930), in The Standard Edition of the Complete Psychological Works of Sigmund Freud, Vol 21. Translated and edited by Strachey J. London, Hogarth Press, 1953, pp 59–145

Fry DP: Intercommunity differences in aggression among Zapotee children. Child Dev 59:1008–1019, 1988

Gersten JC, Langner TS, Eisenberg JG, et al: Stability and change in types of behavioral disturbances of children and adolescents. J Abnorm Child Psychol 4:111–127, 1976

Glueck S, Glueck E: Predicting Delinquency and Crime. Cambridge, MA, Harvard University Press, 1959

Halikas JA, Meller J, Morse C, et al: Predicting substance abuse in juvenile offenders: attention deficit disorder versus aggressivity. Child Psychiatry Hum Dev 21:4955, 1990

Hall WM, Cairns RB: Aggressive behavior in children: an outcome of modeling or social reciprocity. Dev Psychol 20:739–745, 1984

Hamburg DA: An evolutionary and developmental approach to human aggressiveness. Psychoanal Q 42:185–196, 1973

Henn FA, Bardwell R, Jenkins R: Juvenile delinquents revisited. Arch Gen Psychiatry 37:1160–1163, 1980

Hobbes T: Leviathan (1651). New York, Collier, 1962

Hutchings B, Mednick SA: Registered criminality in the adoptive and biologic parents of registered male adoptees, in Genetic Research in Psychiatry. Edited by Fieve R, Rosenthal D, Brill H. Baltimore, MD, Johns Hopkins University Press, 1975, pp 105–116

Hartup W: Aggression in childhood: developmental perspectives. Am Psychol 28:336–341, 1974

Havighurst RJ, Bowman PH, Liddle GP, et al: Growing Up in River City. New York, Wiley, 1962

Joseph E: Aggression redefined: its adaptional aspects. Psychoanal Q 42:197–213, 1973

Kohlberg L, Ricks D, Snarey J: Childhood development as a predictor of adaptation in adulthood. Genetic Psychological Monographs 110:91–172, 1984

Kupersmidt JB, Coie JD: Preadolescent peer status, aggression, and school adjustment as predictors of externalizing problems. Child Dev 61:1350–1362, 1990

Loeber R: The stability of antisocial and delinquent child behavior: a review. Child Dev 53:1431–1446, 1982

Loeber R: Antisocial behavior: more enduring than changeable? J Am Acad Child Adolesc Psychiatry 30:393–397, 1991

Lorenz K: On Aggression. New York, Harcourt, Brace & World, 1966

McCord J: Parental behavior in the cycle of aggression. Psychiatry 51:14–23, 1988

O'Connor M, Foch T, Sherry T, et al: A twin study of specific behavioral problems of socialization as viewed by parents. J Abnorm Child Psychol 8:189–199, 1980

Offord DR: Conduct disorder: risk factors and prevention, in Prevention of Mental Disorders, Alcohol and Other Drug Use in Children and Adolescents (OSAP Monograph-2). Rockville, MD, U.S. Department of Health and Human Services, Office for Substance Abuse Prevention, 1989, pp 273–307

Olweus D: Stability of aggressive reaction patterns in males: a review. Psychol Bull 86:852–875, 1979

Parens H: The Development of Aggression in Early Childhood. New York, Jason Aronson, 1979

Parens H: Toward a reformulation of the psychoanalytic theory of aggression, in The Course of Life, Vol 2: Early Childhood. Edited by Greenspan S, Pollock G. Madison, CT, International Universities Press, 1989, pp 83–121

Patterson GR, DeBaryshe BD, Ramsey E: A developmental perspective on antisocial behavior. Am Psychol 44:329–335, 1989

Quay HC: Psychopathic personality as pathological stimulation seeking. Am J Psychiatry 122:180–183, 1965

Raine A, Venables H, Williams MA: Relationship between central and autonomic measures of arousal at age 15 years and criminality at age 24 years. Arch Gen Psychiatry 47:1003–1007, 1990

Reid JB: Patterns of conduct disorder over time. Paper presented at the NIMH Workshop on Subtypes of Conduct Disorders, Bethesda, MD, June 1986

Richman N, Stevenson J, Graham PJ: Preschool to School: A Behavioral Study. London, Academic Press, 1982

Robins LN: Deviant Children Grown Up: A Sociological and Psychiatric Study of Sociopathic Personality. Baltimore, MD, Williams & Wilkins, 1966

Robins LN: The adult development of the antisocial child. Seminars in Psychiatry 2(4):420–434, 1970

Robins LN: Sturdy childhood predictors of adult outcomes: replications from longitudinal studies, in Stress and Mental Disorder. Edited by Barrett JE, Rose RM, Klerman GL. New York, Raven, 1979, pp 219–233

Robins LN: Epidemiological approaches to natural history research: antisocial disorders in children. Journal of the American Academy of Child Psychiatry 20:566–580, 1981

Rogeness GA, Javors MA, Maas JW, et al: Catecholamine and diagnoses in children. J Am Acad Child Adolesc Psychiatry 29:234–241, 1990

Scott JP: Aggression. Chicago, IL, University of Chicago Press, 1975

Siegel L, Senna J: Juvenile Delinquency, 3rd Edition. St. Paul, MN, West Publishing, 1988

Tinbergen N: Fighting and Threat in Animals. New York, Penguin New Biology, 1953

Uniform Crime Reports 1985: U.S. Department of Commerce, census data, 1986

van der Kolk BA: The compulsion to repeat the trauma: reenactment, victimization, and masochism. Psychiatr Clin North Am 12:389–411, 1989

Wasman M, Flynn JP: Directed attack elicited from hypothalamus. Arch Neurol 6:227–330, 1962

Webster's New Twentieth Century Dictionary (Unabridged), 2nd Edition. William Collins, 1980

Wilson EO: Sociobiology: The New Synthesis. Cambridge, MA, Harvard University Press, 1975

West DJ, Farrington DP: The Delinquent Way of Life. London, Heinemann, 1977

Wolfgang ME, Figlio RM, Sellin T: Delinquency in a Birth Cohort. Chicago, IL, University of Chicago Press, 1972

Wynne-Edwards VC: Animal Dispersion in Relation to Social Behavior. Edinburgh, Oliver & Boyd, 1962

Chapter 4

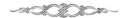

Comorbidity

Kerim Munir, M.D., Sc.D.
David Boulifard, B.A.

I n this chapter we describe the conceptual and practical aspects of psychiatric comorbidity in conduct disorder. The term *conduct disorder* (CD)
refers to children and adolescents who exhibit a persistent pattern (at
least 6 months) of 3 or more of the 13 DSM-III-R (American Psychiatric
Association 1987) criteria (stealing, running away, lying, fire setting, truancy,
breaking and entering, destructiveness, physical cruelty to animals, sexual
coercion, use of a weapon, initiation of physical fights, robbery, or confrontative stealing) and who have associated significant impairments of their everyday functioning at home or school. Although CD is diagnosed when the basic
rights of others, or societal norms or rules, are violated, the CD diagnostic
category is distinguished from *delinquency,* a term referring to a record of
juvenile conviction (Lewis et al. 1984).

In clinical practice, it is unusual for children or adolescents with DSM-
III-R or any other category of CD to seek help of their own volition. Instead,
youngsters with CD are usually brought to clinical attention as a consequence
of unmanageable actions or behaviors reported by parents, teachers, counsel-
ors, psychologists, pediatricians, or other responsible caregivers (Robins
1991).

The complex stages of referral make generalizations about comorbidity
biased in some respects toward cases that are of longer duration or greater
severity, or that have some other unknown or peculiar characteristic
(Achenbach 1991; Caron and Rutter 1991; Cohen and Cohen 1984). De-

This work was supported, in part, by Research Scientist Development Grant MH-00826
(to Dr. Munir) from the National Institute of Mental Health.

spite the recognition of this high level of uncertainty about the nature of the relationship of "discrete" disorders, the concept of comorbidity has come to symbolize a new "code" for DSM psychiatry (Klerman 1990; Sabshin 1991). If we assume that CD, as defined in the DSM, is a valid category that can be diagnosed with adequate precision, the question can then be reduced to the following: What is the nature of the relationship between CD and other psychiatric disorders co-occurring in the same subject? This chapter defines the concept of comorbidity as it is presently envisioned in the psychiatric literature and presents evidence for comorbidity in CD in children and adolescents.

Definitions

Definitions of comorbidity have ranged from "dual diagnosis," when a psychiatric or medical disorder occurs with substance abuse, to increased relative risk (or odds) of one or more disorders in the presence of an index condition (Maser and Cloninger 1990). An examination of the term's epidemiological origins reveals that comorbidity was first formally described by Feinstein (1970), who defined it as "any distinct additional clinical entity that has existed or that may occur during the clinical course of a patient who has the index disease under study" (pp. 456–457).

Comorbidity of psychiatric disorders can occur within an episode of illness assessed cross-sectionally as an elevated prevalence of other disorders (*current comorbidity*) or within the lifespan of an individual as an elevated lifetime prevalence of other disorders (*lifetime comorbidity*) (Klerman 1990; Lewinsohn et al. 1991). Feinstein (1985) also distinguished among 1) *pathogenic comorbidity*, in which an index disease leads to another co-occurring disease that is considered to be etiologically related (e.g., the hypothesis that attention-deficit hyperactivity disorder [ADHD] or another specific developmental disorder may lead to CD); 2) *diagnostic comorbidity*, in which diagnostic criteria are based on symptoms that are not specific to one disorder (e.g., as between oppositional defiant disorder [ODD] and ADHD); and 3) *prognostic comorbidity*, in which the index disease predisposes the individual to develop other conditions (e.g., CD leading to substance abuse and criminality) (Maser and Cloninger 1990).

Assessment

Paying attention to the array of disorders observed in a given patient enables the clinician to be more efficient in selecting appropriate interventions: psychotherapy, family therapy, psychopharmacology, and/or behavior therapy.

Failing to pay attention to comorbidity may thus mean delivering less-effective clinical treatment. From a research perspective, failing to take comorbidity into account may result in making false inferences about risk or causal factors (Maser and Cloninger 1990). Caron and Rutter (1991) have presented two major reasons why comorbidity cannot be ignored: 1) correlates, outcome, and genetic characteristics reported for an index disorder may be attributable to another disorder; and 2) the meaning of an index disorder with and without comorbidity may differ fundamentally.

Assessment of comorbidity is itself a difficult process prone to scientific error. Risk of such error accompanies the benefits of an essentially cross-sectional research structure (Feinstein 1985) based on inadequately "operationalized" diagnostic criteria (Kendall 1975). Furthermore, the criteria are themselves in a state of periodic revision, making the tasks of longitudinal assessment and comparison among studies complicated (Cantwell and Baker 1988; Shaffer et al. 1989).

Other difficulties in assessing comorbidity involve biases owing to differential rates of hospital referral—a circumstance that has led Feinstein (1985), for example, to warn that "studies of coexisting diseases are best conducted in community populations and should be avoided in hospital patients" (p. 472). Whenever less than all possible subjects with an index disorder are referred to a clinic, that sample will always contain disproportionately large numbers of patients with comorbidities (Caron and Rutter 1991). This phenomenon was first noted by Berkson (1946), who reported that the increased probability of referral for a patient with comorbid disorders is a function of the combined probabilities of referral for each disorder.

Caron and Rutter (1991) have qualified these concerns by asserting that clinic data can justifiably be used to assess comorbidity, but only in the rare instances in which the population base rates, clinic referral rates, and idiosyncratic referral biases for the index and comorbid disorders are known to investigators.

Accordingly, if the prevalence rate of CD is 5% and that of ADHD is also 5%, the prevalence of CD and ADHD occurring together (assuming independence of the two disorders) would be the product of the two prevalence rates—i.e., 5% (0.05) × 5% (0.05), or 0.25% (0.0025). If, as in many epidemiological studies, the observed prevalence of comorbid CD and ADHD is significantly higher than the figure that would be expected by chance, then comorbidity is inferred. Differential nonresponse from families with children with one, two, or more comorbid disorders and errors in measuring base rates of disorders further distort inferred disease relationships (Rosenthal and Rosnow 1975).

Epidemiological data have consistently pointed to the co-occurrence of various "categorical" psychiatric disorders in children (Anderson et al. 1987; Bird et al. 1988; Costello 1989; Costello et al. 1988; Kashani et al. 1987; McGee et al. 1984; Rutter 1989; Szatmari et al. 1989). The discussion of comorbidity in CD is particularly important with regard to ADHD, ODD, specific developmental disorders, mood and anxiety disorders (including bipolar disorder and somatization), alcohol and substance abuse, posttraumatic stress disorder (including a history of physical and/or sexual abuse), paraphilia, intermittent explosive disorder, psychosis (including schizophrenia), tics (including Tourette's syndrome), seizure disorder, and organic mental disorder.

Prevalence and Course

CD is one of the most serious mental health problems affecting children and adolescents. The prevalence of CD (various types) has been found to be 1.5% in 4- to 16-year-olds in Puerto Rico (Bird et al. 1988), 2.6% in 7- to 11-year-olds in a pediatric primary care population in the United States (Costello et al. 1988), 3.2% in 10-year-olds in the Isle of Wight, United Kingdom (Rutter et al. 1970), 3.4% in 11-year-olds (Anderson et al. 1987) and 6.9% in 7-year-olds in Dunedin, New Zealand (McGee et al. 1984), and 5.5% in 6- to 13-year-olds in Ontario, Canada (Offord et al. 1987). These epidemiological studies report a preponderance of the disorder in boys (Anderson et al. 1987; Kashani et al. 1989; McGee et al. 1984; Offord et al. 1987). In the Isle of Wight cohort, for example, the high male preponderance of CD was responsible for the overall elevated rate of psychopathology in males (Rutter et al. 1970).

The prevalence of CD in the overall population varies depending on the characteristics of the sample (e.g., age of subjects), the setting (e.g., urban or rural), the sampling method, and the classification instrument used to measure disorders (Costello 1989). Although the incidence of new cases is not known, it is possibly on the rise (Loeber 1991).

The diagnosis of CD in children is seldom made before school age (Robins 1978, 1991). In clinical populations, 50% of children with CD are believed to continue to exhibit antisocial behaviors in adulthood. Early-onset CD (i.e., CD with an onset prior to the advent of puberty) is believed to have a more persistent course than later-onset forms of the disorder (Robins 1966, 1978, 1991).

There is limited information on the population frequency and stability of CD and/or ODD symptoms. Early-onset aggressive behaviors are believed to persist (Loeber 1982). Antisocial behaviors are also believed to be stable, as noted in the Dunedin Longitudinal Study of children from birth to 15 years of age (White et al. 1991). Externalizing behaviors at age 3 were found to predict CD diagnosis at age 13. No association was observed with school problems, intelligence, or ADHD in postpubertal children who first exhibited antisocial behavior around the age of 13 (White et al. 1991).

Implications of Changes in Nosology

The decision to suspend diagnostic hierarchies in DSM-III (American Psychiatric Association 1980) encouraged multiple diagnoses and inherent cross-sectional comorbidity. This tradition was extended in DSM-III-R, which further eliminated some of the remaining DSM-III hierarchies—for example, ADHD could now occur in the presence of mental retardation or schizophrenia (the latter was again changed in DSM-IV [American Psychiatric Association 1994]). Inconsistency in the exclusionary rules also underlies different assumptions about the basic relationships of CD, ODD, and ADHD—for example, CD and ODD are considered mutually exclusive, whereas ADHD can occur with either condition.

The effect of changes in DSM criteria in the prevalence, interrelationships, and validity of disorders has been discussed by Lahey et al. (1990). Robins (1991) has likewise predicted that the more restrictive DSM-III-R criteria for CD will lead to a reduction in the number of diagnosable cases in children, particularly in girls.

DSM-IV also denotes comorbidity by assignment of multiple diagnoses. To date, the distinctions made in DSM-III (*socialized/undersocialized, aggressive/nonaggressive*) and in DSM-III-R (*group/solitary-aggressive/undifferentiated*) have not been useful. The *International Classification of Diseases, 10th Revision* (ICD-10; World Health Organization 1992) has also incorporated the epidemiological evidence of comorbidity by defining CD subcategories in "compound" forms, such as hyperkinetic CD, depressive CD, or "mixed disorders of conduct and emotions."

An important issue contributing to problems in assessing comorbidity has been the cumbersome and complex nature of the diagnostic criteria themselves. The DSM-IV disruptive behavior disorders field trial has therefore explored ways of combining intercorrelated items and eliminating poorly performing ones (American Psychiatric Association 1994). By evaluating the effect of small changes on prevalence, this effort can provide data on appropriate thresholds (Loeber et al. 1991).

One rationale for suspending the hierarchies among disorders was the unavailability of valid inclusion and exclusion criteria. Use of conditional probabilities of child symptoms has enabled systematic examination of the utility of inclusion criteria (ruling in the disorder by their presence) or exclusion criteria (ruling out the disorder by their absence) (Milich et al. 1987). The conditional probability and predictive power methods are expected to help further refine the diagnostic criteria.

Unlike major depression, CD is a "polythetic" diagnostic category—that is, no single item is necessary for the diagnosis; any combination of 3 out of 13 criteria is sufficient to establish the diagnosis (Milich et al. 1987). In this model, each symptom carries an empirical (and imperfect) probability that helps to predict the presence or absence of CD. Furthermore, the criteria do not have a hierarchical order of discriminating power, as has been incorrectly implied (American Psychiatric Association 1987).

Polythetic diagnostic categories (also known as "diagnostic prototypes") are therefore inherently more heterogeneous with regard to constituent symptoms than are classical medical disease models. In the polythetic diagnostic model, a group of children classified as having CD may have met the minimum three criteria required for the diagnosis with completely different symptom combinations, thus complicating symptom homogeneity (Achenbach 1991; Klerman 1990; Maser and Cloninger 1990).

Comorbidity of CD With Specific Disorders

Relationship of CD and Oppositional Defiant Disorders

Hierarchically, DSM-III oppositional disorder (OD) and DSM-III-R ODD are considered to be mutually exclusive of CD. Theoretically, there is no possibility of comorbidity between these disorders and CD. DSM-III OD was conceptualized as a mild condition, characterized by disobedient and negativistic opposition to authority figures (American Psychiatric Association 1980). DSM-III-R ODD requires a higher threshold and greater severity for diagnosis, bringing it closer to the DSM-III conceptualization of CD (American Psychiatric Association 1987).

To date, there have been few empirical investigations of ODD. Some of these have questioned the utility of the ODD diagnosis altogether as being too close to normality in children. In a controlled investigation, Schachar and Wachsmuth (1990) presented evidence suggesting that ODD is a variant of CD rather than of "normality," with high associated rates of comorbid ADHD, specific developmental disorders, and undersocialization, as well as paternal psychiatric history and family, peer, and sibling relationship problems. These findings are consistent with those of Reeves et al. (1987) and Rey et al. (1988), who distinguished ODD children from normal—but not from CD—children.

DSM-IV field trials have contrasted these two options: 1) that ODD and CD are distinct disorders, versus 2) that ODD and CD are a unified disorder with oppositional defiant, moderate, and severe conduct levels (American Psychiatric Association 1991). In investigating the overlap and demarcation of CD and/or ODD with other conditions, Loeber et al. (1991) have likewise emphasized the need to study the age and gender appropriateness, onset, stability, and developmental course of symptoms.

Comorbidity With ADHD

Epidemiological and clinical studies suggest a considerable degree of co-morbidity between CD and/or ODD and attention-deficit disorder (ADD) (Biederman et al. 1991). Anderson et al. (1987), in an epidemiological study of 11-year-old children, reported a comorbidity rate of 47% for DSM-III CD and/or OD in children with ADD compared with a rate of 35% for ADD in children with CD and/or OD. Similarly, in a two-stage probability sample in Puerto Rico, Bird et al. (1988) reported a comorbidity rate of 57% for CD and/or OD in children with ADD compared with a rate of 47% for ADD in children with CD and/or OD.

In a clinic-based study of DSM-III ADD, CD, and ADD + CD in 6- to 12-year boys, the conditional probability of ADD given CD was estimated to be 67% compared with a probability of 37% for CD given ADD (Milich et al. 1987). In a clinical family study of DSM-III ADD with hyperactivity, Faraone et al. (1991) reported a comorbidity rate of 64% in ADD probands with any CD and/or OD, and of 33% in ADD probands with CD only. An earlier family study reported a comorbidity rate of 64% with any CD and/or OD in ADD probands (Biederman et al. 1987; Munir et al. 1987).

Part of the problem in assessing ADHD and CD comorbidity stems from the high intercorrelations between hyperactivity and conduct disorder items (Shaywitz and Shaywitz 1988; Swanson 1988). Loney and Milich (1982) showed that Conners questionnaire Inattention/Overactivity items load on the same factor as Aggression/Defiance items. Furthermore, Inattention/Overactivity items were not exclusively associated with ADD. Shaywitz and Shaywitz (1988) noted that mixed symptoms of Inattention/Overactivity and Aggression/Defiance are overrepresented in clinic-referred samples, presumably reflecting the extreme cases more likely to be sent for treatment. Likewise, whereas Aggression/Defiance items described disruptive behavior, they did not sufficiently predict CD.

Another part of the problem in assessing ADHD and CD comorbidity stems from the fact that the behaviors described as DSM criteria are more typical of adolescents than of children younger than 12 years of age (Swanson 1988). In fact, compared with the CD symptoms in the later DSM-III and DSM-III-R versions, the DSM-II (American Psychiatric Association 1968) symptoms of CD were more characteristic of younger children and tended to correspond closely with the Conners Aggression/Defiance items (Swanson 1988). The correspondence of behavior dimensions to diagnostic categories needs to be studied further (Achenbach 1991; Loney and Milich 1982; Loney et al. 1978; Schachar and Wachsmuth 1990).

No prospective follow-up studies have compared the differences in taxonomy and risk factors for CD and/or ODD and ADHD (Szatmari et al. 1989). Of the numerous existing cross-sectional and case-control studies, inconsistent findings emerge in differences on developmental and cognitive test scores, psychosocial disadvantage, and measures of attention and motor behavior. The literature does not confidently support a different pattern of covariates for the two disorders.

In the Ontario Child Health Study, in which Child Behavior Checklist (Achenbach and Edelbrock 1983) and DSM-III items guided the diagnosis of four disorders (ADD, CD, emotional disorder, and somatization), significant comorbidity was observed between CD and ADD (broadly defined), with a high correlation between their items (Offord et al. 1987).

Analyses by Szatmari et al. (1989) showed that for 4- to 11-year-old boys, the prevalence of ADD was twice that of CD (CD only, 2.6%; ADD only, 5.1%; mixed ADD + CD, 3.7%). For 12- to 16-year-old boys, the prevalence of CD was twice that of ADD (CD only, 6.7%; ADD only, 3.8%; mixed ADD + CD, 2.9%). Developmental problems tended to be more common in ADD than in CD, with difficulty remembering and learning five times more common in ADD than in CD. Adverse familial and demographic factors, including parental ill health, were more common in CD than in ADD. Poverty was 4.2 times and overcrowding 3.9 times more common in CD than in ADD. The mixed CD and ADD group had higher total CD and ADD scores than either the noncomorbid CD group or the noncomorbid ADD group.

The overlap of CD and ADD varied by gender, with the two conditions almost completely overlapping in girls. Four- to 16-year-old girls with ADD were 40 times more likely to have CD, compared with a factor of 14 for boys with ADD in the same age group. The greatest overlap between ADD and CD was for girls who had not experienced developmental problems (51-fold increase in the odds of having CD) (Szatmari et al. 1989).

Based on these findings, Szatmari et al. (1989) hypothesized that ADD in boys was more akin to a developmental disorder, whereas ADD in girls was an early variant of CD. The study supported the expectation that children with CD would be older than children with ADD (Rutter and Giller 1983). These epidemiological findings are also consistent with the hypothesis that ADD children who are psychosocially disadvantaged are more likely to have mixed CD + ADD.

Follow-up studies of simple and mixed groups of CD and ADHD are expected to further test the hypotheses generated by cross-sectional and case-control investigations. Given the age- and gender-biased criteria for CD, studies based on DSM-III-R definitions are likely to find comorbidity of ADHD with ODD in children 5–12 years old, with comorbidity of ADHD with CD emerging in the adolescent years (Robins 1991; Shaywitz and Shaywitz 1988).

Conceptual Framework for Covariation of CD and ADHD

Epidemiological theories may provide a conceptual framework for understanding the co-occurrence of CD and ADHD. Epidemiology considers "exposures," determinants, risk factors, or risk indicators within a broad causal model based on the notion of relative risk (or relative odds) (Rothman 1976, 1986). Categorizing causes descriptively—for example, as necessary or sufficient, direct or indirect—is a helpful paradigm for elucidating the covariation of discrete disorders. In this paradigm, a given risk condition—for example, ADHD—can be envisioned as a risk indicator for an index disorder—for example, CD.

Susser (1991) has described three essential prerequisites for a cause: 1) *association,* which is probabilistic and dependent on strength and consistency; 2) *time order* or *temporal relationship* of the relevant variables, which is dependent on their access to observation, which in turn is dependent on design (e.g., prospective follow-up study); and 3) *direction or consequential change,* which is dependent on consistency (together with replicability), strength, specificity in cause and effect, predictive performance, and coherence in all forms (e.g., theoretical, factual, biological, statistical). In considering a causal association between ADHD and CD, the following are some hypothetical ways in which the two conditions may occur:

1. ADHD may be a risk indicator of CD (association).
2. ADHD and CD may have a common or shared cause (association).
3. CD may be a risk indicator of ADHD (association).
4. CD and ADHD may be classified together by chance alone (no association).

In epidemiological studies, CD is more common among children with ADHD than among those without, supporting the hypothesis that an association does indeed exist between CD and ADHD. The temporal relationship between CD and ADHD suggests that ADHD occurs before CD. ADHD is therefore more likely to be a risk indicator for CD (hypothesis 1). CD is more common among males than among females and among older than among younger children—that is, besides ADHD, gender, age, and other factors (e.g., specific developmental disorder, psychosocial disadvantage) are also risk indicators for CD.

A necessary causal factor may not be *sufficient*—in the absence of other component causes—for a disorder to occur (Rothman 1976). The absence of ADHD as a precursor condition in many cases where CD is observed disqualifies ADHD as a necessary cause (i.e., for ADHD to be considered a necessary causal factor, it must *always* be observed before CD). As a risk indicator or a component cause, ADHD may directly or indirectly interact with other component causes (e.g., psychosocial disadvantage), leading to CD (hypothesis 1 or 2). It is conceivable that ADHD may be a surrogate or correlate of some other vulnerability that may be necessary but as yet unidentified causal factor of CD. These theoretical issues need to be further pursued in follow-up studies that carefully examine a range of developmental risk conditions.

Comorbidity With Specific Developmental Disorders

Specific developmental disorders (SDDs), or "learning disabilities," are prevalent among children and adolescents with CD and/or juvenile delinquency (Cantwell and Baker 1991; Rutter et al. 1970). This is particularly true for specific reading disability and deficits in verbal skills not explicable by poor educational opportunities. For example, the Isle of Wight study found that approximately one-quarter of children with specific reading retardation exhibited antisocial behavior (Rutter et al. 1970). SDD children also have higher rates of ADHD and problems with social skills and relationships.

In many children, SDD may not be associated with or lead to psychiatric disturbance (Cantwell and Baker 1991). The association between CD and SDD is a complex one: certain neurocognitive characteristics may be risk indicators for CD; CD and SDD may share common etiological processes such as familial adversity; and/or CD may arise as a result of cognitive limitations and school failure in conjunction with negative reinforcement from others.

Comorbidity With Alcohol and Substance Abuse

An earlier age of initiation of substance abuse and its greater impact on school performance are particularly noticeable for youngsters living in deprived inner-city neighborhoods. A number of studies have examined the comorbidity of CD with substance abuse and other factors predictive of longer-term substance abuse (Burkstein et al. 1989). In a large-scale epidemiological study, Robins and Przybeck (1985) found that drug abuse before the age of 15 predicted greater severity of CD symptoms. Further analysis indicated that the presence of CD was a powerful predictor of early-onset substance abuse.

The presence of an antisocial or alcohol-abusing close relative is also predictive of early-onset substance abuse, whereas parental separation and race are not (Robins and McEvoy 1991). Family adversity, in particular, is considered to be a major predisposing factor for CD. There is a parallel association between substance abuse and family adversity, social deprivation, and unemployment. Because a high concentration of social and educational disadvantage exists in inner-city environments, the co-occurrence of substance abuse and CD in such areas is not surprising.

Comorbidity With Mood and Anxiety Disorders and With Suicidality

Major depression, dysthymia, and anxiety disorders (including somatization) frequently co-occur with all three types of disruptive behavior disorders (i.e.,

ADHD, CD, and ODD). A significant minority of prepubertal children with depressive disorders meet criteria for CD, suggesting that attention to comorbidity may lead to earlier recognition, more appropriate treatment, and better outcome (Puig-Antich 1982). CD may precede the onset of a depressive disorder. It may also first become evident after the onset of depression and follow a variable course, disappearing or persisting beyond recovery from depression (Kovacs et al. 1988).

In a study of hospitalized patients, children with disruptive behavior disorders and comorbid affective or anxiety disorders exhibited more age-appropriate skills and fewer externalizing behaviors than children without such comorbid disorders, leading the investigators to postulate that inhibition related to anxiety or depression may temper disruptive behavior symptoms (Woolston et al. 1989).

Naturalistic and clinical studies have also reported evidence suggesting a significant overlap of CD with affective/anxiety disorders, with little differences in socioeconomic and demographic characteristics by comorbidity (Anderson et al. 1987; Kovacs et al. 1988; Pfeffer and Plutchik 1989).

CD is among the leading disorders associated with youth suicide and nonfatal suicidal behavior (Pfeffer 1991). In a study of adolescent suicide victims, Shaffer (1974) reported that 57% of the youth had exhibited both antisocial and depressive symptoms, 17% had only antisocial symptoms, 13% had only affective symptoms, and 15% had neither type of symptoms. The presence of antisocial behavior increases the risk for suicide by a factor of 4.4 in males and of 3.2 in females; only major depression and a previous history of suicide attempts exceed this strength as predictors of suicide (Shaffer 1988). Shafii et al. (1985) reported evidence of antisocial behaviors (stealing, physical fights, school suspension, and legal involvements) in 70% of suicide victims compared with 24% of nonsuicidal control subjects. In the San Diego Suicide Study, comorbidity of suicide with antisocial behavior and substance abuse was more frequent in victims younger than 30 years of age—a finding comparable to the frequency found for the comorbidity of suicide with affective disorders in older victims (Pfeffer 1991; Rich et al. 1986).

Comorbidity With Posttraumatic Stress Disorder

Posttraumatic stress disorder (PTSD) in children, like mood and anxiety disorders, may mimic "externalizing" symptoms, thereby leading to superfluous diagnoses of CD or ODD. The longer course and duration of CD or ODD compared with depression (except dysthymia), the presence or absence of disruptive behavior symptoms prior to the onset of depressive or anxiety symptoms, and the occurrence of traumatic events (e.g., emotional, physical, sexual abuse) in PTSD may aid differential diagnosis. Furthermore, traumatic events and life stressors and other hardships may highlight and exaggerate preexisting CD or ODD (Patterson et al. 1989).

Comorbidity With Neurological, Tic, and Medical Disorders

Brain damage (including cerebral palsy and epilepsy) is a strong predictor of psychiatric disorder in children in general (Rutter et al. 1970). However, the presence of brain damage is not associated with a specific type of psychiatric disorder (Kindlon et al. 1988), with the possible exception of SDDs (including coordination), enuresis, and encopresis.

Delinquent youngsters with and without CD are reported to have more accidents, injuries, physical illnesses, and visits to hospital facilities than demographically similar nondelinquent peers (Lewis and Shanok 1977). Although there is a general association of chronic health problems with psychiatric disorder (including disruptive behavior) in children, the specificity of this association with CD and/or ODD has not been established.

Stewart et al. (1981) reported that 32% of subjects with both ADD and Tourette's syndrome also had CD, compared with 26% of those with ADD alone. Comings and Comings (1987) reported less frequent comorbidity with CD in patients with ADD secondary to Tourette's syndrome. ADD secondary to Tourette's syndrome was reported to usually have a later onset (age 7 years) with less "lead time" for the appearance of CD. Unlike CD, obsessive-compulsive behaviors were significantly present in both the ADD + Tourette's syndrome and the ADD-only groups (Comings and Comings 1988).

Comorbidity in High-Risk Studies and Environmental Influences

The families of CD children are traditionally characterized by high rates of psychopathology and an absence of good parental relationships. These family characteristics include paternal alcoholism; parental aggressive behavior, antisocial personality, and criminality; and maternal depression (Patterson 1982). Other characteristics frequently seen in CD families include poverty of parent-child, peer, and interpersonal relationships; diminished affectional bonds; verbal aggression; and intrusiveness (Quay 1986). The relationship to CD of specific aspects of parental care, such as hostility, lack of warmth, inappropriate role modeling, and punitive interactions, has also been highlighted (Patterson et al. 1989).

Shared (or familywide) environmental influences are thought likely to play a major role in the development of CD and/or juvenile delinquency (Rutter and Giller 1983). Information from family and genetic studies can be used to highlight the differential importance of such shared or nonshared contrasting environmental influences (Plomin and Daniels 1987). For example, CD in Huntington's disease is observed as a consequence of family discord, whereas affective disorder may present as an early psychiatric manifestation of Huntington's disease. The complex interaction between genetic and environmental factors varies over critical developmental periods of the life cycle. Genetic factors are especially difficult to study because they may influence susceptibility to environmental exposure as well as affect the choice and/or shaping of environments themselves (Rutter et al. 1990a, 1990b).

Studies have shown that family discord and disruption, parental unemployment, geographic overcrowding, lower socioeconomic status, and inadequate educational opportunities are all associated with development of juvenile delinquency (Rutter and Giller 1983). Overall, socioeconomic status is a much weaker predictor than family variables such as discord, disruption, poor relationships, and poor supervision of children. When family disruption is controlled, an important variable that emerges with respect to geographic area/overcrowding is the climate of schools in terms of their educational philosophy, social management, and structure (Rutter and Quinton 1977).

Earls and colleagues (Earls 1987; Earls et al. 1988) have shown that mental disorders in parents is associated with a wide range of environmental psychiatric risk factors, such as impaired parenting and family discord. High-risk studies of children of alcoholic parents have shown an increased risk of delinquency, truancy, substance abuse, and school dropout. Studies of these children also suggest that they have a higher frequency of DSM-III CD, OD, and ADD (Earls et al. 1988). Other studies have also shown a strong association between parental alcoholism and childhood CD (Steinhausen et al. 1984). Among children characterized by undersocialized behavior, there is also a higher reported rate of alcoholism in parents (Stewart et al. 1981). As a risk factor with or without parental alcoholism, family discord also influences the development of delinquency (Rutter and Giller 1983). One hypothesis is that parental alcoholism may not directly lead to CD but may contribute to the child's risk when other family stressors are present—that is, several stressors may potentiate one another (Rutter 1979).

Comorbidity in Family Genetic Studies

Family genetic studies that use standardized interviews, blind raters, and advanced analytic strategies can help to better define the phenotypic expression of disorders as well as aid in generating hypotheses about risk and protective factors in the development of disorders. There have been few such studies involving "pure" CD and/or ODD probands.

In a clinical family study of DSM-III ADD with hyperactivity, Faraone et al. (1991) reported that 1) the risk for ADD in first-degree relatives (parents and siblings) of children with ADD was 38% among children with ADD + CD, 24% among those with ADD without CD or OD, 17% among those with ADD + OD, and lowest among relatives of psychiatric and nonpsychiatric control subjects (5% for both); and 2) the risk for "any antisocial disorder" (i.e., OD or antisocial personality) in first-degree relatives of children with ADD was 34% among children with ADD + CD, 24% among those with ADD + OD, 11% among those with ADD without CD or OD, 7% among psychiatric control subjects, and 4% among nonpsychiatric control subjects. The interpretation of these findings is complicated by the probands' high rate of overall comorbidity with other DSM-III disorders, including major depression, anxiety, and SDDs; by lack of specificity of familial loading concerning ADD; and by lack of differentiation between environmental and familial factors. The results are in fact more supportive of the hypothesis for increased association of family psychopathology (higher rates of antisocial, affective, and anxiety disorders) in the relatives of ADD probands with CD and/or OD (Biederman et al. 1987).

Categorically defined "levels" of comorbidity—for example, ADHD alone, ADHD with ODD, ADHD with CD—can be envisioned on a continuum of severity in a multifactorial model. *Heritability* owing to genes—that is, the amount of variance in the phenotype explained by the variance in the genotype—represents only one component of liability within such a multifactorial model (Rutter et al. 1990a).

So far, the patterns of disorder identified in genetic studies have not, in practice, been what has emerged from nosological investigations that incorporate DSM or ICD diagnostic schemas. Taylor (1991) has suggested that the study of behavioral phenotypic variation may be limited in practicability. A given behavioral phenotype (e.g., for ADHD, CD, or autism) may include a broad range of neurobehavioral and cognitive characteristics. The uncertainty about the meaning of a behavioral phenotype therefore contributes to the uncertainty inherent in comorbidity. Further problems include the variable expressions of a given genotype and the heterogeneity of psychiatric syndromes that represent various genetic conditions (Rutter et al. 1990a, 1990b).

Although a number of twin and adoptee studies have demonstrated a significant genetic component—with respect to associations between criminality and antisocial personality disorder—in parents and their adopted-away offspring (Cloninger and Gottesman 1987), such studies in children with CD or delinquency have not sufficiently differentiated this risk as genetic or environmental (Robins 1978). It is believed that CD and juvenile crime in children may not necessarily persist in adulthood (Robins 1991), although some studies have reported otherwise (Osborn and West 1979).

Implications for Therapeutic
Intervention and Prevention

Children and adolescents with CD have multiple biological, social, and psychological vulnerabilities. They require early identification, accessible social supports, and multimodal treatments. No single mode of treatment, on its own, is sufficiently effective (Lewis 1990).

The American Academy of Child and Adolescent Psychiatry (AACAP; 1990) has developed practice guidelines for the evaluation and treatment of CD that emphasize the assessment of prenatal, birth, developmental history, and associated medical or neurological conditions (including seizures or head trauma) as well as physical and/or sexual abuse. The AACAP guidelines stress the importance of assessing family history of alcohol and substance abuse, personality disorder (including antisocial behavior and incarceration), and paranoid or psychotic ideation. It is recommended that children and adolescents with possible CD be evaluated with respect to associated risk factors and comorbid conditions. Such an evaluation should include assessment of speech and language, vision, hearing, cognitive, and educational functioning as well as physical and neurological examination and laboratory workup (including screening for substance abuse).

Both evaluative and therapeutic strategies invariably require child and parent cooperation and advocacy resources that may be unrealistic for discordant families or hard-pressed communities. Furthermore, programs for parents and residential programs for youngsters are limited in availability, duration, and continuity of services (Kazdin 1985).

The diagnosis of CD is not a primary indication for initiation of psychopharmacological treatment. Attention to comorbidity in CD, however, may guide appropriate choice of psychopharmacological treatment for component conditions: stimulants or antidepressants for ADHD; antidepressants for affective or anxiety disorders; lithium or carbamazepine for bipolar or seizure disorder; and lithium or propranolol for intermittent explosive disorder or aggressive behavior (Campbell et al. 1982; Evans et al. 1987; Puig-Antich 1982; Williams et al. 1982). The therapeutic rationale must take into account relative and absolute indications and contraindications for using psychoactive agents in co-occurring disorders—for example, in children with CD + ADHD + tics, psychostimulants need to be avoided; in children with CD + ADHD + depression, antidepressants may be the preferred medications. Although it may be necessary, psychopharmacological treatment as a single mode of therapy is not sufficient to address the complex psychoeducational, social, and remedial needs of CD children.

Boyle and Offord (1990) have advocated the implementation of primary prevention demonstration projects for CD and have pointed out the analytic and cost-beneficial advantages of focusing on children in high-risk situations.

One strategy, for example, is to reduce discord by strengthening family functioning—including such factors as communication and responsiveness—in at-risk families (Patterson et al. 1989). Establishing such programs also entails more precise measurement of risk factors and outcomes.

Interventions are needed for early ODD or ADHD precursors of CD symptoms, since there is evidence that such behaviors may become more entrenched and difficult to change as a child grows older (Wolf et al. 1987). For this reason, in presenting evidence for distinct behavioral covariation of symptoms of CD and ODD, Loeber et al. (1991) also argue that "the elimination of ODD in favor of CD as a single entity would preclude early identification and easier modification of disruptive child behavior" (p. 387).

Conclusion

In a given child or adolescent with CD, possible co-occurring conditions include ADHD, SDDs, mood or anxiety disorders (including bipolar disorder and somatization), substance abuse, suicidality, PTSD, intermittent explosive disorder, paraphilia, tics (including Tourette's syndrome), enuresis, encopresis, psychosis (possible prodromal phase of schizophrenia or schizoaffective disorder), neurological disturbances (including seizure disorder), or other medical conditions.

In the decade since Boyd et al. (1984) highlighted the co-occurrence of DSM-III adult psychiatric diagnoses in the Epidemiologic Catchment Area (ECA) study, child and adolescent psychiatric research has entered a new era (Institute of Medicine 1989). Psychiatric disorders of children and adolescents in the general population are unlikely to be independently distributed. Among children who meet criteria for one DSM disorder, a disproportionate number will also meet criteria for two, three, or more disorders.

Challenges continue to confront investigators interested in better understanding the complex natural history, developmental range, and course of CD. Cross-sectional assessment of current functioning does not precisely reflect earlier problems and is prone to reporting errors. Questions about comorbidity, continuity/discontinuity, and course of CD symptoms can best be studied by means of longitudinal designs involving well-defined "homogeneous" populations with respect to age, gender, and ethnicity (Leckman 1989).

Our ability to study children exposed versus those unexposed to posited risk factors and to prospectively follow up outcomes into adolescence and young adulthood is likely to yield a better understanding of these conditions. Principles of philosophy in science dictate that a given psychiatric condition exists because there is some truth or essence about its meaning that demarcates it from other conditions, as predicted by risk factors, course, and outcome. Although the scientific debate on comorbidity is expected to continue, the notation of multiple, differential, primary, or secondary diagnoses related or unrelated to CD will continue to be a useful exercise insofar as such notations lead to better understanding as well as to effective preventive and therapeutic interventions.

References

Achenbach TM: "Comorbidity" in child and adolescent psychiatry: categorical quantitative perspectives. Journal of Child and Adolescent Psychopharmacology 1:271–278, 1991

Achenbach TM, Edelbrock CS: Manual for the Child Behavior Checklist and Revised Child Behavior Profile. Burlington, University of Vermont, Department of Psychiatry, 1983

American Academy of Child and Adolescent Psychiatry: Practice Parameters for the Assessment and Treatment of Conduct Disorders. Washington, DC, AACAP Work Group on Quality Issues, 1990

American Psychiatric Association: Diagnostic and Statistical Manual of Mental Disorders, 2nd Edition. Washington, DC, American Psychiatric Association, 1968

American Psychiatric Association: Diagnostic and Statistical Manual of Mental Disorders, 3rd Edition. Washington, DC, American Psychiatric Association, 1980

American Psychiatric Association: Diagnostic and Statistical Manual of Mental Disorders, 3rd Edition, Revised. Washington, DC, American Psychiatric Association, 1987

American Psychiatric Association: DSM-IV Options Book: Work in Progress (9/1/91). Washington, DC, American Psychiatric Association, 1991

American Psychiatric Association: Diagnostic and Statistical Manual of Mental Disorders, 4th Edition. Washington, DC, American Psychiatric Association, 1994

Anderson JC, Williams S, McGee R, et al: DSM-III disorders in preadolescent children: prevalence in a large sample from the general population. Arch Gen Psychiatry 44:69–78, 1987

Berkson I: Limitations of the application of fourfold table analysis to hospital data. Biometrics 2:47–53, 1946

Biederman J, Munir K, Knee D: Conduct and oppositional defiant disorder in clinically referred children with attention deficit disorder: a controlled family study. J Am Acad Child Adolesc Psychiatry 26:724–727, 1987

Biederman J, Newcorn J, Sprich S: Comorbidity of attention deficit hyperactivity disorder with conduct, depressive, anxiety and other disorders. Am J Psychiatry 148:564–577, 1991

Bird HR, Canino G, Rubio-Stipec M, et al: Estimates of the prevalence of childhood maladjustment in a community survey in Puerto Rico. Arch Gen Psychiatry 45:1120–1126, 1988

Boyd JH, Burke ID, Gruenberg E, et al: Exclusion criteria of DSM-III. Arch Gen Psychiatry 41:983–989, 1984

Boyle MH, Offord DR: Primary prevention of conduct disorder: issues and prospects. J Am Acad Child Adolesc Psychiatry 29:227–233, 1990

Burkstein OG, Brent DA, Kaminer Y: Comorbidity of substance abuse and other psychiatric disorders in adolescents. Am J Psychiatry 146:1131–1141, 1989

Campbell M, Cohen IL, Small AM: Drugs in aggressive behavior. Journal of the American Academy of Child Psychiatry 21:107–117, 1982

Cantwell DP, Baker L: Issues in the classification of child and adolescent psychopathology. J Am Acad Child Adolesc Psychiatry 27:521–533, 1988

Cantwell DP, Baker L: Psychiatric and Developmental Disorders in Children With Communication Disorder. Washington, DC, American Psychiatric Press, 1991

Caron C, Rutter MP: Comorbidity in child psychopathology: concepts, issues and research strategies. J Child Psychol Psychiatry 32:1063–1080, 1991

Cloninger CR, Gottesman I: Genetic and environmental factors in antisocial behavior disorders, in Causes of Crime: Non-Biological Approaches. Edited by Mednick SA, Moffitt TE. Cambridge, UK, Cambridge University Press, 1987, pp 92–109

Cohen P, Cohen J: The clinician's illusion. Arch Gen Psychiatry 41:1178–1182, 1984

Comings DE, Comings BG: A controlled study of Tourette syndrome, II: conduct. Am J Hum Genet 41:742–760, 1987

Comings DE, Comings BG: Tourette's syndrome and attention deficit disorder, in Tourette Syndrome and Tic Disorders. Edited by Cohen DJ, Bruun RD, Leckman IF. New York, Wiley, 1988, pp 120–135

Costello EJ: Developments in child psychiatric epidemiology. J Am Acad Child Adolesc Psychiatry 28:836–841, 1989

Costello EJ, Costello AI, Edelbrock C, et al: Psychiatric disorders in pediatric primary care: prevalence and risk factors. Arch Gen Psychiatry 26:57–63, 1988

Earls F: On the familial transmission of child psychiatric disorder. J Child Psychol Psychiatry 28:791–801, 1987

Earls F, Reich W, Lung KG, et al: Psychopathology in children of alcoholic and antisocial parents. Alcohol Clin Exp Res 12:481–487, 1988

Evans RW, Clay TH, Gualtieri CT: Carbamazepine in pediatric psychiatry. J Am Acad Child Adolesc Psychiatry 26:2–8, 1987

Faraone SV, Biederman J, Keenan K, et al: Separation of DSM-III attention deficit disorder and conduct disorder: evidence from a family genetic study of American child psychiatric patients. Psychol Med 21:109–121, 1991

Feinstein AR: The pre-therapeutic classification of comorbidity in chronic disease. Journal of Chronic Diseases 23:455–469, 1970

Feinstein AR: Scientific decisions in choosing groups, in Clinical Epidemiology: The Architecture of Clinical Research. Philadelphia, PA, WB Saunders, 1985, pp 458–499

Institute of Medicine (National Academy of Sciences): Report of a Study of the Committee of the Division of Mental Health and Behavioral Medicine: Research on Children and Adolescents with Mental, Behavioral and Developmental Disorders. Washington, DC, National Academy Press, 1989

Kashani JH, Beck N, Hoeper EW, et al: Psychiatric disorders in a community sample of adolescents. Am J Psychiatry 144:584–589, 1987

Kashani JH, Orvaschel H, Rosenberg TX, et al: Psychopathology in a community sample of children and adolescents: a developmental perspective. J Am Acad Child Adolesc Psychiatry 28:701–706, 1989

Kazdin AE: Treatment of Antisocial Behavior in Children and Adolescents. Homewood, IL, Dorsey Press, 1985

Kendall RE: The Role of Diagnosis in Psychiatry. Oxford, UK, Blackwell Scientific, 1975

Kindlon D, Sollee N, Yando R: Specificity of behavior problems among children with neurological dysfunctions. J Pediatr Psychol 13:239–247, 1988

Klerman GL: Approaches to the phenomena of comorbidity, in Comorbidity of Mood and Anxiety Disorders. Edited by Maser JD, Cloninger CR. Washington, DC, American Psychiatric Press, 1990, pp 13–37

Kovacs M, Paulauskas SL, Gatsonis C, et al: Depressive disorders in childhood, III: a longitudinal study of comorbidity with and risk for conduct disorders. J Affect Disord 15:205–217, 1988

Lahey BB, Loeber R, Stouthamer-Loeber M, et al: Comparison of DSM-III and DSM-III-R diagnoses for prepubertal children: changes in prevalence and validity. J Am Acad Child Adolesc Psychiatry 29:620–626, 1990

Milich R, Widiger TA, Landau S: Differential diagnosis of attention deficit and conduct disorders using conditional probabilities. J Consult Clin Psychol 55:762–767, 1987

Leckman JF: Genetics and child psychiatry (editorial). J Am Acad Child Adolesc Psychiatry 29:174–176, 1989

Lewinsohn PM, Rohde P, Seeley JR, et al: Comorbidity of unipolar depression, I: major depression with dysthymia. J Abnorm Psychol 100:205–213, 1991

Lewis DO: Conduct disorders, in Psychiatric Disorders in Children and Adolescents, Edited by Garfinkel BD, Carlson GA, Weller EB. Philadelphia, PA, WB Saunders, 1990, pp 193–209

Lewis DO, Shanok SS: Medical histories of delinquent and non-delinquent children: an epidemiological study. Am J Psychiatry 134:1020–1035, 1977

Lewis DO, Lewis M, Unger I, et al: Conduct disorder and its synonyms: diagnoses of dubious validity and usefulness. Am J Psychiatry 141:514–519, 1984

Loeber R: The stability of antisocial and delinquent child behavior: a review. Child Dev 53:1431–1446, 1982

Loeber R: Antisocial behavior: more enduring than changeable? J Am Acad Child Adolesc Psychiatry 30:393–397, 1991

Loeber R, Lahey BB, Thomas C: Diagnostic conundrum of oppositional defiant disorder and conduct disorder. J Abnorm Psychol 100:379–390, 1991

Loney J, Milich R: Hyperactivity, inattention, and aggression in clinical practice, in Advances in Developmental and Behavioral Pediatrics, Vol 2. Edited by Wolraich M, Routh DK. Greenwich, CT, JAI Press, 1982, pp 113–147

Loney J, Langhorne IF, Paternite CE: An empirical basis for subgrouping the hyperkinetic/minimal brain dysfunction syndrome. J Abnorm Psychol 87:431–441, 1978

Maser JD, Cloninger CR: Comorbidity of anxiety and mood disorders: introduction and overview, in Comorbidity of Anxiety and Mood Disorders. Edited by Maser JD, Cloninger CR. Washington, DC, American Psychiatric Press, 1990, pp 3–12

McGee R, Silva PA, Williams S: Behavior problems in a population of seven-year-old children: prevalence, stability, and types of disorder—a research note. J Child Psychol Psychiatry 25:251–259, 1984

Milich R, Widiger TA, Landau S: Differential diagnosis of attention deficit and conduct disorders using conditional probabilities. J Consult Clin Psychol 55:762–767, 1987

Munir KM, Biederman I, Knee D: Psychiatric comorbidity in patients with attention deficit disorder: a controlled study. J Am Acad Child Adolesc Psychiatry 26:844–848, 1987

Offord DR, Boyle MH, Szatmari P, et al: Ontario Child Health Study, II: six-month prevalence of disorder and rates of service utilization. Arch Gen Psychiatry 44:832–836, 1987

Osborn SG, West DJ: Conviction records of fathers and sons compared. British Journal of Criminology 19:120–133, 1979

Patterson GR: Coercive Family Processes. Eugene, OR, Castalia, 1982

Patterson CJ, Cohn DA, Kao BT: Maternal warmth as a protective factor against risks associated with peer rejection among children. Development and Psychopathology 1:21–38, 1989

Pfeffer CR: Suicide and suicidality, in Textbook of Child and Adolescent Psychiatry. Edited by Wiener JM. Washington, DC, American Psychiatric Press, 1991, pp 507–514

Pfeffer CR, Plutchik R: Co-occurrence of psychiatric disorders in child psychiatric patients and non-patients: a circumplex model. Compr Psychiatry 30:275–282, 1989

Plomin R, Daniels D: Why are children in the same family so different from one another? Behavioral and Brain Sciences 10:1–15, 1987

Puig-Antich J: Major depression and conduct disorder in prepuberty. Journal of the American Academy of Child Psychiatry 21:118–128, 1982

Quay HC: Conduct disorders, in Psychopathological Disorders of Childhood, 3rd Edition. Edited by Quay HC, Werry JS. New York, Wiley, 1986, pp 35–72

Reeves JC, Werry JS, Elkind GS, et al: Attention deficit, conduct, oppositional and anxiety disorders in children, II: clinical characteristics. J Am Acad Child Adolesc Psychiatry 26:144–155, 1987

Rey JM, Bashir MR, Schwartz M, et al: Oppositional disorder: fact or fiction? J Am Acad Child Adolesc Psychiatry 27:157–162, 1988

Rich CL, Young D, Fowler RC: San Diego Suicide Study, I: young versus old subjects. Arch Gen Psychiatry 43:577–582, 1986

Robins LN: Deviant Children Grown Up: A Sociological and Psychiatric Study of Sociopathic Personality. Baltimore, MD, Williams & Wilkins, 1966

Robins LN: Sturdy childhood predictors of adult outcomes: replication from longitudinal studies. Psychol Med 8:611–622, 1978

Robins LN: Conduct disorder. J Child Psychol Psychiatry 32:193–212, 1991

Robins LN, McEvoy LT: Conduct problems and substance abuse, in Straight and Devious Pathways From Childhood to Adulthood. Edited by Robins LN, Rutter MP. Cambridge, Cambridge University Press, 1991

Robins LN, Przybeck TR: Age of onset of drug use as a factor in drug and other disorders, in Etiology of Drug Abuse: Implications for Prevention (NIDA Res Monogr #56). Rockville, MD, National Institute on Drug Abuse, 1985

Rosenthal R, Rosnow RL: The Volunteer Subject. New York, Wiley-Interscience, 1975

Rothman KJ: Causes. Am J Epidemiol 104:587–592, 1976

Rothman KJ: Modern Epidemiology. Boston, MA, Little, Brown, 1986

Rutter MP: Protective factors in children's responses to stress and disadvantage, in Social Competence in Children. Edited by Kent MW, Rolf JE. Hanover, NH, University Press of New England, 1979, pp 49–74

Rutter MP: Isle of Wight revisited: twenty-five years of child psychiatric epidemiology. J Am Acad Child Adolesc Psychiatry 28:633–653, 1989

Rutter MP, Giller H: Juvenile Delinquency: Trends and Perspectives. New York, Guilford, 1983

Rutter MP, Quinton D: Psychiatric disorder: ecological factors and concepts of causation, in Ecological Factors in Human Development. Edited by McGurk H. Amsterdam, Elsevier North Holland, 1977, pp 173–187

Rutter MP, Tizard J, Whitmore K (eds): Education, Health and Behavior. London, Longman, 1970

Rutter MP, Bolton P, Harrington R, et al: Genetic factors in child psychiatric disorders, I: a review of research strategies. J Am Acad Child Adolesc Psychiatry 31:3–37, 1990a

Rutter MP, MacDonald M, Le Couteur A, et al: Genetic factors in child psychiatric disorders, II: empirical findings. J Am Acad Child Adolesc Psychiatry 31:39–83, 1990b

Sabshin M: Comorbidity: a central concern of psychiatry in the 1990s (editorial). Hosp Community Psychiatry 42:345, 1991

Schachar R, Wachsmuth R: Oppositional disorder in children: a validation study comparing conduct disorder, oppositional disorder and normal control children. J Child Psychol Psychiatry 31:1089–1102, 1990

Shaffer D: Suicide in childhood and early adolescence. J Child Psychol Psychiatry 15:275–291, 1974

Shaffer D: The epidemiology of teen suicide: an examination of risk factors. J Clin Psychiatry 49 (No 9, suppl):36–41, 1988

Shaffer D, Campbell M, Cantwell D, et al: Child and adolescent psychiatric disorders in DSM-IV: issues facing the work group. J Am Acad Child Adolesc Psychiatry 28:830–835, 1989

Shafii M, Carrigan S, Whittinghill JR, et al: Psychological autopsy of completed suicide in children and adolescents. Am J Psychiatry 142:1061–1064, 1985

Shaywitz SE, Shaywitz BE: Attention deficit disorder: current perspectives, in Learning Disabilities: Proceedings of the National Conference. Edited by Kavanagh IF, Truss TJ. Parkton, MD, York Press, 1988, pp 369–523

Steinhausen H, Gobel D, Nestler Y: Psychopathology in the offspring of alcoholic parents. Journal of the American Academy of Child Psychiatry 23:465–471, 1984

Stewart MA, Cummings C, Singer S, et al: The overlap between hyperactive and unsocialized aggressive children. J Child Psychol Psychiatry 22:35–45, 1981

Susser M: What is a cause and how do we know one? a grammar for pragmatic epidemiology. Am J Epidemiol 133:635–648, 1991

Swanson JM: Discussion, attention deficit disorder: current perspectives, in Learning Disabilities: Proceedings of the National Conference. Edited by Kavanagh IF, Truss TJ. Parkton, MD, York Press, 1988, pp 532–546

Szatmari P, Boyle M, Offord DR: ADDH and conduct disorder: degree of diagnostic overlap and differences among correlates. J Am Acad Child Adolesc Psychiatry 28:865–872, 1989

Taylor E: Developmental neuropsychiatry. J Child Psychol Psychiatry 32:2–47, 1991

White J, Moffitt TE, Earls F, et al: Preschool predictors of conduct disorder. Criminology 28:507–533, 1991

Williams DJ, Mehl R, Yudofsky S, et al: The effect of propranolol on uncontrolled rage outbursts in children and adolescents with organic brain dysfunction. Journal of the American Academy of Child Psychiatry 21:128–138, 1982

Wolf MM, Braukmann CJ, Ramp HA: Serious delinquent behavior may be part of a significantly handicapping condition: cures and supportive environments. J Appl Behav Anal 20:347–359, 1987

Woolston IL, Rosenthal SL, Riddle MA, et al: Childhood comorbidity of anxiety/affective disorders and behavior disorders. J Am Acad Child Adolesc Psychiatry 28:707–713, 1989

World Health Organization: ICD-10 Classification of Mental and Behavioural Disorders: Clinical Descriptions and Diagnostic Guidelines. Geneva, World Health Organization, 1992

Chapter 5

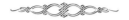

Rating Scales

Karen C. Wells, Ph.D.

Numerous methods exist for describing and measuring behavior and emotions in children, among them clinical and structured interviews, rating scales, observational methods, and measures of psychophysiological and biological functions. Of these methods, rating scales are assessment methods with a long and venerable history. Their modern origin in the behavioral sciences is commonly ascribed to Sir Francis Galton, who in the late 19th century developed an eight-category scale for measuring the "vividness" of visual imagery (Galton 1908).

Twentieth-century history of experimental psychology is replete with investigations using scaling methods in the study of sensory and perceptual responses. Paralleling these developments, World Wars I and II and the educational movement in the United States prompted much activity in the areas of educational measurement and personnel selection. Many of the principles of scale construction and analysis were developed during this time. More recent years have seen these principles and methods generalized to the arenas of adult and child psychiatry.

It is the purpose of this chapter to provide a brief review of the use of rating scales in a very specific area of child and adolescent psychiatry—that is, the area of conduct disorder. Before beginning, however, it is necessary to clarify terminology as it will be used in this chapter.

The term *conduct disorder* (CD) has been used in the psychiatric and psychological literature to reflect a specific diagnostic category, which in the current nosologic system has three subtypes: solitary aggressive type, group type, and undifferentiated type (American Psychiatric Association 1987). This diagnostic label is given to children and adolescents who violate the basic rights of other persons or the rules of society through serious antisocial actions.

The term CD has also been used in the literature in a generic sense to describe children and adolescents who exhibit aggression. This is a broader and more general use of the term that encompasses children who engage in interpersonal and physical aggression as well as in community rule violations.

When a diagnosis of CD is required, the appropriate assessment method is more likely to be the structured psychiatric interview, which reflects a *categorical approach* to classifying human behavior. Rating scales tend to reflect a *dimensional approach* to the study of behavior in children. They assess the dimension of aggressive conduct rather than the diagnosis of CD. As such, rating scales measuring aggression have been used in studies of patient populations as well as in normative studies and epidemiological samples. Because rating scale methodologies historically have been based on a dimensional approach, the term *CD* will be used in this chapter in the generic sense to describe children who display an aggressive behavior pattern, alone or in addition to other disturbances of emotions or behavior.

Rating scales have many uses in studies of child CD. Their results can be used to inform the diagnostic process. They can be used to compare a child's position on an aggressive behavior dimension with that of other children from either normative or clinical samples. They can be used to track the progress of treatment or to provide a measure of treatment outcome. They can be used to measure long-term follow-up of treatment as well as to track the developmental process of aggression.

In addition to their many uses, rating scales offer several advantages over other methods of assessment. They are efficient in terms of their brevity and cost. Most scales do not require training of the raters. They permit the assessment of covert or low-frequency behaviors that are difficult to measure with observational methods. They incorporate the observations of significant individuals in the child's life who have access to the child in natural environments. They can be used to sample across relevant settings in the child's daily life (i.e., home, school, community). Despite some generally acknowledged methodological pitfalls and potential sources of error in rating scales, their many uses and advantages have made them central among the methods of assessment in child and adolescent psychiatry.

Psychometric Properties of Rating Scales

A multitude of behavioral rating scales have been developed for assessing child behavior disorders, many of which include factors or dimensions reflecting CD. However, the most frequently used rating scales—and the ones that will be reviewed in this chapter—are those with research demonstrating their psychometric properties. Because any rating scale must be evaluated in the context of the adequacy of its psychometric properties, a very brief overview of these principles is provided below. This discussion is necessarily limited, and those readers familiar with psychometric theory may wish to skip ahead to the next section.

_____

Reliability

As applied to rating scales, *reliability* refers to the consistency, reproducibility, or accuracy of scale results. A basic notion in the concept of reliability is that of measurement error. This refers to the fact that ratings are subject to two sources of influence: the hypothetical "true" value that can never be determined with perfect accuracy and the error inherent in estimating that true value. The smaller this error, the more reliable the data. When a rating scale is assessed to have adequate or good reliability, it is, in general, one that has been found to accurately and consistently measure a particular dimension, state, or trait. Several indices of reliability are important to consider in evaluating rating scales:

Interrater reliability.   This index of reliability reflects the agreement among two or more raters of the same children. With regard to rating scales, indices of interrater reliability (e.g., agreements between ratings by parents and teachers) are frequently lower than other reliability indices because they can be subject to the influence of situational variations.

Test-retest reliability.   This index reflects the stability of a rating scale by correlating ratings made using the same scale at different times (e.g., with the lapse of 1 month). Test-retest reliability is optimally assessed in situations in which behavior change is not expected, so that the stability of the scale is not confounded with changes in behavior. For example, test-retest reliability should not be assessed in the context of an active treatment program because the resulting correlation coefficient might be distorted by changes occurring as a function of treatment.

Internal consistency indices.   These indices are estimates of how well the items in a scale agree with respect to the characteristic that they presume to measure. "Split half" consistency coefficients are computed by dividing all of the items within a scale (or factor) into two sets (first half, second half; or odd versus even-numbered items; or randomly determined halves) and examining the correlation between the two sets. This method may not be suitable for scales that contain only a small number of items.

Intraclass reliability coefficient.   This reliability coefficient ignores rater identity and considers agreements among all raters interchangeably. The intraclass reliability coefficient is valuable in situations in which there are two or more ratings for each child that are not made by the same set of raters. In these cases, it is not possible to compute a correlation coefficient between any pair of raters.

Judging Reliability Estimates

The question of how large a reliability coefficient should be to justify use of a scale has no precise answer; rather, it depends on how the ratings will be used, the nature of the index, and so on. For questions of classification or treatment planning for a single individual, in which reasonable accuracy is desired, one might want to see reliabilities as high as 0.80 or greater. For research purposes, when one is testing hypotheses with large numbers of cases, lower reliabilities may be acceptable. In fact, if significant differences are obtained using scales with reliabilities as low as .40 or .50, one may interpret that result as evidence of the robust nature of the experimental effect. However, if differences are not obtained using a less-reliable scale, one cannot ascertain whether that result is due simply to the weakness of the instrument.

Validity

The concept of validity addresses the question "Is this scale measuring what it purports to be measuring?" One cannot simply ask, "How valid is this scale?" The concept of validity is evaluated in the context of the question being asked; for example, "How valid is this scale for differentiating between aggression and other behavior disorders?" or "How valid is this scale for predicting response to treatment A?" In this regard, four types of empirical validity can be distinguished:

Construct validity.   Construct validity is usually associated with theoretical research; it answers the question, "How well does this test reflect the construct presumed to underlie performance on the test?" The interest is not in direct sampling of behavior, but rather in measuring a hypothesized theoretical state. Although it is of theoretical interest, construct validity but has less utility in the clinical setting than the other three indices of validity.

Content validity.   This form of validity answers the question "How well does this scale measure the behavioral dimension that I am interested in?" With regard to the topic of this chapter, the question is "How well does a particular scale in fact measure the dimension of aggression in children?"

Predictive validity.   Predictive validity is oriented toward a criterion or outcome in which an investigator is interested. One form of predictive validity (sometimes called *discriminative validity*) refers to the question of whether a scale can detect differences between conditions or treatments. Another form of predictive validity refers to the question of how well the scale's results relate to future performance (e.g., How well does a score of X on a CD scale predict future involvement with the police?).

Concurrent validity.   Predictive validity and concurrent validity differ only with regard to time. Concurrent validity refers to the comparability of two sets of measures at the same point in time (e.g., Does a short rating scale of aggression compare with a lengthy, more expensive rating scale?).

Factor Analysis

Many of the rating scales discussed in the next section are actually multidimensional scales containing several subscales or factors, one or more of which are CD factors. To obtain a CD factor, a statistical procedure called *factor analysis* is applied to data obtained from many respondents on the entire scale. Factor analysis is a complex set of arithmetical operations that allows an evaluation of the simultaneous interrelationship among all of the items in a scale. Such evaluation, in turn, enables the investigator to identify items that cluster together (i.e., factors) within the overall rating scale. The investigator provides labels for the factors that seem to reflect the basic behavioral dimension addressed by the items that make up each factor. For example, a factor analysis may be conducted on a rating scale with 100 items filled out by 500 informants, revealing that six factors account for or explain the observed relationships among all the items. For the purposes of this chapter, rating scales that have at least one CD or aggression factor embedded within them will be reviewed.

Rating Scales

Child Behavior Checklist

The Child Behavior Checklist (CBCL; Achenbach and Edelbrock 1983) is a 113-item rating scale sampling a broad range of child and adolescent behavioral and emotional symptoms as well as behavioral competencies. The scale is designed for use with youths ranging from 2 to 16 years of age. One advantage of the CBCL is that it has been analyzed separately for different sexes and age levels so that a child can be evaluated relative to his or her same-age and same-sex peers. A potential disadvantage of this approach is that the factors vary across sexes and age levels. The CBCL has parallel forms for parents, teachers, youths, and observers, with the most complete data being available for the parent and teacher forms.

Once a parent has completed the entire scale (which takes approximately 15 minutes to complete), the scores are summarized on the Revised Child Behavior Profile for 4- to 16-year-olds or on the Child Behavior Profile for 2- to 3-year-olds. Both profiles compare the child's scores with relevant norms on broad-band (Internalizing and Externalizing) syndromes as well as on several narrow-band factors. Three narrow-band factors reflect CDs in the Externalizing syndrome: Aggressive, Delinquent, and Cruel (Achenbach and Edelbrock 1983). The Aggressive factor is found for both sexes at each of three age levels (4–5, 6–11, and 12–16 years). The Delinquent factor is found for each level except 4- to 5-year-old girls. The Cruel factor is found only for girls at ages 6–11 and 12–16 years.

The CBCL has been subjected to extensive examination of its psychometric properties (Achenbach and Edelbrock 1983). Reliability information indicates 1-week test-retest coefficients of .95 (behavior problems) and .99 (social competence) by the intraclass method. Test-retest reliability coefficients over a 3-month interval were .84 (behavior problems) and .97 (social competence). Pearson coefficients ranged from .61 to .96 across factors and age and sex groupings. Stability coefficients of .53 for clinicians' reports and of .59 for mothers' reports over a 6-month period have been noted. Interparent agreement across the entire scale in a clinical sample of children was .985 for behavior problems. The range of agreement between parents was .26–.78 across factors on the Behavior Problems profile.

Concurrent validity has been established by demonstrating significant correlations of like factors between the CBCL and the Diagnostic Interview Schedule for Children—Parent Report (Costello et al. 1984), the Conners Parent Rating Scale, and the Quay Revised Behavior Problem Checklist (Barkley 1988). The CBCL has shown adequate discriminant validity in distinguishing between clinic-referred and non-clinic-referred children (Achenbach and Edelbrock 1983). Kazdin and Heidish (1984) found that parents of 6- to 11-year-old boys with diagnoses of CD reported significantly greater problems on the Aggressive and Delinquent factors of the CBCL as well as on the broad-band Externalizing scale than did parents of children with other diagnoses. When each of these scales was used, 94%–99% of the boys diagnosed with CD were correctly identified, thereby indicating a high degree of sensitivity for the CBCL. The CBCL is also sensitive to changes brought aboutas a result of family-based treatment of CD (Webster-Stratton 1984, 1985).

The adequacy of its psychometric properties is only one reason recommending the use of the CBCL in studies and treatment of CD. Other advantages are that it is one of the few scales to assess behavioral and social competencies as well as symptoms, and that it provides equivalent forms for different informants, thereby maximizing the amount of relevant information that can be gathered about a child. Users can focus only on the scales reflecting CD or can use the entire scale to screen for comorbid conditions as well.

Conners Parent and Teacher Rating Scales

The Conners Parent Rating Scale (CPRS) and Conners Teacher Rating Scale (CTRS) were devised to measure a broad range of children's behavioral and emotional symptoms in two settings: home and school (Conners 1969, 1970, 1973). The original CPRS and CTRS contain 93 and 39 items, respectively. Conners revised the original rating scales in 1978, reducing the number of items in the CPRS to 48 and in the CTRS to 28 (Goyette et al. 1978). Those items assessing internalizing symptoms were reduced in number, with the result that the revised versions are more useful for assessing conduct problems and hyperactivity than for evaluating anxiety or psychosomatic symptoms.

Because much of Conners's own research has been in the area of attention-deficit hyperactivity disorder (ADHD), the Conners scales tend to be viewed as instruments for use in ADHD treatment and research. However, the scales have been used extensively in general child psychopathology research as well as in the study of aggressive behavior, with or without hyperactivity. The CPRS 48-item and the CTRS 39-item and 28-item versions all have a factor—Conduct Problem—that assesses a dimension of aggressive behavior. The CPRS 93-item scale has two factors assessing aggressive behavior: Conduct Problem and Antisocial. Thus, the 93-item questionnaire might be used when a more fine-grained analysis of aggression is needed.

There are vast amounts of normative data from use of the Conners scales in many countries, including the United States (Goyette et al. 1978; Kupietz et al. 1972; Ullman et al. 1985), New Zealand (Sprague et al. 1974), Germany (Sprague et al. 1977), Australia (Glow 1979), Italy (K. D. O'Leary et al. 1985), and England (Taylor and Sandberg 1984). A large sample of normative data was collected in Canada based on CTRS data on more than 9,500 Canadian schoolchildren (Trites et al. 1982). Because of the extensive research on these instruments, they have become the most widely used rating scales in research on child psychopathology to date (Barkley 1988).

The Conners scales have a substantial research literature on their psychometric properties. Studies have demonstrated good test-retest reliabilities for both the CPRS (O'Conner et al. 1980) and the CTRS (Conners 1973) for intervals ranging from 1 month to 1 year. Interrater agreement (teachers) across the Externalizing factors ranged from .44 to .53 (Trites et al. 1982) and was .92 for the entire scale (Vincent et al. 1977). Good agreement between teachers and trained classroom observers (mean of .51 across factors) has also been reported (Kazdin et al. 1983). Declines in factor scores from first to second administration have been reported, suggesting a possible practice effect (Ullman et al. 1985; Werry and Sprague 1974). This has prompted Conners to suggest that the scale be administered twice before being used in assessing treatment outcome to reduce the confounding of treatment effects with practice effects (Conners 1989).

The concurrent validity of the Conners scales has been amply demonstrated by studies showing significant correlations with other scales. For the CPRS, significant correlations have been found with the Child Behavior Checklist (Achenbach and Edelbrock 1983), with the Behavior Problem Checklist (Arnold et al. 1981), and with ratings of parent-reported stress and self-esteem (Mash and Johnston 1983). Similar findings regarding concurrent validity have been reported for the CTRS (Arnold et al. 1981; Campbell and Steinert 1978). With regard to CD, several studies have demonstrated discriminant validity of the scales in differentiating between children with CD and other child populations (Conners 1970; Taylor and Sandberg 1984). The scales are also quite useful in measuring treatment effects with a variety of treatment approaches (Abikoff and Gittelman 1984; Cantwell and Carlson 1979; S. G. O'Leary and Pelham 1978). Research on the reliability and validity of the revised CPRS and CTRS is less extensive than for the original forms because of their more recent development. However, since the items for the Conduct Problem and Hyperactivity factors are similar to those in the original scales, it is likely that the revised scales also have satisfactory reliability and validity.

Two brief rating scales are derived from subsets of items on the CPRS and CTRS that are relevant to the assessment of CD. The Conners Abbreviated Symptom Questionnaire (ASQ) consists of the 10 items most frequently endorsed by the parents and teachers of hyperactive children. Because of the strong concurrence of hyperactivity and CD, items from both of these dimensions are represented in the scale along with items from other dimensions. The ASQ is an appropriate measure to employ when identification or treatment of children with features of both hyperactivity and CD is required. As with the other versions of the Conners scales, there are abundant data demonstrating the reliability and validity of the parent and teacher versions of the ASQ (Brown and Wynne 1982; Edelbrock and Reed 1984; Milich et al. 1980; Sprague and Sleator 1977).

In an attempt to more clearly discriminate between aggressive and hyperactive dimensions of behavior, Loney and Milich (1982) developed the Iowa-Conners Teacher Rating Scale (I-CTRS). This scale also consists of 10 items, but the items are derived solely from the Hyperactivity and Conduct Problem factors (five items from each factor). This was done to allow for the identification of children who are purely aggressive, who are purely hyperactive, or who have a mixed syndrome. Norms and cutoff scores for boys and girls at three grade levels are available (Murphey et al. 1985), and the discriminant validity of this version of the Conners scale has been demonstrated.

Quay's Revised Behavior Problem Checklist

The original Behavior Problem Checklist (BPC) was revised by Quay and Peterson in 1983, and the revised version is the only version now distributed by Quay. The Revised Behavior Problem Checklist (RBPC) has 89 items and consists of six factors, two of which reflect aggressive behavior: Conduct Disorder and Socialized Aggression. Although much of the extensive work indicating satisfactory psychometric properties was done on the original BPC, correlations between similar scales of the BPC and RBPC allow one to generalize with some confidence to the RBPC. In addition, the psychometric data that do exist on the RBPC are promising. Test-retest coefficients for the revised version have ranged between .49 and .83, interteacher agreements have ranged between .52 and .85, and interparent agreements have ranged between .55 and .93 (Quay and Peterson 1983). Support for various types of validity is also promising. Teacher ratings on the Conduct Disorder factor correlate significantly with peer nominations for aggression and with observations of initiated aggression in peer interactions (Quay and Peterson 1983). The scale also discriminates significantly between clinic-referred and non-clinic-referred children (Aman and Werry 1984). Unlike the Child Behavior Checklist and the Conners Parent Rating Scale, the RBPC has not been shown to predict treatment outcome.

Achenbach-Conners-Quay Questionnaire

In a collaboration supported by the American Psychological Association, Achenbach, Conners, and Quay have recently combined their considerable knowledge and expertise in the area of rating scales and have devised a scale to comprehensively assess dimensions of behavioral and emotional disturbance in children and adolescents. The resulting rating scale is known as the Achenbach-Conners-Quay Questionnaire (ACQ). By expanding the number of items relative to other rating scales (ACQ = 216 Problem Behavior items and 23 Competence items), the ACQ was designed to provide data on a much wider array of problems and competencies than have previously been assessed with other scales.

Analyses of the ACQ on a national sample of 5,200 children revealed eight empirically derived factors, two of which reflect aggressive behavior. Achenbach et al. (in press) labeled these factors Aggressive Behavior and Delinquent Behavior (Table 5–1). Initial analyses reveal evidence for good test-retest and interrater reliability and good concurrent validity. In addition, the ACQ significantly discriminates between clinic-referred and non-clinic-referred populations. The ACQ might be chosen when the user's need is to assess the widest possible array of problems and competencies.

Eyberg Child Behavior Inventory

The Eyberg Child Behavior Inventory (ECBI) is the only rating scale that was designed exclusively for the assessment of CD. It consists of 36 items that sample primarily overt forms of aggressive behavior. Factor analyses have confirmed that the ECBI is a unidimensional aggressive behavior scale (Eyberg and Robinson 1983; Robinson et al. 1980).

The ECBI can be used for children 2–16 years of age and yields two scores: an Intensity score, reflecting the sum of the ratings, and a Problem score, composed of the number of items endorsed as a problem by the parent.

Normative data are available for two age groups: 2–12 years (Robinson et al. 1980) and 3–16 years (Eyberg and Robinson 1983). Adequate test-retest,

Table 5–1. Achenbach-Connors-Quay Questionnaire (ACQ) delinquent and aggressive behavior dimensions

Delinquent behavior	Aggressive behavior
Cheats	Argues
Doesn't feel guilty	Brags
Hangs around kids who get in trouble	Bullies; is mean to others
Lies	Destroys others' things
Runs away from home	Demands attention
Sets fires	Destroys own things
Steals at home	Disobedient at home
Steals outside home	Disobedient at school
Swears; uses obscene language	Jealous
Talks or thinks about sex too much	Irritable
Truancy	Loud
Uses alcohol	Physically attacks people
Uses drugs	Screams
Vandalizes with others	Shows off or clowns
Prefers older kids	Starts fights
	Stubborn
	Sudden mood changes
	Talks too much
	Teases other kids
	Temper tantrums
	Threatens

Source. Reprinted from Achenbach TM, Howell CT, Quay HC, et al: "Problems and Competencies Reported by Parents for National Normative and Clinical Samples of 4- to 16-Year-Olds." *Monographs of the Society for Research in Child Development* (in press). Used with permission.

split-half, and internal consistency reliability indices have been reported (Eyberg and Robinson 1983; Robinson et al. 1980), and scores on both dimensions discriminate between children with CD, other clinic-referred children, and nonreferred children. The ECBI also discriminates between treatment and nontreatment conditions (Eyberg and Robinson 1982; Eyberg and Ross 1978; Webster-Stratton 1984).

The ECBI is a very useful rating scale for situations in which the focus is on identification and treatment of CD. The fact that it is a unidimensional scale—measuring CD only—restricts its usefulness as a screening instrument and does not allow for assessment of co-occurring behavioral disturbances.

Summary

There are many rating scales available for assessment of CD and other psychopathological conditions in children and adolescents. This review has focused on scales that are most commonly used and that have the greatest evidence attesting to the adequacy of their psychometric properties.

The choice of a particular instrument depends on the specific purpose(s) intended by the user. When the purpose is to discriminate clinical from nonclinical populations or CD from non-CD populations, scales with the strongest evidence for discriminant validity might be chosen (e.g., Child Behavior Checklist, Conners Parent Rating Scale, Conners Teacher Rating Scale, Quay Revised Behavior Problem Checklist, Eyberg Child Behavior Inventory). When the purpose is to predict or measure treatment effects, scales with good evidence for predictive validity might be chosen (e.g., Child Behavior Checklist, Conners Parent Rating Scale, Conners Teacher Rating Scale, Eyberg Child Behavior Inventory). When brevity and efficiency are important issues, the shorter rating scales might be chosen (e.g., Conners Abbreviated Symptom Questionnaire, Conners Parent Rating Scale, Conners Teacher Rating Scale, Eyberg Child Behavior Inventory, Iowa-Conners Teacher Rating Scale). Certainly, when multiple or repeated measures of behavior over time are an issue (e.g., tracking treatment or developmental effects over time), a shorter rating scale would be indicated. If there is a need to assess behavioral competencies as well as behavioral problems, the Child Behavior Checklist should be chosen.

In some settings (e.g., a general child psychiatry clinic), screening for a wide array of presenting problems, including CD, might be important. In such a setting, a multidimensional scale that assesses the presence of CD as well as other psychopathological conditions might be used (e.g., Achenbach-Conners-Quay Questionnaire, Child Behavior Checklist, Conners Parent Rating Scale, Conners Teacher Rating Scale, Quay Revised Behavior Problem Checklist). A multidimensional scale might also be used when it is important to assess the presence of conditions that co-occur with CD (e.g., ADHD). In other settings (e.g., a CD specialty clinic), a unidimensional scale such as the Eyberg Child Behavior Inventory might be sufficient for verifying the presence of a CD and tracking treatment effects over time. The main point is that the choice of a rating scale should be based on an evaluation of the adequacy of the scale for the specific purpose(s) of the assessment.

References

Abikoff H, Gittelman R: Does behavior therapy normalize the classroom behavior of hyperactive children? Arch Gen Psychiatry 41:449–454, 1984

Achenbach TM, Edelbrock CS: Manual for the Child Behavior Checklist and Revised Child Behavior Profile. Burlington, University of Vermont, Department of Psychiatry, 1983

Achenbach TM, Howell CT, Quay HC, et al: Problems and competencies reported by parents for national normative and clinical samples of 4- to 16-year olds. Monogr Soc Res Child Dev (in press)

Aman MG, Werry JS: The Revised Behavior Problem Checklist in clinic attenders and nonattenders: age and sex effects. Journal of Clinical Child Psychology 13:237–242, 1984

American Psychiatric Association: Diagnostic and Statistical Manual of Mental Disorders, 3rd Edition, Revised. Washington, DC, American Psychiatric Association, 1987

Arnold LE, Barnebey NS, Smeltzer DJ: First grade norms, factor analysis, and cross-correlation for Conners, Davids, and Quay-Peterson behavior rating scales. Journal of Learning Disabilities 14:269–275, 1981

Barkley RA: Child behavior rating scales and checklists, in Assessment and Diagnosis in Child Psychology. Edited by Rutter M, Tuma AH, Lann IS. New York, Guilford, 1988, pp 113–155

Brown RT, Wynne ME: Correlates of teacher ratings, sustained attention, and impulsivity in hyperactive and normal boys. Journal of Clinical Child Psychology 11:262–267, 1982

Campbell SB, Steinert Y: Comparisons of rating scales of child psychopathology in clinic and nonclinic samples. J Consult Clin Psychol 46:358–359, 1978

Cantwell DP, Carlson G: Stimulants, in Pediatric Psychopharmacology. Edited by Werry J. New York, Brunner/Mazel, 1979, pp 171–207

Conners CK: A teacher rating scale for use in drug studies with children. Am J Psychiatry 126:884–888, 1969

Conners CK: Symptom patterns in hyperkinetic, neurotic, and normal children. Child Dev 41:667–682, 1970

Conners CK: Rating scales for use in drug studies with children. Psychopharmacol Bull 9:24–84, 1973

Conners CK: Conners' Rating Scales Manual: Instruments for Use With Children and Adolescents. North Tonawanda, NY, Multi-Head Systems, 1989

Costello EJ, Edelbrock CS, Dulcan MK, et al: Testing of the NIMH Diagnostic Interview Schedule for Children (DISC) in a clinical population. Contract No. DB-81-0027, final report to the Center for Epidemiological Studies, National Institute for Mental Health. Pittsburgh, PA, February 1984

Edelbrock CS, Reed ML: Reliability and Concurrent Validity of the Teacher Version of the Child Behavior Profile. Pittsburgh, PA, University of Pittsburgh, April 1984

Eyberg SM, Robinson EA: Parent-child interaction training: effects on family functioning. Journal of Clinical Child Psychology 11:130–137, 1982

Eyberg SM, Robinson EA: Conduct problem behavior: standardization of a behavioral rating scale with adolescents. Journal of Clinical Child Psychology 12:347–354, 1983

Eyberg SM, Ross AW: Assessment of child behavior problems: the validation of a new inventory. Journal of Clinical Child Psychology 7:113–116, 1978

Galton F: Memories of My Life. London, Methuen, 1908

Glow RA: Cross-validity and normative data on the Conners Parent and Teacher Rating Scales, in Psychosocial Aspects of Drug Treatment for Hyperactivity. Edited by Gadow K, Loney J. Boulder, CO, Westview Press, 1979

Goyette CH, Conners CK, Ulrich RF: Normative data on revised Conners Parent and Teacher Rating Scales. J Abnorm Child Psychol 6:221–236, 1978

Kazdin AE, Heidish IE: Convergence of clinically derived diagnoses and parent checklists among inpatient children. J Abnorm Child Psychol 12:421–436, 1984

Kazdin AE, Esveldt-Dawson K, Loar LL: Correspondence of teacher ratings and direct observations of classroom behavior of psychiatric inpatient children. J Abnorm Child Psychol 11:549–564, 1983

Kupietz SS, Bialer I, Winsberg BG: A behavior rating scale for assessing improvement in behaviorally deviant children: a preliminary investigation. Am J Psychiatry 128:1432–1436, 1972

Loney J, Milich RS: Hyperactivity, inattention, and aggression in clinical practice, in Advances in Developmental and Behavioral Pediatrics, Vol 2. Edited by Wolraich M, Routh DK. Greenwich, CT, JAI Press, 1982, pp 113–147

Mash EJ, Johnston C: Parental perceptions of child behavior problems, parenting self-esteem, and mothers' reported stress in younger and older hyperactive and normal children. J Consult Clin Psychol 51:68–99, 1983

Milich R, Loney J, Whitten P: Two-year stability and validity of playroom observations of hyperactivity. Paper presented at the annual meeting of the American Psychological Association, Anaheim, CA, August 1980

Murphey DA, Pelham WE, Milich RS: Normative and validity data on the Iowa Conners Teacher Rating Scale. Paper presented at the annual meeting of the Association for the Advancement of Behavior Therapy, Houston, TX, November 1985

O'Conner M, Foch T, Sherry R, et al: A twin study of specific behavioral problems of socialization as viewed by parents. J Abnorm Child Psychol 8:189–199, 1980

O'Leary KD, Vivian D, Nisi A: Hyperactivity in Italy. J Abnorm Child Psychol 13:485–500, 1985

O'Leary SG, Pelham WE: Behavior therapy and withdrawal of stimulant medication in hyperactive children. Pediatrics 61:211–217, 1978

Quay HC, Peterson DR: Interim Manual for the Revised Behavior Problem Checklist. Miami, FL, University of Miami, March 1983

Robinson EA, Eyberg SM, Ross AW: The standardization of an inventory of child conduct problem behaviors. Journal of Clinical Child Psychology 9:22–28, 1980

Sprague RL, Sleator EK: Methylphenidate in hyperkinetic children: differences in dose effects on learning and social behavior. Science 198:1274–1276, 1977

Sprague RL, Cohen MN, Werry J: Normative Data on the Conners Teacher Rating Scale and Abbreviated Scale. Urbana, University of Illinois, January 1974

Sprague RL, Cohen MN, Eichlseder W: Are there hyperactive children in Europe and the South Pacific? Paper presented at the annual meeting of the American Psychological Association, San Francisco, CA, August 1977

Taylor E, Sandberg S: Hyperactive behavior in English schoolchildren: a questionnaire survey. J Abnorm Child Psychol 12:143–156, 1984

Trites RL, Blouin AG, Laprade K: Factor analysis of the Conners Teacher Rating Scale based on a large normative sample. J Consult Clin Psychol 50:615–623, 1982

Ullman RK, Sleator EK, Sprague RL: A change of mind: the Conners abbreviated rating scales reconsidered. J Abnorm Child Psychol 13:553–565, 1985

Vincent JP, Williams BJ, Harris GE, et al: Classroom observations of hyperactive children: a multiple validation study. Paper presented at the annual meeting of the American Psychological Association, San Francisco, CA, August 1977

Webster-Stratton C: Randomized trial of two parent-training programs for families with conduct-disordered children. J Consult Clin Psychol 52:666–678, 1984

Webster-Stratton C: Comparisons of behavior transactions between conduct-disordered children and their mothers in the clinic and at home. J Abnorm Child Psychol 13:169–184, 1985

Werry JS, Sprague RL: Methylphenidate in children: effect of dosage. Aust N Z J Psychiatry 8:9–19, 1974

Chapter 6

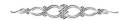

Homicidal Behavior

Balkozar S. Adam, M.D.
Richard Livingston, M.D.

onduct disorder is among the most common diagnoses treated by child and adolescent psychiatrists. Violation of the basic rights of others, a basic characteristic of conduct disorder, may lead in some instances to homicide—the ultimate violation of another's basic rights. Zenoff and Zients (1979) described the developmental background of homicidal children whose mothers seemed incapable of providing minimal psychological nurturance essential to the establishment of object constancy. Clinically, these children are divided into two groups, according to the pattern of their aggressive behavior. Those displaying the solitary aggressive pattern are characterized as socially isolated children who come from small families. Those displaying the group aggressive pattern are described as having warm relationships with their peers and a great desire to be part of the peer group; they usually come from large families and had warm relationships with their mothers when younger. Juveniles in both of these groups are described as impulsive and lacking in moral development.

The families of homicidal children with conduct disorder are frequently characterized by low socioeconomic status. Their home environments are usually chaotic; marital discord also prevails. The presence of an antisocial or alcoholic father, of a stepfather, or of multiple father figures (e.g., foster, adoptive, mother's boyfriend) is common. A history of abuse and neglect is frequently reported in homicidally aggressive juveniles. Identification with the aggressor, the availability of an aggressive role model, the organic effects of abuse, and the child's defense against loss of control are among the identified bases of these juveniles' aggressive homicidal behavior. Substance abuse and the availability of weapons also facilitate the commission of such acts.

News reports of homicide by older adolescents are unfortunately not rare. The Federal Bureau of Investigation (1987) has released the following alarming figures: of all the murder arrests in 1986, 9% were of persons younger than 18 years, and 33% were of persons 18–24 years of age. A trend toward an increasing prevalence of murders among younger people has also been noted in other parts of the world (de Castro 1991). Despite this increase in prevalence, we are still startled when we hear of children or young adolescents accused of murderous acts.

In this chapter we provide an overview of the problem of homicidal aggression in youths and use case material as a basis for discussing the psychiatric evaluation, legal disposition, and treatment of these children, as well as the implications of the conduct disorder construct as applied to these cases.

It has been suggested that violent and destructive behaviors should be viewed as a continuum rather than as separate entities of homicide, assault, suicide, and self-mutilation. A relationship between homicide and suicide has been described by several investigators. Holinger and colleagues (1987), in a study of violent death, found significant positive correlations between the suicide and homicide rates for 15- to 24-year-olds and the proportion of 15- to 24-year-olds in the United States population from 1933 to 1982. However, negative correlations were found for most adults 35–64 years of age. Holinger (1981) described the concept of a continuum of self-destructiveness in adolescents as follows:

> Self-destructive behavior appears to range from covert (from ways in which one subtly sabotages one's efforts daily, to excessive risk-taking, to thoughts of suicide) to overt manifestations (from self-mutilation to actual suicide). Suicide, homicide, and accidents can be seen as various dimensions of this self-destructive continuum. (p. 281)

This concept is interesting and should be empirically tested at both the individual and the population level, particularly as it relates to the identification of individuals at risk and to the possibility that the violent behavior of young people differs in some fundamental way from that of adults.

Tonken (1987) acknowledged the existence of a general agreement that violence in adolescence is occurring at unprecedented and unacceptably high levels. A number of hypotheses have been offered to account for this increase. Rydelius (1988) investigated the relationship of antisocial behavior and the incidence of "sudden, violent death" in young people. Of 1,056 adolescents admitted to Swedish probationary schools during the period 1967–1985, he found that 13% of the boys and 10% of the girls had died by 1986. Furthermore, of the deceased, 88% of the boys and 77% of the girls had died a "sudden, violent death"—accidents, suicides, death from uncertain causes, murder/manslaughter, or death as a direct result of alcohol or drug abuse. Rydelius also reported that in both sexes the most frequent single causes of death were uncertain cause and suicide, and that death as a direct result of alcohol and drug abuse occurred only in boys. These data offer some support for the hypothesized link between childhood environment, the development of antisocial behavior, and sudden, violent death at an early age.

Lewis et al. (1985) recognized a combination of five variables that most strongly distinguish murderers from other delinquents: 1) severe neuropsychiatric impairment, 2) presence of close relatives who were psychotic and/or had been psychiatrically hospitalized, 3) history of severe physical abuse, 4) serious violent behavior exhibited long before murder was committed, and 5) psychotic symptoms, especially paranoid ideation. Violent behavior alone or a history of abuse did not strongly distinguish murderers from other delinquents. Busch et al. (1979), in their study of 71 delinquent and homicidal adolescents, found that the presence of criminally violent family members, gang membership, severe alcohol abuse, and serious educational difficulties was especially common in the homicidal group compared with the nonviolent delinquents. Zagar et al. (1979) reported a similar constellation of symptoms. Stark (1990), in an investigation of possible misperceptions related to homicide, challenged the claim that most homicides are motivated either by uncontrollable passion or by some combination of environmental stress and personal deficits. That author also perceived a general failure to recognize the historical and social character of most interpersonal violence, and emphasized the need to intervene before assault occurs.

Cornell et al. (1987) studied 72 juvenile murderers and separated them into three groups based on differing circumstances of offense: psychotic, conflict, and crime. Compared with the adolescents charged with nonviolent offenses, the homicidal adolescents scored higher (i.e., exhibited more problems) on composite measures of school adjustment, childhood symptoms, criminal activity, and psychiatric history. One explanation for the finding that the adolescents charged with homicide came from relatively less-troubled backgrounds was that homicide defendants are referred for pretrial evaluation because of the seriousness of the offense, even in the absence of a background that might support pursuit of the insanity defense.

Case reports have provided more detailed descriptions of the reasons and motivations behind violent crimes. For example, Marohn et al. (1982) explored the life history and reviewed the writings of John Wesley Hardin, who was known for killing 42 people in 8 years, and described the emergence of Hardin's narcissistic behavior disorder. Ratner (1985) noted the case of a 19-year-old single teenager who had been charged with attempted murder, child abuse, assault, and intent to murder after she abandoned her newborn infant as a result of feeling rejected by her own mother.

Adolescence is considered a unique developmental phase in which, according to Erikson (1963), the life task of identity formation must be addressed. Blos (1983) described a second individuation process to represent the adolescent task of achieving independence. These internal processes account for much of the emotional turbulence of adolescence. The tasks may proceed either noisily and agitatedly or calmly and silently. Blos also reported that adolescents frequently exhibit affective states and forms of behavior that are considered abnormal or bizarre, and that may be transient or irreversible, depending on the adolescent's psychic restructuring.

Although several investigators have reported associations of psychiatric disorders, including conduct disorder, with homicidal behavior in young people, other problems and symptoms have been linked with conduct disorder as well. Malmquist (1990) described a mixed symptom picture in a sample of 6,500 alleged delinquents and—depending on which group of symptoms is emphasized—overlapping diagnostic possibilities. The symptoms and findings of the agitated disturbed adolescents in Malmquist's study could lead to their classification as a variety of conduct disorders (group or solitary aggressive), with a depressive affect often part of the picture. He also suggested that the conduct disorder diagnosis overlaps with affective disorder in this age group and that the two are difficult to differentiate—a view that remains controversial.

Myers and Kemph (1990) studied the DSM-III-R (American Psychiatric Association 1987) classification of murderous youth and reported a wide range of diagnoses in conjunction with conduct disorder. DSM-III-R diagnoses in this population also included mood disorders, psychoactive substance use and dependency disorders, anxiety disorders, and several other diagnoses; however, no diagnoses of psychotic disorder were described in their report.

Conceptual View of Conduct Disorder

In general, United States classification systems for psychiatric disorders of children have "split" what British classifications have "lumped." DSM-IV (American Psychiatric Association 1994) recognizes three disruptive behavior disorders as overlapping but separate: attention-deficit hyperactivity disorder (ADHD), oppositional defiant disorder (ODD), and conduct disorder (CD). The latter category is reserved for children and adolescents who violate major societal rules and the rights of others. CD is further rated as mild, moderate, or severe. Comparative studies suggest that the current classification is superior to its immediate predecessor in several ways (Adam et al. 1991).

Robins (1966) showed that the CD diagnosis in childhood predicts continuing difficulty in adulthood, although the difficulty is not uniformly of a criminal nature. Lewis et al. (1984) have questioned the validity and appropriateness of the CD diagnosis—particularly as applied to the most violent youths, whom they frequently find to be so neurologically damaged and impaired in reality testing that the CD diagnosis is misleading and incomplete.

Criterion symptoms for CD include several varieties of violent behavior: initiating physical fights outside the household, engaging in stealing that involves confronting the victim, using weapons in fights, forcing someone into sexual activity, and being physically cruel to animals. Nonpersonal violence in the forms of vandalism and fire setting is also included.

Principles for Evaluation of Children Accused of Homicidal Acts

Psychiatric advice may be sought for children accused of murder for several reasons. Sometimes there is a specific request, based upon a plea of not guilty by reason of mental disorder or a question of competence to stand trial in juvenile or adult court. Frequently, however, it seems that psychiatric evaluation is sought because, given the fact that it is so unusual for the very young to kill, there is an underlying assumption of psychological disturbance.

Whatever precipitates the evaluation, two fundamental issues must be faced by the evaluation team. The first involves legal concerns; the second, treatment or disposition. The forensic aspects require a basic knowledge of the relevant juvenile or general laws applicable to the case, which vary among states. The need to respect the rights of the accused, confidentiality concerns, security issues, regional politics, staff reactions to the crime, media coverage, and other factors can complicate these evaluations. Caution, thoroughness, and clear goals are the psychiatrist's best buffers.

The more purely psychiatric issues should be approached with the initial understanding that a psychiatric diagnosis alone is unlikely to provide sufficient basis for answering the questions that someone ultimately must attempt to answer about a child who has killed or attempted to kill another person: What should be done about it? Can treatment help? Will this child kill again? The latter question cannot be answered with any certainty, but some sense of the probabilities and the prognosis is essential to adequately answer the first two questions.

A complete routine history and examination of the child in both a family and a developmental context is, of course, essential. Detailed accounts of the crime as reported by the child and as documented in police reports must be obtained. Especially important in the evaluation of violent youth are the following:

— The presence of neurological abnormalities as evidenced by lateralizing or localizing signs, paroxysmal or seizure phenomena, neurological se-

quelae of physical abuse or head injury, signs of neurodevelopmental immaturity, or cognitive impairments
— The child's degree of superego development and enhancement of prosocial behavior as evidenced by statements of guilt or remorse, impulse control in usual situations, response to positive and negative reinforcers and punishers, stated ideals, heroes and ambitions, and roles adopted in play or imagination
— A family history of psychiatric disorders in general and of alcoholism, sociopathy, and somatization (a common familial cluster associated with criminality), neurological disorders, other substance abuse, mania, and psychosis in particular
— When the child knew the victim, a thorough understanding of the interpersonal dynamics
— The child's environment at home, in the community, and at school; specifically, the stressors present and the models available to the child for dealing with anger, aggressive impulses, and interpersonal conflict
— The presence of other problems that may be seen concurrently with violence (not necessarily implying causality), such as hallucinations, delusions, substance abuse, reading or language disability, and ADHD

Ancillary examinations may be required to provide satisfactory assessment of these areas: electroencephalogram (EEG), head imaging, bone scan (for old fractures from abuse), psychological tests, and inpatient observation can all contribute information. In addition to clinical interviews, parent and child versions of structured diagnostic interviews may be helpful to the extent that they ensure that psychiatric symptoms of all major disorders have been pursued.

After the information is obtained and carefully documented, a multiaxial diagnosis and biopsychosocial formulation for the child's psychopathology, the crime, and the child's current developmental and situational status will provide the foundation for a comprehensive approach to treatment. The forensic parameters within which treatment must be provided should be specified and any questions of competence that precede the trial or delinquency hearing answered.

Illustrative Cases

Martin

At age 12, Martin had the body of a 15-year-old. His father was a con-artist evangelist who had begun that year to use Martin as a "greeter" at revival meetings. Martin and the other greeters would meet people and find out their names and their concerns; later during the meeting the preacher would call their names and appear to know things about them by divine inspiration, which would, he hoped, increase his evening's donations. Martin cooperated a few times, then declined to do it any more. He felt too guilty "even though the people who could be fooled by him were so stupid." Even more distressing to Martin was the fact that his father dated women who came to his meetings. His mother had gone on the revival trips more frequently in the past, but was staying home more because the children were in school and also because of her numerous physical complaints, which included nervous stomach, chest pains, back pain, and "female problems."

Martin's father had kept a large stack of pornographic magazines in a closet. Martin expressed relief when his mother burned them all, but the stack immediately began to grow again. As his father explained to his mother, "Sex is 90% of marriage; I need that to keep me stimulated for you." It was about this time that Martin began exercising "to get strong enough to kill him [his father], to help everybody and stop all his deceit and the damage he did." He considered shooting or poisoning, but eventually decided on stabbing.

On the day of his father's return from a series of revivals, Martin followed him into the bedroom and stabbed him 13 times. Immediately, he said, "I knew I had done wrong, I had been so sure it was good but I felt so bad." He was charged with murder in juvenile court and referred for inpatient psychiatric evaluation.

Martin was the product of a "difficult" but uncomplicated pregnancy, and his early development was not remarkable. As he grew, he proved to be athletic and generally above average in academic achievement. There were no instances of fighting, truancy, stealing, or school discipline problems and no significant illnesses or injuries.

About a year before the murder, Martin began showing some emotional intensity. He threatened to kill himself if he had to stay with his grandparents half the time while his mother and father traveled; this was another reason his mother had stopped going on the revival trips. About 3 months before the climactic incident, his mother said, "I began to think Martin needed more attention so I gave him more. Like I would tuck him in at night and kiss him like a baby and he loved it, he would just giggle."

On examination, it was determined that Martin was completely developed sexually (Tanner stage IV), but no endocrinological abnormalities were found after consultation and further evaluation. There was no evidence of abnormal perceptions, affective states, or flow of thought, and he was cognitively quite intact. Verbal IQ was 114, performance was 101, and reading was 3 years above the expected level, with other achievement measures at grade level.

Projective tests revealed some idiosyncratic thinking but no frank psychosis. Themes of violence and sexual seduction were common in responses to the cards of the Thematic Apperception Test. On the Diagnostic Interview for Children and Adolescents (DICA; Welner et al. 1987), there were isolated symptoms but no areas in which symptoms endorsed even came close to criterion level for any syndrome. Neurological examination and EEG were normal.

In response to a hypothetical situation in which he sees a $50 bill fall out of a man's pocket unnoticed, Martin said, "If it was a rich man I would keep it, if he was poor I'd give it back." He was confident he could tell the difference: "The rich look underworked and well dressed. They have all this gold. My dad had all kinds of gold bracelets and everything." Several weeks after his father's death he showed some remorse but still maintained that his father was evil and thought overall that perhaps he had done the world a service.

Three child psychiatrists evaluated Martin. All felt that his oedipal rage and distorted value development were inevitable products of his family situation and heritage and that regardless of guilt (which was not contested), long-term treatment in a normalizing setting was needed. Despite this testimony and none to the contrary, he was found guilty of murder, adjudicated delinquent, and sentenced to the reformatory. His only formal diagnosis was childhood antisocial behavior, which was used descriptively and applied only in reference to his patricide.

William

Fourteen-year-old William answered questions readily but with little affect as he described his commando-style killing of his mother, sister, and grandfather and wounding of his younger brother. His account of the events was dry: "I just did it. I was only thinking one thought at a time. All sounds were muffled, things just seemed different." He had never before had any kind of dissociative experience. He did not remember being angry at anyone, but maybe "irritated"; the word "irritate" peppered his speech and described all his favorite activities—irritating girls, irritating the neighbors, and irritating birds (by shooting at them with an air rifle). He could not, however, recall any special irritations from these family members. "Something just snapped."

Behavioral symptoms elicited on the DICA included frequent lying, several instances of cruelty to cats and birds, and three episodes of threatening someone with a weapon. He denied all other symptoms except for occasional ideas of reference (thinking other kids were talking about him) and two brief spells of feeling sad and embarrassed after girls made remarks he took as insulting. In general, William associated only with his small circle of friends, a group of boys who saw themselves as different and socially separate, although he objected to the term "nerds." Their primary activity when together was war games. Occasionally they played "Dungeons and Dragons," during which William invariably chose to assume the character called "Berserker."

William said that he coped by not thinking about the murders: "I just turn it off. I can control my thinking by a kind of automatic lockback." He thought his father would be all right after a while: "He copes by staying busy." No one in the family had a history of psychiatric problems or of violent or odd behavior, alcoholism, criminality, or somatization.

Apart from his tendency to daydream in school from first grade onward, William's early development was not unusual in any respect. A tonsillectomy at age 6 and occasional allergic rhinitis (not treated) constituted his entire medical history. He had been hit on the head with a stick a year before, with no loss of consciousness and no noted sequelae. The last school year, he made A's and B's in regular classes.

Physical and neurological examinations were unremarkable, as were two EEGs and a CT scan of the head. He was not cooperative with projective testing, and the psychologist who attempted to test him speculated that William was worried about what might be discovered. Mental status was considered remarkable for constricted affect and somewhat monotonous speech, and there were several subtle indicators of paranoid feelings. Detailed cognitive exams revealed no deficits. Although William's stated interests were primarily in aggressive fantasy activities, there was no evidence that he was unable to separate reality from fantasy. Minimization and isolation of emotions were evidently long-used defense mechanisms.

Two child psychiatrists evaluated William independently. One concluded that his dissociative state during the killings was such that he was unaware of the quality of his actions and unable to control his behavior at that time; the second evaluator thought that the acts of murder and assault were consistent with William's long-standing internal and fantasy states, and that the dissociative phenomenon was nonpsychotic in nature and did not cause enough impairment to render him unable to appreciate the wrongfulness of his act or to change his behavior. The second evaluator also asserted that although William's symptom picture did not fit precisely with any available DSM diagnosis, there was definitely something wrong with him and the diagnostic picture would probably become clearer in time.

William was charged as an adult with premeditated murder. He was allowed to plead guilty to a lesser felony, and an arrangement was made in cooperation with correctional mental health personnel that he would be incarcerated only in the mental health treatment unit of the state prison, where reasonable protection as well as treatment could be anticipated.

Edward

On one of many truant days, 12-year-old Edward and his friend James broke into an old house in search of money for the arcade or something they could steal and sell. There was no car outside, and the boys assumed that no one was home. In the kitchen, the first room they entered, they found a lot of $1 and $5 bills in a drawer. After stuffing their pockets, they decided to cover their tracks and set fire to the window curtain. The entire house burned rapidly and the elderly owners, apparently asleep in the bedroom, died in the blaze. Edward was charged in juvenile court with theft, arson, and murder. A juvenile court worker felt that Edward's apparent lack of emotional response to his situation indicated possible psychiatric disorder, and because Edward had a history of an outpatient psychiatric visit, the judge ordered hospitalization for evaluation and specifically requested to know whether any disposition other than reformatory was indicated.

Edward's one previous psychiatric contact had been 3 years earlier, when his third-grade teacher suggested that an evaluation might be warranted because of Edward's constant disruptive behavior and his lack of academic achievement. Behaviors noted as frequently observed at school included fighting, lying, stealing, and intimidating younger children. Edward was usually suspended from school several times each year. In sixth grade he was regularly truant. Each year he did just enough schoolwork to pass.

Edward's household consisted of himself, his mother, and one younger brother. His father was a drug abuser and had disappeared when Edward was 3. His mother worked in a local factory; she acknowledged not supervising Edward closely enough, saying he could not be controlled anyway and that she was too tired to try. Edward did not generally misbehave very badly at home and was not verbally defiant toward her, but simply ignored her instructions. When the outpatient psychologist had recommended weekly sessions for behavior management 3 years earlier, Edward's mother had felt unable to take off work each week and had never followed up or pursued other possibilities.

Edward freely described the break-in and theft but contended that it was unreasonable to hold him responsible for the deaths of the occupants: "They shouldn't have been sleeping that late . . . at least they should've figured out something was wrong and got out." He acknowledged that breaking into houses was exciting for him and that he might do it again but would not set any more fires.

Examination revealed a boy at 70th percentile for height and 95th for weight, with no signs of physical illness or neurological abnormality. Edward's verbal IQ of 78 was significantly lower than his performance IQ of 104; the lowest subscales were information, vocabulary, and picture arrangement. Educational achievement tests showed reading, spelling, and arithmetic standard scores in the same range as verbal IQ. Responses to Rorschach and TAT cards were concrete and were performed "mechanically, with so little engagement [that] interpretation cannot be reliable." A language consultant concluded that Edward's language difficulties were not indicative of a specific learning disability and that although he was capable of expanding his vocabulary, he was entirely unmotivated. On the DICA, he endorsed enough items to satisfy DSM-III (American Psychiatric Association 1980) criteria for CD and denied virtually all other symptoms.

Edward's appearance was unkempt and he slouched in his chair throughout each psychiatric evaluation visit, which he described as "the only thing more boring than school." He was not particularly distracted and actually appeared euthymic but sluggish in movement and speech; with the children on the ward, he appeared much more animated. He participated in all ward activities and was compliant with most rules, although he occasionally attempted to cheat at a game or to intimidate another child with a threatening gesture he thought the staff did not see. There were no signs of psychosis or brain syndrome. EEG was interpreted as normal but having "more slow wave activity than is usual at this age"; none of it was paroxysmal or localized. CT of the head was normal.

A diagnosis of CD was made. The report to the court included the suggestion that although Edward's behavior could be easily kept within acceptable bounds in a sufficiently structured setting, his prognosis for lasting change with active treatment did not seem great. He was adjudicated delinquent and sent to reformatory.

Stephanie

Ten-year-old Stephanie showed no emotion as she described stabbing her sister to death. Although the 7-year-old had been physically aggressive with Stephanie, the reverse was not evident until one day while the girls were alone a few minutes after school. Police and court officials requested psychiatric evaluation primarily because of the child's lack of emotional response.

Both Stephanie and her parents denied that she had any of the psychiatric symptoms that were asked about, and reported a completely unremarkable developmental course. The family's only major life change had occurred 3 years before, when the father's job was relocated from a larger city to a rural area. Stephanie had previously gone to private school and had numerous friends, but since the move she said she disliked her school and thought that even the children in her classes for the gifted and talented were stupid. Her primary leisure activity was reading. Her only notable preoccupation was a particular fascination with the television miniseries "V," about extraterrestrials that initially seem benign but are revealed to be dangerous. (In the authors' opinion, some explicit and fairly shocking violent scenes in "V" would warrant parental concern, and the network that showed the series made announcements to that effect.)

Despite her superiority to her sister as a student, Stephanie showed an intensely competitive attitude. The younger girl beat Stephanie on the back when angry and often called her "stupid." Stephanie was not well liked by the town children in general. Court personnel reported that the parents' defensive attitude toward Stephanie following her sister's death had generated ill will among the local adults as well.

During her inpatient evaluation, Stephanie was from the beginning bossy with and aloof from the other children. Psychological tests confirmed superior intellectual functioning (full-scale IQ = 124), and projectives showed a remarkable degree of egocentricity and a tendency to ruminate or obsess. Fairy-tale fantasy themes were common, but reality testing was not impaired. Her final psychiatric diagnosis was an Axis II notation of significant personality traits in the narcissistic, antisocial, and obsessive-compulsive areas.

This emerging personality disorder was considered serious enough to warrant a recommendation for long-term treatment. After considerable discussion, residential treatment was prescribed; this would remove Stephanie from the hostility of the small community and from the superego lacunae of her parents for a time, during which the family could be treated with a goal of creating a more suitable environment for her continuing development. It was further recommended that she be required to perform community and family service of some sort to "discharge her debt" to family and society.

Rusty

Rusty's father and the father's family were all well known in the state penal system. His paternal grandmother had been convicted of theft and fraud; his father and his brothers each had multiple convictions for burglary, drug violations, and auto theft. Rusty was the first, however, to show dangerous violence. Before school age as well as in the earliest grades of school, he frequently fought, kicked, and bit other children. These early incidents seemed mostly impulsive and reactive.

At age 10, a more calculated violence emerged. Rusty began setting fires. He built a primitive bomb with which he planned to blow up his grandmother's car. At 11 he sharpened a pair of scissors and took them to school to use against another child. At the same time, his reactive violence also escalated, and he was admitted to the hospital after choking another child and threatening the life of a pregnant teacher.

Rusty's parents had divorced when he was 7, remarried the same year, and divorced again when his father went back to prison. When Rusty was 9, his father was released and Rusty visited him most weekends after that. Four months before his hospitalization, his mother remarried and his father initiated a custody battle. Rusty acknowledged being continually upset about the custody fight.

For about 2 years, Rusty received psychotherapy (attended sporadically) and was prescribed methylphenidate for attention-deficit disorder, with some benefit. He required resource room intervention in reading, and his school grades vacillated wildly, ranging from A's to D's, despite average verbal and performance IQ scores. In the hospital, his extensive medical and neurological examinations failed to show even "soft signs" of neurological dysfunction, and his EEG was unremarkable. Specific mood disorder, anxiety, and psychotic symptoms were absent.

Diagnostically, CD symptoms (solitary aggressive type) had been evident for years. The temporal course suggested strongly that recent exacerbations of behavioral symptoms were related to stressors, and this was noted in the case formulation.

Rusty came across as being more receptive to therapy than his history had led some staff to expect; to some extent, his more outrageous behaviors seemed ego-dystonic. Brief inpatient therapy was directed primarily toward helping him develop and practice an acceptable repertoire of anger management methods. It was clear to hospital personnel that both his temper and his attention span were better controlled when he was taking methylphenidate than when he wasn't. The recommendation to the court was for continuing intensive treatment on an outpatient basis, including parent guidance, medication, and individual therapy, as well as continuing family supervision by the local social service agency.

Charles

School and law enforcement employees suspected Charles of gang involvement when he was 9 years old. He seemed to prefer the company of older boys known to have gang affiliations, and he was already showing the kind of behavior problems more typical of older youths. Although he fought frequently and had made numerous threats with knives and ice picks, he had not used these weapons until he stabbed his 5-year-old sister with frank homicidal intention.

Charles's aggression was not directed only outward, however; he had also threatened suicide and on one occasion had turned on an unlit gas burner while both he and his family were in the house.

Charles was the fourth of six children born to an impoverished single mother and a transient alcoholic father. His mother had always found Charles difficult to manage and had tried letting him live with her brother in Los Angeles. He fared no better there, with eight school suspensions in 18 months, and returned to his home state 8 months before the incident that led to his hospitalization, accusing the uncle of physically abusing him. During the months before he stabbed his sister, Charles threw a chair at his teacher and cut a dog with a knife.

It became evident that Charles was not closely affiliated with any gang, nor did he have any identifiable friends at all. The symptom pattern was classic for solitary aggressive type CD. His evaluation also showed several neurodevelopmental problems: moderately severe expressive and receptive language disorder, poor visual-motor integration, numerous neurological "soft signs," and academic performance in all areas far below that predicted by his low-average IQ.

His mother was concerned but felt powerless and unable to control his behavior. Long-term guidance and support for her were clearly essential. Because the severity and chronicity of Charles's violent behavior was considered to pose a distinct and continuous danger for serious harm to others and to himself, he was referred for residential treatment. His behavior problems in school had previously been the focus of attention in that setting to such an extent that his neurodevelopmental problems had gone unrecognized; therefore, specific remediation was recommended as part of the residential program.

Carl

Carl lived in the most violent housing project in town and at age 12 was considered one of its more dangerous residents. Over a 2-year period, he had stabbed two boys, beat several others with sticks, destroyed property, and broken into apartments. He was hospitalized for evaluation after stabbing an older youth in the lung three times with nearly fatal results. For 7 weeks after admission, he required repeated seclusion or restraint for attacking staff and other children. Suicide threats, often accompanied by medically nonserious attempts (e.g., putting a sock around his neck and pulling on the ends, always with others in eyesight), persisted for several weeks as well.

Carl's mother seemed preoccupied with her own problems, which included an unconfirmed history of seizures, dizzy spells, and other physical complaints. His father was said to be alcoholic and was not involved. Maternal aunts had histories of seizures, alcohol problems, and felony convictions. The immediate household included Carl and four half-siblings, one of them a mentally retarded younger boy with severe behavior problems of his own. Social agency involvement with this family extended back at least 6 years.

Carl's physical and neurological exams, including CT of the head and EEG, were unremarkable. His verbal, performance, and full-scale IQs were 84, 106, and 93, respectively. Neuromotor development was intact. He and his mother denied his having any mood disorder symptoms except irritability, which they both admitted was present to an extreme degree. Psychotic symptoms were also denied. Impulsiveness and the antisocial behaviors described were the only symptoms acknowledged. CD (solitary aggressive type) was the principal diagnosis.

Initially, behavior modification alone failed to produce any appreciable decrease in Carl's assaultive behavior. The respective additions of methylphenidate and lithium added nothing. Finally, a trial of thioridazine was instituted and his assaults and overreactions to provocations decreased to a point that discharge to a residential facility could safely be tried.

Discussion

These cases illustrate several factors. Martin's history of an antisocial father is a pattern commonly seen in histories of homicidal children and children with CD. His sexual maturity and the sexual tone of his interaction with his mother, in addition to his oedipal rage toward his father, are components of the psychodynamic background of some homicidal acts by children.

William's story comes the closest to the psychotic/dissociative background of homicidal children described by Lewis et al. (1985). However, symptoms of CD are also clearly apparent (e.g., DICA results).

Edward's story fits the well-known model of homicide during the course of another crime. CD behaviors appear frequently in his history, and he endorsed most of these symptoms on the DICA. His lower cognitive ability is also congruent with other reports in the literature.

Many features of Stephanie's case resemble those described in Ewing's (1990) characterization of preteen children who commit homicide. Immaturity, impulsivity, and the presence of the victim and the perpetrator at the wrong place at the wrong time are demonstrated. Neurological impairment and psychotic background, which were described by Lewis et al. (1985), are not evident. Abuse history is also absent in this case.

Rusty's history indicates behavior that violated societal norms and rules, as well as poor anger control, starting at an early age. The behavior gradually worsened and led to the homicide attempt. Family and marital discord are also demonstrated. Family histories of antisocial behavior and child abuse are obvious. Many years of involvement with the juvenile justice system and the presence of a learning disability are also observed in Rusty's case.

Charles's history is consistent with that of a child with CD who has multiple behavioral problems. Both the chaotic family background and the history of abuse also conform to the profile described in the literature. Academic and neuromotor delays, which are frequently present in homicidal children, are observed in Charles's case as well.

Carl's history is also consistent with descriptions of homicidal nonempathic children with CD in the literature. A family history of alcoholism, antisocial behavior, and seizure disorders is commonly found in such children.

Homicidal Behavior and Conduct Disorder

CD was among the diagnoses in four of the seven homicidally violent children we have described. Clearly, the constellation of symptoms, personality characteristics, and familial patterns associated with CD accounts for some of the risk for committing fatal violence. In perspective, however, it is notable that these four cases represented the most lethal or nearly lethal of about 160 children with CD from about 1,000 admissions to Arkansas Children's Hospital psychiatric unit over a period of 8 years. Further explanation is required: Why these particular children?

Edward's situation is sadly reminiscent of adult criminals whose mundane felonies turn lethal. Rusty's extreme and combative reactions seem to be at the more severe end of the violence spectrum but within the usual range of CD/ADHD behaviors. With Charles, we encounter a more alarming pattern of homicidal violence in repeated episodes with knives and ice picks as well as self-directed violence and stronger indications of neurological dysfunction. Carl, likewise, had a more extreme pattern of violence toward others and himself and showed some indications of psychosis. These more extreme cases illustrate the kinds of additional factors described by Lewis et al. (1985).

It is not difficult to generate hypotheses about how CD increases the risk for violent behavior with a fatal outcome. Fundamental personality traits—genetic, constitutional, or learned—such as impulsiveness, overreactiveness, and poor frustration tolerance may inherently increase risks. Being a victim of physical abuse—exposed to violent behavior at home as well as to inconsistent discipline by parents who alternate between undersupervising and over-punishing—certainly could contribute, and all are characteristic of the family situations of children with CD. Perhaps the CD substrate is such that in the presence of additional risk factors, such as neurological damage or poor reality testing, the sensitivity to frustration becomes dangerously high. In any case, it is clear from the literature and from clinical experience that CD is sometimes associated with lethal violence; however, the presence of CD alone may or may not account satisfactorily for the origins of such violence.

We suggest, therefore, that it is logical to treat homicidal children with the models we use for CD only when CD seems to account for the violent behavior. This principle has implications not only for individual cases but also for policy making as it pertains to juvenile justice, state service arrays, and—when these children are charged as adults—adult judicial and correctional systems. For example, reformatories may be inadequately staffed and equipped to treat children with neurological problems or psychotic symptoms—and thus may, in some cases, actually be countertherapeutic for such children.

Treatment Principles

Because homicidal children form a heterogeneous group, treatment must be individualized. However, the violent nature of this crime dictates that certain specific treatment issues be addressed:

— What is the best setting in which treatment can occur, and what options are available with each possible forensic disposition?
— Are special security measures necessary to provide for the safety of others?
— What safe and effective treatments are available to decrease the child's murderous impulses in frequency or intensity?
— What interpersonal and intrapersonal sequelae are expected that may require psychotherapy (individual or family) currently and at different periods of development?
— What interventions are indicated for comorbid conditions? To what extent can these be pursued within the forensically determined limits applied to this child?

What is the best setting in which treatment can occur, and what options are available with each possible forensic disposition? After a child or an adolescent commits a homicidal act, a detention center is usually the landing facility. Initial evaluation takes place during this period; however, neither the child nor the detention center staff is ready for in-depth therapy. Therefore, treatment usually starts there but continues elsewhere, depending on the disposition of the juvenile by the court.

Outpatient treatment is usually recommended when the juvenile is not thought of as a high risk and the community is relatively safe.

Hospitalization was suggested by Pfeffer (1980) as often the best first phase of intervention. The proposed goals of hospitalization include redirecting homicidal impulses, strengthening ego functioning, and reducing conflicts for the child and family. The suggested treatment modalities offered by the hospital include individual, group, and family therapy; school remediation; and psychopharmacology. Pfeffer also noted that the hospital milieu promotes social skills and strengthens ego functioning. The same author reported the successful outcome of a holistic treatment approach that included extensive evaluation of factors such as constitutional vulnerability, environmental stress, intrapsychic conflict, and state of the child's ego functioning.

Long-term residential treatment is often recommended for juveniles with homicidal impulses. This is usually arranged in conjunction with the court, where communication about the juvenile's progress in treatment and disposition status to a less restrictive environment is frequently evaluated. In such an environment, the juvenile is reasonably shielded from the bias of society, gains insight into the seriousness of his or her crime, and works on learning new coping skills.

Contrarily, if the juvenile is criminally charged and incarcerated as an adult, treatment may or may not take place. Unfortunately, all too frequently, placement in such a setting only increases the likelihood that the juvenile will be exposed to further antisocial behavior and learn better how to manipulate the system.

Are special security measures necessary to provide for the safety of others?
When the juvenile is detained at or admitted to any of the above-mentioned facilities, staff members may be very alarmed because of the seriousness of the crime. This apprehension necessitates a high level of security and vigilance. The juvenile continues to be watched closely, and his or her past history remains vivid in the eyes of the caretakers. However, as the staff members begin to feel less anxious, as the juvenile refrains from exhibiting aggressive behavior, and especially as he or she expresses remorse about the crime, the perceived need for security gradually diminishes. A great deal of hesitancy commonly accompanies such a decision.

The initial release of the juvenile to the community (through passes or other arrangements) is especially anxiety provoking. A high level of supervision is required until the juvenile and the professional staff develop a comfortable level of trust. The probation division of the juvenile court may play an active part in supervising the juvenile when his or her level of freedom increases.

What safe and effective treatments are available to decrease the child's murderous impulses in frequency or intensity?   The use of several psychopharmacological agents for controlling aggressive/violent episodes has been described (Stewart et al. 1990). However, because homicidal children and adolescents are not a homogeneous entity, no single, specific psychopharmacological medication is universally helpful in this population. Lithium has been prescribed for children and adolescents with aggressive/violent behavior and poor impulse control. It may be especially effective when such behavior in children and adolescents represents early bipolar disorder.

The use of psychostimulants (e.g., methylphenidate, magnesium pemoline, or dextroamphetamine) is also helpful and has been reported to decrease aggressive behavior. These medications are especially beneficial in homicidal children with CD who have underlying ADHD.

Carbamazepine has also been recommended for use in aggressive/violent children. It is helpful for children with CD who have an underlying seizure disorder, particularly complex partial seizure disorder.

Although tricyclic antidepressants have not been demonstrated to be unequivocally effective for depressive disorders in children, clinical experience suggests that they are beneficial in appropriately selected individuals with significant symptoms of depression—particularly the neurovegetative symptoms of altered sleep and appetite, irritability, and melancholic retardation of thought and activity. The efficacy of these agents in ADHD is better documented.

Neuroleptic medications are commonly used in the treatment of aggressive and/or violent children and adolescents. This group of medications could be especially beneficial in the treatment of children with CD who have neuropsychiatric impairment (Lewis et al. 1985). However, because safer medications are available, and because of the long-term side effects of neuro-leptics, their risks and benefits need to be evaluated thoroughly prior to their use.

Other medications have been described in the treatment of aggres-sive/violent children and adolescents, including beta-blockers, anticonvul-sant medications, and clonidine. As stated earlier, however, medication should be used not as the sole mode of treatment, but rather in combination with several modalities in a comprehensive treatment plan.

What interpersonal and intrapersonal sequelae are expected that may require psychotherapy (individual or family) currently and at different periods of development? Although the recidivism rate of homicide in children and adolescents is relatively low (Cormier and Markus 1980), treat-ment is often indicated not only for risk reduction but also for the "larger" psychopathology of which violence may be only one symptom.

In the initial aftermath of a juvenile homicide, both the child and his or her family are in a state of shock. A long period of time usually elapses before the child expresses guilt or remorse (average of 3–5 years). This delay may represent the child's way of coping with the seriousness of the act and may constitute a protective mechanism against suicide. Depression usually accompanies the expression of guilt and remorse, and the professional staff need to be aware of the possibility of self-harming behavior, which could take place during this period.

Beres (1952) suggested the following guidelines when one is dealing with homicidal children and adolescents:

1. Promoting opportunities to develop relationships with adults with whom the youngster can identify may rectify a problematic relationship from an earlier period of life that contributed to a disturbed ego development.
2. Integrating the expression of aggressive and libidinal impulses with inten-sive psychotherapy may help resolve ambivalent and predominantly sado-masochistic relationships.
3. Providing education and parental guidance to enforce realistic limits while promoting independence and ego development ultimately will increase the youngster's capability to tolerate frustration.

Beres emphasized that treatment is not meant to abolish aggressive impulses, but rather to promote sublimation of—and decrease the destructive compo-nent of—such impulses.

Cormier and Markus (1980), in their longitudinal study of adolescent murderers, acknowledged the difficulty in treating this age group, especially because of adolescents' frequent lack of empathy, remorse, and guilt feelings. However, the authors noted the great potential for recovery from acute crisis in adolescents when they enter maturity.

Another treatment approach involves teaching problem-solving skills, which help the juvenile find ways of dealing with anger other than through violent aggression.

Family therapy/involvement could also play a role in dealing with homicidally aggressive/violent adolescents. In the initial stage, therapy helps the family to deal with the fact that one of its members has committed a crime and to accept the consequences of that action (MacLeod 1982). It also fosters a continuing relationship/attachment and helps the juvenile feel accepted by the family. This support, in turn, is important as the child deals with guilt, remorse, and suicidal feelings. Finally, if the juvenile is found not guilty and is preparing for discharge, family therapy can help smooth the transition and enhance parental skills.

When the juvenile who attempted or successfully committed a homicide returns home, the family is usually ambivalent about his or her return. Such ambivalence seriously affects the subsequent life of other family members. Although they may wish to trust the child, they have no assurance that the violent behavior will not be repeated. The family usually manifests increased vigilance and watch the juvenile closely, especially when he or she is first united with the family. Close supervision, continued observation of the juvenile's behavior, and clear communication in regard to expected behavior, as well as persistent communication with the therapist and probation officer concerning the juvenile's progress, are critical to the success of the process of reintegration into the family and the community.

What interventions are indicated for comorbid conditions? To what extent can these be pursued within the forensically determined limits applied to this child? Academic delays, impaired social development, comorbid ADHD, and at times problems in speech/language and motor skills are frequently observed in juvenile murderers. Educational remediation is especially important when these children are being kept in an institution for a relatively long time. As already mentioned, many such juveniles have been academically delayed for some time before the homicidal act. In fact, several authors indicate that the academic delays are a risk factor for the development of CD and destructive aggression in these children. One observation by educators dealing with child/adolescent murderers while they are institutionalized is these juveniles' great need to achieve and to take every opportunity to learn (Cormier and Markus 1980). Away from the biases of society, educational remediation can best be accomplished during the period these children spend in a correctional institution or in a long-term residential treatment program.

Special speech/language therapy, occupational therapy, and physical therapy are also indicated for a number of these juvenile murderers. However, these specific treatment modalities may not be readily available in all treatment/detention settings, especially in the detention/reform institutional setting. Some access to educational remediation and medication management is available in most settings.

As mentioned previously, psychostimulants are especially helpful for treating underlying ADHD, which is often a comorbid condition in homicidal adolescents with the diagnosis of CD.

Petti and Davidman (1981) emphasized the need for this group of children and adolescents to master and develop appropriate social and academic skills. It is also important to realize that adolescent murderers will suffer a social lag when it is time for them to be discharged into society. Thus, every effort should be made to help them reintegrate into society and to learn new coping skills for dealing with anger, frustration, impulsivity, humiliation, and low self-esteem without resorting to violent behavior. Achieving this goal will require providing them with social support, opportunities, and continuous supervision.

Outcome Studies of Younger Murderers

We know of no long-term studies of homicidal preadolescents. Russels (1965), in his study of 15 adolescent murderers, indicated that 6 of these juveniles made good adjustments, 4 made borderline adjustments, and 5 were considered unchanged and as maintaining possible potential for murderous aggression.

Cormier and Markus (1980), in their study of 29 adolescent murderers, found that only one of these individuals committed a second murder in adulthood, and that was followed by suicide. They concluded that the recidivism rate for homicidal juveniles is low, and possibly lower than that of adults who commit homicidal acts.

Zenoff and Zients (1979) discriminated between the appropriate legal actions for different types of adolescent murderers and suggested that because "nonempathic" murderers—those who kill strangers either in the course of a robbery or for no apparent reason—have a poor prognosis and are at greater risk for further violence, the court system should treat them differently from adolescents who murder an acquaintance in the course of self-defense or an accident. New research to differentiate these two groups psychologically and developmentally would ensure a more equitable legal disposition in cases of fatal violence.

Prevention

The identification of risk factors is essential to prevention. The biopsychosocial constellation described by Lewis et al. (1985) identifies several such factors. Early detection and treatment of learning disabilities, ADHD, and emerging conduct problems may enhance prevention. Stark (1990) suggests that professional failure to respond appropriately to aggression is a major reason that assault becomes fatal, and that appropriate response to such behavior could prevent further fatal violence. Stark also theorized that half of all homicides could be prevented if an international strategy could be applied—one combining sanctions against interpersonal assault, gun control, and empowerment of survivors. The American Academy of Child and Adolescent Psychiatry has always emphasized the danger of having guns within reach of youngsters.

References

Adam BS, Kashani JH, Shulte JE: The classification of conduct disorders. Child Psychiatry Hum Dev 21:3–26, 1991

American Psychiatric Association: Diagnostic and Statistical Manual of Mental Disorders, 3rd Edition. Washington, DC, American Psychiatric Association, 1980

American Psychiatric Association: Diagnostic and Statistical Manual of Mental Disorders, 3rd Edition, Revised. Washington, DC, American Psychiatric Association, 1987

Beres D: Clinical notes on aggression in children. Psychoanal Study Child 7:241–263, 1952

Blos P: The contribution of psychoanalysis to the psychotherapy of adolescents. Adolesc Psychiatry 11:104–124, 1983

Busch KG, Zagar R, Hughes JR, et al: Adolescents who kill. J Clin Psychol 46:472–485, 1979

Cormier BM, Markus B: A longitudinal study of adolescent murderers. Bull Am Acad Psychiatry Law 8:240–260, 1980

Cornell DG, Benedek EP, Benedek DM: Juvenile homicide: prior adjustment and a proposed typology. Am J Orthopsychiatry 57:383–393, 1987

de Castro EF, Pimenta F, Martins I: Who kills whom in Portugal? Acta Psychiatr Scand 83:92–98, 1991

Erikson E: Childhood and Society, 2nd Edition. New York, WW Norton, 1963

Ewing C: Children who kill, in When Children Kill. Edited by Ewing C. Lexington, MA, DC Heath, 1990, pp 91–100

Federal Bureau of Investigation: Uniform Crime Report. Washington, DC, FBI, 1987

Holinger PC: Self-destructiveness among the young: an epidemiological study of violent deaths. Int J Soc Psychiatry 27:277–283, 1981

Holinger PC, Offer D, Ostrov E: Suicide and homicide in the United States: an epidemiologic study of violent death, population changes and the potential for prediction. Am J Psychiatry 144:215–219, 1987

Lewis DO, Lewis M, Unger L, et al: Conduct disorder and its synonyms: diagnoses of dubious validity and usefulness. Am J Psychiatry 141:514–519, 1984

Lewis DO, Moy E, Jackson LD, et al: Biopsychosocial characteristics of children who later murder: a prospective study. Am J Psychiatry 142:1161–1167, 1985

MacLeod R: A child is charged with homicide: his family responds. Br J Psychiatry 141:199–201, 1982

Malmquist CP: Depression in homicidal adolescents. Bull Am Acad Psychiatry Law 18:23–36, 1990

Marohn RC, Locke E, Rosenthal R, et al: Juvenile delinquents and violent death. Adolesc Psychiatry 10:147–170, 1982

Myers WC, Kemph JP: DSM-III-R classification of murderous youth: help or hindrance? J Clin Psychiatry 51:239–242, 1990

Petti TA, Davidman L: Homicidal school-age children: cognitive style and demographic features. Child Psychiatry Hum Dev 12:82–89, 1981

Pfeffer CR: Psychiatric hospital treatment of assaultive homicidal children. Am J Psychother 34:197–207, 1980

Ratner RA: A case of child abandonment: reflections on criminal responsibility in adolescents. Bull Am Acad Psychiatry Law 13:291–301, 1985

Robins LN: Deviant Children Grown Up: A Sociological and Psychiatric Study of Sociopathic Personality. Baltimore, MD, Williams & Wilkins, 1966

Russels DH: A study of juvenile murderers. Journal of Offenders Therapy 9(3):235–239, 1965

Rydelius PA: The development of antisocial behaviour and sudden violent death. Acta Psychiatr Scand 77:398–403, 1988

Stark E: Rethinking homicide: violence, race, and the politics of gender. Int J Health Serv 20:3–26, 1990

Stewart JT, Myers WC, Burket RC, et al: A review of the pharmacotherapy of aggression in children and adolescents. J Am Acad Child Adolesc Psychiatry 29:269–277, 1990

Tonken RS: Adolescent risk-taking behavior. Journal of Adolescent Health Care 8:213–220, 1987

Welner Z, Reich W, Herjanic B, et al: Reliability, validity, and parent-child agreement studies of the Diagnostic Interview for Children and Adolescents. J Am Acad Child Adolesc Psychiatry 26:649–653, 1987

Zagar R, Arbit J, Sylvies R, et al: Homicidal adolescents: a replication. Psychol Rep 67:1235–1242, 1979

Zenoff EH, Zients AB: Juvenile murders: should the punishment fit the crime? Int J Law Psychiatry 2:533–553, 1979

Chapter 7

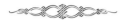

Sexual Abuse Perpetration

Jeffrey L. Metzner, M.D.
Gail D. Ryan, M.A.

R eports of child sexual abuse have increased dramatically during the past decade. There is a growing recognition that a significant proportion of perpetrators of child sexual abuse are adolescents (Krugman 1986). In the recent past, juvenile perpetrators were often not held accountable for their sexually exploitative behaviors, which were often minimized as being part of an adolescent adjustment reaction, or as representing experimental or situational events. Legal interventions were infrequent and consequences were minimal. Mental health intervention might have been recommended for juveniles when violence was associated with the sexual behavior. It has only been during the last 15 years that the criminal justice and human service systems have reviewed these practices and specialized intervention has evolved for juvenile sex offenders (National Task Force on Juvenile Sexual Offending 1988; Ryan et al. 1990).

Despite the growing recognition of issues related to adolescent sex offenders, the societal desire to take remedial action has far outpaced advances in knowledge (Davis and Leitenberg 1987). The psychiatric research literature on adolescent sex offenders is relatively sparse, although we do know that many of these adolescents have symptoms consistent with conduct disorder (CD) and histories of sexual victimization. This chapter provides an overview of the adolescent sex offender and summarizes relevant evaluation and treatment principles.

Definition of Sexual Abuse

The legal definition of sexual abuse is fairly straightforward but quite narrow in scope. *Sexual abuse of a child* is generally defined by statute as involving sexual assault against a minor and often specifies a minimum age difference between the victim and perpetrator, such as 4 or 5 years. *Sexual assault* is usually defined as knowingly inflicting sexual penetration, intrusion, or contact on a victim under conditions of physical force, threat, or other means of coercion. The severity of the felony charge is often increased if the perpetrator is a person in a position of trust with respect to the victim.

Kempe (1980) defined *sexual abuse* as the involvement of dependent, developmentally immature children and adolescents in sexual activities that they do not fully comprehend, to which they are unable to give informed consent, or that violate the social taboos of family roles. Reviewing various studies concerning the prevalence of sexual abuse is helpful in further understanding the clinical conceptualization of sexual abuse, which is less restricted than the legal definition (Salter 1988). For example, one study asked the subjects, "Before the age of 15, did you encounter any incident connected with sex, which shocked or greatly disgusted you at the time?" (Terman 1938). Another study defined sexual abuse as "sexual aggression" by an older boy, adult, or family member (Landis 1940). Researchers have generally required that sexual experiences be unwanted, forced, or coercive in order to be categorized as sexually abusive (Peters et al. 1986).

Three elements of operational definitions for child sexual abuse were described by Peters et al. (1986) in their review of sexual abuse prevalence studies. Most of these studies placed an upper limit on the victim's age at the time of the abuse that ranged from 15 to 17 years. The second characteristic was the type of sexual behavior included in each definition, which was divided into noncontact abuse (e.g., exhibitionism) and contact abuse (e.g., some type of "hands-on" sexual behavior). A third element was the criteria used to define a sexual encounter as abusive; such criteria generally focused on the differences in age between the perpetrator and victim, although several studies assessed the victim's perception of the sexual experience.

Sexual abuse of children by adults is usually easy to define based on the nature of the behaviors and age differences, although assessment is frequently difficult due to factual disputes. However, when sexual interactions involve youths under the age of 18 years, age and behavior are often inadequate in determining the presence or absence of sexual abuse, and further evaluation is needed. It is clear that an older adolescent having sexual activity with a small child constitutes sexual abuse, but health care professionals have had difficulty in distinguishing between "normal" sexual experimentation and sexually abusive behaviors among similarly aged children or adolescents, especially when the behaviors are characterized by minimal intrusiveness and/or aggressiveness. Evaluation under the latter circumstances requires a thorough assessment of issues related to consent and the dynamics of the relationship between the two youths (Ryan 1991a).

Informed consent in this context usually requires that a person be adequately informed and competent to make a decision about participating in the sexual activity, and that the decision be made in a voluntary fashion. Legally, various ages have arbitrarily been assigned as indicating presumed competence to make a decision about engaging in sexual relationships. The issue of voluntariness is often difficult to evaluate because of the wide variety of coercive techniques used by perpetrators in sexual abuse situations. Sexual activity occurring through mutual agreement and negotiation is very different from sexual behavior that is the result of deception, enticement, entrapment, intimidation, or physical force. Sexually abusive behavior is often characterized by a significant lack of equality in the relationship between the juveniles. Factors to be considered in assessing that equality include the physical, cognitive, and emotional development of each child.

The type of sexual activity involved and the circumstances of the sexual contact are important factors to consider when attempting to determine whether sexual abuse has occurred. Sexual acts that appear to reflect more advanced knowledge or experience than would be expected from the age of the involved persons may be a sign of sexual abuse. Sexual activity perceived as a way of hurting, embarrassing, degrading, punishing, or controlling someone should raise suspicion concerning probable abuse (Groth and Loredo 1981). Sexual interactions in which one individual disregards the needs and desires of the other individual are usually experienced as abusive. Bolton et al. (1989) have proposed an "abuse of sexuality" model that emphasizes psychosocial and sociocultural experiences that may also be experienced as sexual victimization even in the absence of overt sexual contact.

Scope of the Problem

The 1990 Uniform Crime Reports indicated that 15% of the arrests for forcible rape (excluded by definition are statutory rape without force and other sex offenses) were committed by youths younger than 18 years old (Federal Bureau of Investigation 1990). Youths under 15 years old accounted for 5% of the arrests for forcible rapes during 1990. Sixteen percent and 8% of all sex offenses, excluding forcible rape and prostitution, were committed by youths younger than age 18 and age 15 years, respectively. Abel et al. (1986), in reviewing the records of 20 paraphilic patients seen before the age of 18, found that these patients had averaged 7.7 attempted or completed sexual crimes per offender against an average of 6.7 victims.

The National Center on Child Abuse and Neglect indicated in 1987 that the reported cases of child sexual abuse had tripled since 1980, resulting in an incidence rate of 2.5 children per 1,000 per year (National Center on Child Abuse and Neglect 1987). Salter (1988) reviewed 13 recent prevalence studies of sexual abuse in nonclinical populations and found rates ranging from 7.7% to 38%. Peters et al. (1986) also reviewed and assessed the available research on the incidence and prevalence of child sexual abuse and concluded that no statistics yet exist that provide an accurate national estimate.

Studies of adult offenders reveal that a significant proportion of individuals with paraphilic disorders developed their deviant sexual arousal patterns before the age of 18 (Abel et al. 1986; Longo and Groth 1983; Marshal et al. 1991). Groth (1977) refuted earlier findings that tended to minimize the deviant sexual behavior of male adolescents as reflecting either experimentation or innocent sexual activity. Findings by Becker et al. (1986a), and a report by Becker et al. (1986b) that the mean onset of nondeviant genital sexual behavior preceded the onset of deviant sexual behavior in 22 adolescent males, support the assessment that deviant sexual behaviors are not the explorations of the inexperienced.

Showers et al. (1983) found that 50% of boy victims and at least 15% of girl victims evaluated at their hospital had been molested by teenagers. Deisher et al. (1982) reviewed the statistics from two large programs serving child victims of sexual assault. Forty-two percent of the more than 1,000 child victims had been assaulted by adolescents. Davis and Leitenberg (1987) summarized the various reasons that arrest statistics underestimate the extent of juvenile sexual offending; these reasons include failure to report sexual offenses to the police and exclusion of adolescent sexual offenses in various arrest statistics because victims under the age of 12 are often excluded.

The number of sexual offenses committed by an offender dramatically increases as adulthood is reached. In a study of 240 adult offenders, all of whom had developed their deviant sexual arousal patterns before the age of 18, it was reported that each offender averaged 581 attempted or completed deviant sexual acts. The average of 380 victims per offender for these adult sexual offenders was more than 56 times the number of victims per offender for adolescent sex offenders (Abel et al. 1986). Longo and Groth (1983) found evidence that at least one of every three convicted adult rapists or child molesters showed progression from nonviolent sex crimes during adolescence to more serious sexual assaults as adults. Weinrott and Saylor (1991) report that adult sex offenders also have a high frequency of participation in minor nonsexual offenses (e.g., public intoxication, petty theft).

Characteristics of the Adolescent Sex Offender

Ryan et al. summarized information obtained from the National Adolescent Perpetrator Network Uniform Data Collection System, which contains data for more than 1,600 juveniles referred for evaluation and/or treatment to 90 sex offender–specific programs in 30 states (G. Ryan, T. Miyoshi, J. Metzner, R. Krugman, G. Fryer, "Trends in a National Sample of Juvenile Sexual Abusers," January 1991 [submitted for publication]). Ninety percent of these subjects were between the ages of 10 and 18 years. Males represented 97% of the sample, and race, income, and religion were reflective of the general population. Most were living in a parent's home (85%), although only 28% were living with both natural parents, which is consistent with the findings of other studies (Becker et al. 1986a; Fehrenbach et al. 1986). Parental loss was a common experience for this population because of out-of-home placements (34%), death of one or both parents (12%), and other permanent disruptions in the parent-child relationship.

A large number of these youths were known to have truancy, learning disabilities, and/or behavioral problems at school. Only 28% reported no problems at school. These results are similar to those of other studies (Davis and Leitenberg 1987; Fehrenbach et al. 1986; Kahn and Chambers 1991).

Forty-two percent of the subjects had a history of physical abuse, 39% were known to have been sexually abused, and 26% had documented neglect. More than 22% of the perpetrators who had been sexually abused reported that the abuse was done by a female, and only 10% were abused by strangers. Twenty-five percent of the sexually abused subjects indicated that their perpetrator was less than 5 years older. Fewer than 17% of the physical abuse cases and only 37% of the sexual abuse complaints led to legal action (i.e., adjudication). Forty percent reported having had an "age appropriate" sexual relationship at some time. Over 60% of the youths had witnessed some form of family violence in the home, 28% had some history suggesting substance abuse, and 46% had previously been referred for some type of psychotherapy.

Sixty-three percent of the youths had a known nonsexual offense on record at the time of referral, and 28% had a history of more than three nonsexual offenses, which included the full range of delinquent behaviors. These results are consistent with those of other smaller studies of adolescent sex offenders, which have demonstrated a history of nonsexual offenses in their sample populations ranging from 44% to 63% (Becker et al. 1986b; Fehrenbach et al. 1986; Shoor et al. 1966). Abel et al. (1986) reported that approximately 29% of adult sex offenders have antisocial personality disorders. It is certainly possible that the juveniles with multiple nonsexual offenses are at high risk for becoming the adults with antisocial personality disorders who also commit sex offenses.

There were indications that a significant percentage (approximately 25%) of those referred after age 12 had engaged in some sexually abusive behaviors prior to age 12. However, only 7.5% of the sample had previously been charged with a sexual offense. Eighty-three percent of the alleged perpetrators were charged in juvenile court, with 47% being found guilty as charged. The subjects frequently accepted little or no responsibility for their sexual offense, and most expressed little or no empathy for the victim. One-third of the subjects blamed the victims for the sexual abuse.

Ninety-one percent of the sexual abuse victims were between 3 and 16 years of age. Twice as many of the referring offenses involved female victims compared with male victims. The average number of known victims per offender at the time of intake was 7.7, with 39% being blood relatives of the young offender and from the same household. Sexual abuse of a peer accounted for 10% of the offenses, and sexual victimization of strangers, only 6%; only 4.5% of the sexual abuse victims were adults. These findings are consistent with those reported by Becker et al. (1986a) and Fehrenbach et al. (1986). Almost 70% of the referring offenses involved anal or vaginal penetration and/or oral-genital contact.

Kavoussi et al. (1988) determined the psychiatric characteristics of 58 outpatient, mainly inner-city, male adolescent sex offenders by using structured interview instruments and information obtained from the subjects' families and referral sources. Forty-eight percent of this population met diagnostic criteria for CD, with the majority of those being classified as socialized nonaggressive. Thirty-five percent of the adolescents had some evidence for the presence of an attention-deficit disorder. A larger percentage of adolescents who had raped or attempted to rape adult women (75%) met criteria for CD than of adolescents who had committed other sexual offenses (38%).

Awad and Saunders (1989) reported in their study of 29 adolescent sex offenders that one-third had been diagnosed as suffering from emotional problems prior to committing a sexual offense, 87% were found to meet criteria for a DSM-III (American Psychiatric Association 1980) diagnosis, and one-third had received outpatient psychiatric treatment prior to their referral to the court clinic. In their sample, there was an overlap between serious psychopathology and both antisocial and sexually deviant behavior.

Becker et al. (1991) assessed depressive symptomatology in a sample of 246 outpatient male juvenile sex offenders with the Beck Depression Inventory (Beck 1978). Forty-two percent of their sample attained scores consistent with appreciable depressive symptomatology. The severity of the depressive symptoms correlated with a history of sexual or physical abuse. Other studies described substance use in adolescent sex offenders at the time of perpetration as ranging from 6% to 11% (Fehrenbach et al. 1986; Groth 1977; Wasserman and Kappel 1985). Becker et al. (1986a) reported that 97% of their 67 adolescent male sexual offender subjects had never been hospitalized for a psychiatric illness.

Most of the literature on juvenile sex offenders has focused on the adolescent male offender. Studies indicate that from 2% to 5% of identified adolescent sexual offenders are female (Brown et al. 1984; Davis and Leitenberg 1987; Fehrenbach et al. 1986; Wasserman and Kappel 1985). Finkelhor and Russell (1984) reported that women constitute about 5% of the perpetrators in known cases of sexual abuse of girls and about 20% in cases of abuse of boys. Arrest statistics summarized in the 1990 Uniform Crime Reports indicated that 0.2% of the total arrests for forcible rape and slightly over 1% of the total arrests for sex offenses (excluding forcible rape and prostitution) were for cases committed by females less than 18 years old (Federal Bureau of Investigation 1990). Female offending is likely to be underreported because of the dissonance of such behavior with society's expected role of females. Further research is needed to adequately understand issues related to adolescent female offenders; however, clinical impressions suggest more similarities than differences between male and female offenders (Lane 1991).

There is little information concerning mentally retarded adolescent sex offenders, although preliminary data indicate that such offenders tend to have fewer victims and to victimize males more often as compared with non-retarded adolescent offenders (Gilby et al. 1989; Griffiths et al. 1985). Swanson and Garwick (1990) provide a concise historical review concerning the mentally retarded sex offender and describe a treatment program for this population. Treatment modifications for such individuals place an emphasis on concrete, practical, and action-oriented components (Gilby et al. 1989).

Evaluation

The assessment of adolescent sex offenders is a time-consuming process because of both clinical and legal issues. There are currently no validated instruments for classifying adolescent sex offenders, although a variety of useful guidelines for evaluation and treatment have been published (Groth and Loredo 1981; Otey and Ryan 1985; Wenet and Clark 1984). The National Task Force on Juvenile Sexual Offending (1988) has summarized guidelines for the following types of evaluations:

1. Pretrial (investigative)
2. Presentencing (dangerousness/risk; placement/prognosis; treatment issues/modes)
3. Treatment needs (planning and progress in treatment)
4. Release/termination from treatment (community safety and successful application of treatment tools)
5. Monitoring and follow-up

The nature of the assessment depends on the referral questions to be answered. In this section we focus on issues related to pretrial and presentence evaluations.

The assessment during the pretrial phase is frequently a good opportunity to obtain an accurate, relevant history from the alleged offender and his or her family. Referrals for evaluation during this period are generally precipitated by the initial involvement with social services and/or the police. Because this experience often constitutes a crisis situation for the adolescent and his or her family, they are likely to be more open during the evaluation if they perceive that openness and cooperation with treatment providers may help the adolescent avoid incarceration. However, the adolescent and/or the family often deny or minimize the adolescent's participation in inappropriate sexual behaviors for a variety of reasons, including attempts to avoid the consequences for those behaviors. Assessments obtained under such circumstances may not be particularly helpful because of the unreliability of the history obtained from the offender and/or the family (Ryan et al. 1990).

More factual information should be available from the criminal justice system concerning the sexual offense when the evaluation is being performed for presentencing purposes. A guilty verdict may decrease the adolescent's denial and result in his or her providing more useful information. Presentence evaluations should supply the court with information concerning the adolescent's diagnosis, prognosis, potential dangerousness, and treatment recommendations, including issues related to treatment setting. The treatment setting should be the least restrictive environment that allows for community safety. Out-of-home placement is initially required, except in unusual circumstances, when the victim is living in the perpetrator's home.

The risks these youths pose both for peers and for younger vulnerable children often cause dilemmas in making placement recommendations. These risks should be addressed to minimize the possibility of further victimization and liability (Freeman-Longo and Ryan 1990). Comprehensive assessments are the first step in risk management. Table 7–1 lists the factors to be considered in such assessments.

An assessment for either pretrial or presentencing purposes requires multiple interviews with the adolescent offender and should also include interviews with parents. It is essential that the limits of confidentiality be thoroughly explained to the adolescent and his or her family at the beginning of these evaluations. Relevant documents must be obtained and reviewed, including reports from the police, social services, courts, and other involved agencies, as well as past medical/mental health records and school reports. Discrepancies between the offender's self-report and information from other sources need to be explored.

The setting for these evaluations will generally depend on community safety requirements, the adolescent's clinical state, and his or her legal status. Although inpatient evaluation is occasionally desirable to allow a comprehensive evaluation to be completed within a relatively brief period, such evaluations, which are fairly time-consuming and complex, are generally best performed over longer time frames for a variety of reasons, including the time required to gather information from other agencies and to establish a working relationship with the adolescent and his or her family. Evaluations conducted in a residential treatment setting offer many of the advantages of an inpatient psychiatric unit without the associated costs.

Table 7–1. Factors to be considered in risk assessment of adolescent sex offenders

1. Victim's statements (as obtained from police and social services reports, mental health professionals, and similar sources)
2. Background information (including family, educational, medical, psychosocial, and developmental histories)
3. Categories of deviant sexual interests
4. Progression of sexually aggressive behavior over time
5. Reported use of sexually deviant fantasies
6. Intensity of sexual arousal during the time surrounding each offense
7. Dynamics/process of victim selection
8. Use of coercion, force, violence, or weapons
9. Behavioral warning signs
10. Identifiable triggers leading to inappropriate sexual behaviors
11. Thinking errors (e.g., cognitive distortions, irrational thinking)
12. Spectrum of injury to victim (i.e., violation of trust, fear, physical injury)
13. Sadistic elements
14. Ritualistic characteristics
15. Deviant nonsexual interests
16. History of assaultive behaviors
17. Issues related to separation/loss
18. Antisocial characteristics
19. Psychiatric diagnosis (e.g., disruptive behavior disorders, affective disorders, developmental disorders, personality disorders, posttraumatic stress disorder, substance abuse disorder, organic mental disorder)
20. Ability to accept responsibility
21. Degree of denial or minimization
22. Understanding of wrongfulness of actions
23. Concern for injury to victim
24. Quality of social, assertive, and empathic skills
25. Family's response (e.g., denial, minimization, support, ability to intervene appropriately)
26. Exposure to pornography
27. History of victimization (sexual, physical, or emotional)
28. Reported ability to control deviant sexual interests
29. Knowledge and expression of appropriate sexual desire
30. Mental status examination

Source. Adapted from National Task Force on Juvenile Sexual Offending 1988; Groth and Loredo 1981; Ryan et al. 1990; Stevenson and Wimberley 1990.

Evaluation of sexual interests with the use of plethysmography may be useful in the assessment and treatment of adolescent sex offenders, although controversy exists about this issue (Travin et al. 1988). Other areas of disagreement involve the process of obtaining informed consent for such testing; concerns about exposing adolescents to deviant sexual stimuli; and uncertainty as to the reliability, validity, and predictive power of phallometric testing (Murphy et al. 1984; National Task Force on Juvenile Sexual Offending 1988; Saunders and Awad 1988). Initial plethysmographic assessments can, however, provide a baseline of the adolescent's sexual arousal patterns, which can aid both the clinician and the adolescent in understanding the role of sexual interest in the offending behaviors as well as provide a measure of change over the course of treatment. Such testing is often not obtained due to the cost involved or to the unavailability of appropriate laboratories. The Association for Treatment of Sexual Abusers (1993) has issued a policy statement regarding the use of plethysmography with juveniles; this statement discourages the use of visual stimuli and limits usage with youth under the age of 14.

A wide range of psychological tests can be helpful in assessing the needs of specific offenders. However, it is generally agreed that adolescent sexual offending behavior does not constitute a single homogeneous class of behavior (Smith et al. 1987). Rorschach testing reveals more similarities than differences between adolescent sex offenders and adolescents who commit nonsexual crimes (McGraw and Pegg-McNab 1989). Tarter et al. (1983) found no systematic group differences among 73 juvenile violent, nonviolent, and sexual offenders measured across a broad range of intellectual, neuropsychological, and psychoeducational parameters. However, psychological tests that measure personality characteristics (Minnesota Multiphasic Personality Inventory [Hathaway and McKinley 1970], Thematic Apperception Test [Murray 1943]), social skills (Matson Evaluation of Social Skills in Youngsters [Matson et al. 1983]), intellectual functioning (Wechsler Intelligence Scale for Children—Revised [Wechsler 1974]), and sexual arousal (Abel and Becker Sexual Interest Cardsort [Abel and Becker 1985]) can provide useful information about an individual offender.

The family's involvement in the evaluation process is crucial. Developmental history concerning the adolescent and each parent should be obtained during interviews with the parents. Family attitudes about sexual issues, each parent's perception of the adolescent's deviant sexual behaviors, and attitudes about the need for treatment are important factors to assess in this evaluation. Other family issues to assess include the degree to which the parents can control the adolescent's access to victims or potential victims, how family decisions are made, the roles of each family member, and rules within the family. It is common to find a history of sexual abuse within the adolescent's family as well as problems in decision making, expression of emotions, family secrets, role reversals, boundary problems, and various intrafamilial alliances

(Otey and Ryan 1985; Ryan et al. 1990; Thomas 1991).

These evaluations frequently structure the goals and plans for the initial phase of treatment. Ongoing evaluation during the treatment process is required to reformulate the treatment plan as more is learned about the adolescent. The range of the adolescent's deviant sexual behavior and levels of violent ideation are often not fully disclosed until much later in the treatment process.

Etiological Theories

There are numerous theories that attempt to explain the development of deviant sexual behaviors in adolescents. Many of these theories were developed to explain deviant sexual behavior by adults and later adapted for adolescent offenders. Psychodynamically oriented clinicians conceptualize paraphilias as being symptomatic of intrapsychic conflict, arrested development, mastery of trauma through repetition, or identification with the aggressor (Fuller 1989). Behaviorists emphasize the importance of operant conditioning in the development of deviant sexual behaviors (Knopp 1984). Modeling has also been hypothesized to explain aspects of deviant sexual development. Sociological theory hypothesizes the importance of cultural factors, male socialization to dominance, impact of exposure to pornography, and the role of social values (Finkelhor 1984). Other theories focus on a sexual assault cycle (Lane and Zamora 1984), biological factors (Berlin and Meinecke 1981), an addictions model (Carnes 1983, 1990), an obsessive-compulsive model (Coleman 1990), and cognitive distortions (Abel et al. 1986; Yochelson and Samenow 1976).

Araji and Finkelhor (1985) reviewed the empirical research concerning explanations of pedophilia and organized the multiple theories into a four-factor model: 1) emotional congruence—attempts to explain the reasons the adult pedophile has an emotional need to relate to a child; 2) sexual arousal—attempts to understand why an adult could become sexually aroused by a child; 3) blockage—attempts to provide reasons that alternative sources of sexual and emotional gratification are not available; or 4) disinhibition—attempts to explain why an adult is not deterred from such an interest by normal prohibitions. This model can be modified to apply to the adolescent sex offender.

Unfortunately, because of significant methodological problems in outcome research, it is very difficult to formulate unambiguous conclusions about factors leading to paraphilias (Araji and Finkelhor 1985). Kilmann et al. (1982) concluded, after a thorough review of the literature concerning outcome studies, that a single, comprehensive theory to explain the development of paraphilic behavior had not yet emerged.

Treatment Issues

Treatment of sex offenders continues to evolve and is characterized by a multidisciplinary and multimodal approach. Treatment methods include psychodynamic, behavioral, cognitive, educational, and biological approaches. The goals of the treatment process are 1) to clearly define sexual abuse (i.e., lack of consent, inequality, use of coercion); 2) to aid the offender in understanding the process that leads to his or her offending behaviors; 3) to provide tools for the offender to intervene in this process; 4) to motivate the offender to use these tools; and 5) to increase empathic foresight. Achieving these goals will help the offender gain control over his or her deviant sexual behavior and will increase the protection for persons in the community from further victimization.

There is broad consensus that treatment for adolescent sex offenders should use a specialized offense-specific group treatment approach (National Task Force on Juvenile Sexual Offending 1988). Denial is more effectively confronted by peers with similar patterns of sexually aggressive behavior. Co-therapists, preferably male and female, are recommended when treating this population to decrease the stress and frustration of dealing with the different transference issues elicited by the therapist's gender. The duration of treatment generally ranges from 12 to 36 months. Table 7–2 lists the primary issues to be addressed in the treatment of adolescent offenders.

Lane and Zamora (1984) identified five distinct phases of treatment for adolescents placed in a treatment unit for violent juvenile offenders: 1) penetrating the denial concerning the sexually abusive behaviors, 2) identifying the adolescent's sexual abuse cycle, 3) helping the adolescent deal with unresolved emotional issues, 4) providing retraining in the areas of skill deficits, and 5) facilitating the adolescent's reentry into the community.

Becker et al. (1988) have described a community based treatment program consisting of the following components: 1) verbal satiation designed to decrease the arousal to deviant sexual fantasies, 2) cognitive restructuring designed to confront rationalizations that justify participation in deviant sexual behavior, 3) covert sensitization designed to disrupt the progression antecedent to the offender's actually coming into contact with his victim, 4) social skills training, 5) anger control training, 6) sex education and values clarification, and 7) relapse prevention.

Effective treatment intervention requires intersystem cooperation and, generally, the support of the legal system. Many clinicians believe that a mandatory treatment model is the most effective way to intervene with this population because of the offender's reluctance to change and the need for external controls from the juvenile court, parents, or protective services system. Involvement with the court system reinforces the principle that the adolescent is accountable for his or her offending behaviors. Mandated treatment can result from diversion programs, conditions of probation, or treatment plans related to dependency and neglect proceedings. Court-ordered treatment provisions should be enforceable for at least 2 years because of the length of time required for adequate treatment and the frequent occurrence of premature termination when treatment is not mandated by the court. Self-motivation for treatment need not be a prerequisite for entrance into a treatment program, but may eventually be a requirement for continuation in treatment.

It is not unusual for offenders to initially appear remorseful and motivated to participate in treatment during the initial crisis following discovery of the abuse. This early motivation for treatment is usually related to minimizing the consequences for the offender and has little to do with empathy for the victim. The motivation for treatment significantly decreases over time as the offender begins to be confronted with a variety of painful treatment issues, including understanding more fully the victim's pain and often dealing with his own victimization issues. It is during these times that premature treatment terminations often occur when the treatment is not court ordered.

The concept of a sexual assault cycle, as described by Lane (1991), has been found helpful for juvenile offenders in dealing with many of the treatment issues. Situational, affective, cognitive, and behavioral factors are all considered in order to understand the individual's pattern of offending behaviors and to help establish appropriate interventions. This cycle is trig-

---

Table 7–2. Issues to be addressed in the treatment of adolescent offenders

1. Acceptance of responsibility for behavior
2. Identification of pattern or cycle of offense behavior
3. Effective interventions to interrupt the sexual abuse cycle
4. Victimization (e.g., sexual abuse) and issues for the offender
5. Capacity for empathy with others, especially past victims
6. Interpersonal power and control issues
7. Role of sexual arousal in offenses
8. Sexual identity
9. Consequences of offending
10. Family issues that support offending behaviors
11. Cognitive distortions related to offending behaviors
12. Expression of feelings
13. Skill deficits (social and academic)
14. Substance use/abuse
15. Relapse prevention
16. Management of concurrent psychiatric disorders

Source. Adapted from National Task Force on Juvenile Sexual Offending 1988.

gered by some current situation that is perceived by the adolescent in a manner that contributes to his feeling diminished in some way. This feeling in turn contributes to the adolescent's expecting something bad to occur, which often results in his feeling threatened emotionally and/or physically. It is common for the offender to become reclusive during such times in an attempt to avoid the anticipated negative occurrence. During this isolation, anger builds and the offender attempts to compensate for the perceived threat by attempting to control others. Fantasies may be retaliatory (How can I get back at others—make others feel as bad as I do?) or compensatory (How can I feel better?) and often become the basis for the decision to engage in sexual behavior. When the motivation is retaliatory, the behaviors may be deliberately abusive, accompanied by a conscious desire to inflict pain, whereas the compensatory motive may simply disregard the victim's needs and fail to anticipate the abusive impact of the behavior (Ryan et al. 1987).

Most of the literature concerning the pharmacological treatment of adult sex offenders has focused on the use of antiandrogenic medications (medroxyprogesterone acetate [MPA], cyproterone acetate [CPA]); there have also been some recent reports concerning the use of fluoxetine (Berlin 1989; Berlin and Meinecke 1981; Bradford 1983, 1985; Kiersch 1990; Melella et al. 1989; Perilstein et al. 1991). There is general agreement that MPA and CPA decrease sexual drive, although they do not change the object of the sexual drive. They may, however, aid some offenders in developing a less sexualized lifestyle.

Unfortunately, little has been written about the use of antiandrogenic medication in the treatment of adolescent sex offenders. Knopp and Lane (1991) describe a survey of identified sex offender treatment programs in the United States during 1988. A total of 574 responses were received, 323 of these from programs treating juvenile sex offenders. Twenty-three (7%) of these juvenile sex offender programs reported that MPA was used as a treatment tool within their program when indicated. MPA and CPA are generally used only with older adolescent sex offenders who have participated in violent crimes, who experience significant deviant sexual obsessions, and who request medications to help them manage deviant sexual arousal. Studies have demonstrated that CPA can prevent the onset of puberty in prepubertal rats as well as affect the epiphyseal closure (Bradford 1985), which raises concern about use of these medications with younger adolescent offenders.

Other pharmacological considerations include appropriate management of coexisting disorders such as attention-deficit hyperactivity disorder (ADHD), anxiety disorders, and affective disorders. For a significant minority of offending youths, failure to successfully participate in required treatment may result from unmanageable mood swings, affective flooding, and/or ADHD. Proper diagnosis and treatment of these conditions may greatly improve the prognosis.

Rules of confidentiality are significantly different for adolescent sex offenders than for most other mental health patients. Most specialized treatment providers include a waiver of confidentiality in the treatment contract so that they can communicate with staff from the courts, the department of social services, the probation department, the school, the residential care facility, the victim's therapist, parents, and others involved in the care and supervision of these offenders. The adolescent and parents (or legal guardians) should obviously be informed of this provision prior to treatment. They are generally reassured when learning from other patients and families that the therapist's discretion concerning what information to reveal has not been abused or harmful to the patient. Adolescent perpetrators have used secrecy and manipulation to commit offenses. The therapeutic value of taking these strategies away from the offender is necessary to provide needed external controls as well as to eliminate the secrecy surrounding abuse issues and encourage honest communication (Metzner 1987; Ross 1986).

Family involvement is generally essential to the treatment process. The offender's use of denial and rationalization is often reflective of a family coping pattern (Stevenson et al. 1990; Thomas 1991). Family treatment needs to address dynamics that support or contribute to the adolescent's offending patterns. Treatment includes helping the family protect the offender and victims from circumstances that are potentially compromising, both psychologically and physically. The family should be able to identify the adolescent offender's sexual assault cycle in the same way that families of children with chronic illness must be aware of signs leading up to a potential crisis (Stevenson and Wimberley 1990). It may be contraindicated to return the juvenile to the home setting if the family treatment is unable to successfully identify and resolve these issues.

Videotaping treatment groups can be a very effective tool in this work. Videotapes capture the dynamics of group interactions and can be used to review sessions with consultants and/or supervisors as well as be shown to group members to clarify and confront distortions and patterns of denial.

Case Example

The following case summary illustrates the treatment of an adolescent offender in a sex offender–specific setting that uses the sexual assault cycle conceptualization.

Joe, a 14-year-old, was referred for treatment following the discovery that he had sodomized his 6-year-old male cousin and engaged in sexual intercourse and oral/genital contact with his 10-year-old sister. Victim statements reflected physical force in the abuse of his cousin, whereas the abuse of his sister appeared more seductive and verbally coercive. Joe did not deny that the behavior had occurred, but attributed both assaults to sexual confusion, stating that he was trying to determine whether he was homosexual or heterosexual.

Joe's history revealed lifelong abuse and neglect by his alcoholic mother and stepfather that included being thrown through a window, waiting by the window all night to see if his mother would return, and fleeing the house to escape parental and spousal violence. The whole family described him as the primary caregiver and protector of his sister, and he was clearly his mother's favorite child. He had been violently sodomized by a 15-year-old cousin at the age of 7, which he had disclosed to his mother at the time. As a result, the cousin had been banned from the home—only to return later to live with them again.

Joe was treated in a residential treatment facility that included offense-specific group treatment twice weekly, other general group counseling, and family therapy. His father had effectively abandoned the family during the process of the sibling incest disclosure and had remained estranged. Joe's mother stopped drinking and was able to comply with Antabuse maintenance. His previously compliant sister began acting out at home and school, exhibiting chronic self-mutilating behaviors, and went through numerous failed treatment attempts. Enmeshment and symbiosis were immediately apparent in the mother-son relationship. Court orders for treatment included no contact between the siblings during the early phases of treatment.

Initially, Joe showed poor impulse control and would become cognitively irrational and disorganized when angered, shutting down completely and being unable to communicate. Low dosages of antipsychotic medications were used on an as-needed basis for several months to help manage these periods of disorganization and overwhelming affect. Working on the mother-son relationship was slow and painful because of the pervasive lack of trust and the family's belief that the expression of anger was unsafe. Joe was initially extremely reluctant and unwilling to explore issues related to the sexual abuse of his sister, although he was open about his sexual confusion and reported discomfort regarding recurrent abusive homosexual thoughts.

The reenactment of his own sexual abuse in the sexual assault on his younger male cousin was more accessible in treatment. He was reassured by understanding that his fantasies were not uncontrollable and that he could choose to dwell on and reinforce those thoughts that were congruent with consensual heterosexual interactions. As his own homophobia diminished, he became more able to interact with male peers without sexualizing those relationships.

For Joe, the triggers that set the dysfunctional cycle in motion were clearly related to the pervasive sense of helplessness he had experienced in a violent and neglectful home. His self-centeredness and lack of empathy were protective mechanisms—his major defense against the posttraumatic flooding he experienced in response to perceived threats. Anger and abusive behavior were congruent with his view of the world. He felt like a victim and would leap to conclusions, expecting the worst and attributing malicious intent to the actions of others. Appearances of remorse or guilt were always associated with negative consequences for him, and he had no interest or tolerance for the needs of others. His disorganized thought processes were symptomatic of his frantic attempts to explain his anxiety in order to feel safe.

Living in a safe, predictable environment and exploring new ways to interact without abuse, he became able to redefine and manage his affect. Empathy was slow in developing, but by the end of his second year in treatment, he was able to express his rage regarding his inadequate parenting and began to disclose much more about his own abusive behaviors against other persons. His resentment regarding the family's expectation that he care for his sister surfaced, along with reports of his chronic physical and emotional abuse of her. He reported violence that included attempts to strangle her as well as voyeuristic behavior prior to the sexual molestation.

The reintegration of Joe back into his home was a slow, cautious process. Constant monitoring for regression into earlier dysfunctional patterns will be a long-term need.

Assessing Treatment Progress

Treatment of sex offenders generally focuses on management and control of the inappropriate sexual behaviors rather than cure. Stevenson and Wimberley (1990) developed a pilot questionnaire designed to help identify variables that assess responses to various types of treatment for adolescent sex offenders. This questionnaire provides a structure for collection of data emphasizing the adolescent's pattern of sexually offensive behavior, the degree of responsibility and denial demonstrated by the adolescent concerning such behaviors, the sexual knowledge and the level of social skills demonstrated by the adolescent, and the family's involvement in treatment. Table 7–3 lists some indicators of treatment progress.

Offender self-reports are important in treatment progress assessments but must be corroborated by information obtained from family, teachers, treatment staff, probation officers, and other relevant persons. Completion of treatment requires consistent demonstration of changes in managing behavior and consideration of the needs of others. Patients must be held accountable for treatment outcomes by demonstrating their ability to apply the knowledge they have gained to their daily activities.

Future Directions

Despite the rapid expansion of treatment programs offering specialized interventions for juvenile sex offenders, there continues to be great disparity in the handling of individual cases as well as in systemic responses in various jurisdictions. As the body of clinical knowledge and experience grows, research must continue to validate and correct the hypotheses guiding current interventions.

A valid taxonomic system for juvenile sexual offenders is needed because of the complexity of the etiological factors involved and the heterogeneous nature of the population that manifests sexually abusive behavior (Knight and Prentky 1993). Research in progress has already begun to confirm some of the developmental factors (Gilgun 1988; Prentky et al. 1989) as well as to define the role of various aspects of the offending syndrome (Becker et al. 1989). The effect of various systemic and behavioral treatment modalities and techniques is also being measured (Borduin et al. 1990; Hunter and Santos 1990).

As is frequently the case, psychodynamic interventions and the role of new life experiences and relationships will be harder to measure. Developmental competence in seemingly irrelevant aspects of the maturation process may affect the course of development of paraphilic disorders, and typological discrimination of offender types may depend on an improved ability to discern the nature of various offense patterns (National Task Force on Juvenile Sexual Offending 1988). Longitudinal follow-up will be needed to assess the impact of intervention.

Similarly, sparse data exist about children younger than 13 years of age who exhibit sexually abusive behaviors. However, it is clear that such children

---

Table 7–3.   Indicators of treatment progress

1. Acknowledgment of responsibility for offense without denial, minimization, or projection of blame
2. Observable efforts designed to achieve treatment goals (e.g., completion of homework assignments, active verbal participation in group sessions)
3. Ability to identify contributing factors of the offending cycles
4. Making effective interventions concerning contributing factors to sexually assaultive behavior
5. Exhibiting empathy for others (including the victim)
6. Increased self-esteem
7. Healthier interactions with family and significant persons
8. Openness in examining thoughts, fantasies, and behavior
9. Recognition of cognitive distortions and institution of effective interventions
10. Identification and avoidance of high-risk situations
11. Improved communication and assertiveness skills
12. Resolution of loss and personal victimization issues
13. Ability to experience pleasure in normal activities

Source. Adapted from National Task Force on Juvenile Sexual Offending 1988.

exist, and more research needs to be conducted to develop the most appropriate treatment modalities for this special population (Cavanaugh-Johnson 1988).

At the same time, prevention efforts are under way. Curricula have been developed for direct education with adolescents regarding sexually abusive attitudes and coercive interpersonal relationships (Strong et al. 1986). Specialized interventions targeting early behavioral manifestations in childhood and "at risk" groups of children are also being explored (Ryan 1991b).

Conclusion

The evaluation and treatment of juvenile sex offenders is a difficult, long-term process that requires offense-specific interventions. Successful treatment generally calls for family intervention, court-mandated treatment for the adolescent, interagency cooperation, and a multimodal approach in a group therapy setting. The amount of scientifically based information accumulated about this population remains quite limited. Efforts must continue to focus on developing more effective early interventions with juvenile sex offenders to minimize the likelihood of their continued offending in adulthood.

References

Abel G, Becker J: Abel and Becker Sexual Interest Cardsort. Atlanta, GA, Behavioral Medicine Institute of Atlanta, 1985

Abel G, Rouleau J, Cunningham-Rathner J: Sexually aggressive behavior, in Psychiatry and Psychology: Perspectives and Standards for Interdisciplinary Practice. Edited by Curran W, McGarry A, Shah S. Philadelphia, PA, FA Davis, 1986, pp 289–314

Abidin RR: Parenting Stress Index Manual. Charlottesville, VA, Pediatric Psychology Press, 1983

Achenbach TM, Edelbrock CS: Manual for the Child Behavior Checklist and Revised Child Behavior Profile. Burlington, University of Vermont, Department of Psychiatry, 1983

American Psychiatric Association: Diagnostic and Statistical Manual of Mental Disorders, 3rd Edition. Washington, DC, American Psychiatric Association, 1980

Araji S, Finkelhor D: Explanations of pedophilia: review of empirical research. Bull Am Acad Psychiatry Law 13:17–37, 1985

Association for Treatment of Sexual Abusers: Policy statement on the use of plethysmography with juveniles. Portland, OR, ATSA, 1993

Awad GA, Saunders EG: Adolescent child molesters: clinical observations. Child Psychiatry Hum Dev 19:195–206, 1989

Beck AT: Depression Inventory. Philadelphia, PA, Philadelphia Center for Cognitive Therapy, 1978

Becker JV, Cunningham-Rathner J, Kaplan MS: Adolescent sexual offenders: demographics, criminal and sexual histories, and recommendations for reducing future offenses. Journal of Interpersonal Violence 1:431–445, 1986a

Becker JV, Kaplan MS, Cunningham-Rathner J, et al: Characteristics of adolescent incest sexual perpetrators: preliminary findings. Journal of Family Violence 1:85–97, 1986b

Becker JV, Kaplan MS, Kavoussi R: Measuring the effectiveness of treatment for the aggressive adolescent sexual offender. Ann N Y Acad Sci 528:215–222, 1988

Becker JV, Hunter J, Stein R, et al: Factors associated with erection in adolescent sex offenders. Journal of Psychopathology and Behavioral Assessment 2:353–362, 1989

Becker JV, Kaplan MS, Tenke CE, et al: The incidence of depressive symptomatology in juvenile sex offenders with a history of abuse. Child Abuse Negl 15:531–536, 1991

Berlin FS: The paraphilias and depo-provera: some medical, ethical, and legal considerations. Bull Am Acad Psychiatry Law 17:233–238, 1989

Berlin FS, Meinecke CF: Treatment of sex offenders with antiandrogenic medication: conceptualization, review of treatment modalities, and preliminary findings. Am J Psychiatry 138:601–607, 1981

Bolton FG, Morris LA, MacEachron AE: Males at Risk: The Other Side of Sexual Abuse. Newbury Park, CA, Sage, 1989

Borduin CM, Blaske DM, Henggeler SW, et al: Multisystemic treatment of adolescent sexual offenders. International Journal of Offender Therapy and Comparative Criminology 35:105–114, 1990

Bradford JMW: The hormonal treatment of sexual offenders. Bull Am Acad Psychiatry Law 11:159–169, 1983

Bradford JMW: Organic treatments for the male sexual offender. Behavioral Sciences and the Law 3:355–375, 1985

Brown EJ, Flanagan TJ, McLeod M (eds): Sourcebook of Criminal Justice Statistics—1983. Washington, DC, Bureau of Justice Statistics, 1984

Carnes PJ: Out of the Shadows: Understanding Sexual Addiction. Minneapolis, MN, CompCare, 1983

Carnes PJ: Sexual addiction: progress, criticism, challenges. American Journal of Preventive Psychiatry and Neurology 2:1–8, 1990

Cavanaugh-Johnson T: Child perpetrators—children who molest other children: preliminary findings. Child Abuse Negl 12:219–229, 1988

Coleman E: The obsessive-compulsive model for describing compulsive sexual behavior. American Journal of Preventive Psychiatry and Neurology 2:9–14, 1990

Cunningham C, MacFarlane K: When Children Molest Children. Orwell, VT, Safer Society Press, 1991

Dancu CV, Riggs DS, Rothbaum BO, et al: A clinician-administered vs self-report instrument to measure post-traumatic stress symptoms: the PTSD Symptom Scale. Paper presented at the 25th annual convention of the Association for the Advancement of Behavior Therapy, New York, NY, November 14–21, 1991

Davis GE, Leitenberg H: Adolescent sex offenders. Psychol Bull 101:417–427, 1987

Deisher RW, Wenet GA, Paperny DM, et al: Adolescent sexual offense behavior: the role of the physician. Journal of Adolescent Health Care 2:279–286, 1982

Derogatis LR: SCL-90: Administration, Scoring and Procedures Manual for the Revised Version. Baltimore, MD, Clinical Psychometric Research, 1977

Derogatis LR, Melisaratos N: The Brief Symptom Inventory: an introductory report. Psychol Med 13:595–605, 1983

Division of Children, Youth and Family Services: Family Centered Case Management With Sexually Aggressive Youth. Olympia, Washington State Department of Social and Health Services, 1987

Exner JE: The Rorschach: A Comprehensive System, 2nd Edition, Vol 1. New York, Wiley, 1986

Federal Bureau of Investigation, U.S. Department of Justice: Uniform Crime Reports for the United States. Washington, DC, U.S. Government Printing Office, 1990

Fehrenbach PA, Smith W, Monastersky C, et al: Adolescent sexual offenders: offender and offense characteristics. Am J Orthopsychiatry 56:225–233, 1986

Finkelhor D, Russell D: Women as perpetrators, in Child Sexual Abuse: New Theory and Research. Edited by Finkelhor D. New York, Free Press, 1984, pp 171–187

Freeman-Longo R, Ryan G: Tort liability in treatment of sexually abusive juveniles. Interchange (Cooperative Newsletter of the National Adolescent Perpetrator Network), October 1990, pp 1–8

Friedrich WN: Psychotherapy of Sexually Abused Children and Their Families. New York, WW Norton, 1990

Friedrich WN, Luecki WJ: Young school-age sexually aggressive children. Professional Psychology: Research and Practice 19(2):155–164, 1988

Friedrich WN, Damon L, Hewitt SK, et al: The Child Sexual Behavior Inventory: normative and clinical comparison. Psychological Assessment 4:303–311, 1992

Fuller AK: Child molestation and pedophilia: an overview for the physician. JAMA 261:602–606, 1989

Gilby R, Wolf L, Goldberg B: Mentally retarded adolescent sex offenders: a survey and pilot study. Can J Psychiatry 34:542–548, 1989

Gilgun J: Factors which block the development of sexually abusive behavior in adults abused as children. Paper presented at the National Conference on Male Victims and Offenders, Minneapolis, MN, October 1988

Griffiths D, Hingsburger D, Christian R: Treating developmentally handicapped sexual offenders: the York Behavior Management Services treatment program. Psychiatric Aspects of Mental Retardation Reviews 4:49–54, 1985

Groth AN: The adolescent sex offender and his prey. International Journal of Offender Therapy and Comparative Criminology 21:249–254, 1977

Groth AN, Loredo CM: Juvenile sexual offenders: guidelines for assessment. International Journal of Offender Therapy and Comparative Criminology 25:31–39, 1981

Harter S: The perceived competence scale for children. Child Dev 53:87–97, 1982

Harter S: Manual for the self-perception profile for children. Denver, CO, University of Denver, 1985

Harter S, Pike R: Procedural manual to accompany the Pictorial Scale of Perceived Competence and Social Acceptance for Young Children. Denver, CO, University of Denver, 1983

Harter S, Pike R: The pictorial scale of perceived competence and social acceptance for young children. Child Dev 55:1969–1982, 1984

Hathaway SR, McKinley JC: Minnesota Multiphasic Personality Inventory, Revised. Minneapolis, University of Minnesota, 1970

Hibbard RA, Hartman G: Genitalia in human figure drawings: childrearing practices and child sexual abuse. J Pediatr 116:822–828, 1990

Hodges K, Stern L, Cytryn L, et al: The development of a child assessment interview for research and clinical use. J Abnorm Child Psychol 10:173–189, 1982

Hudson WW: The Clinical Measurement Package: A Field Manual. Homewood, IL, Dorsey Press, 1982

Hunter JA, Santos DR: The use of specialized cognitive-behavioral therapy in the treatment of adolescent sexual offenders. International Journal of Offender Therapy and Comparative Criminology 34:239–248, 1990

Johnson TC, Berry C: Children who molest: a treatment program. Journal of Interpersonal Violence 4:185–203, 1989

Kahn TJ, Chambers HJ: Assessing reoffense risk with juvenile sex offenders. Child Welfare 70:333–345, 1991

Kaufman AS, Kaufman NL: Manual for the Kaufman Brief Intelligence Test (K-BIT). Circle Pines, MN, American Guidance Service, 1990

Kavoussi RJ, Kaplan M, Becker JV: Psychiatric diagnosis in adolescent sex offenders. J Am Acad Child Adolesc Psychiatry 27:241–243, 1988

Kempe CH: Incest and other forms of sexual abuse, in The Battered Child, 3rd Edition. Edited by Kempe CH, Helfer RE. Chicago, IL, University of Chicago Press, 1980, pp 198–214

Kiersch TA: Treatment of sex offenders with Depo-Provera. Bull Am Acad Psychiatry Law 18:179–187, 1990

Kilmann PR, Sabalis RF, Gearing ML, et al: Treatment of sexual paraphilias: a review of the outcome research. The Journal of Sex Research 18:193–252, 1982

Kiresuk TJ, Sherman RE: Goal Attainment Scaling: a general method for evaluating community mental health programs. Community Ment Health J 4:443–453, 1968

Knight RA, Prentky RA: Exploring characteristics for classifying juvenile sex offenders, in The Juvenile Sex Offender. Edited by Barbaree HE, Marshall WL, Hudson SM. New York, Guilford, 1993, pp 45–83

Knopp FH: Retraining Adult Sex Offenders: Methods and Models. Syracuse, NY, Safer Society Press, 1984

Knopp FH, Lane S: Program development, in Juvenile Sexual Offending: Causes, Consequences, and Correction. Edited by Ryan GD, Lane SL. Lexington, MA, Lexington Books, 1991, pp 21–37

Krugman RD: Recognition of sexual abuse in children. Pediatrics in Review 8:25–30, 1986

Landis C: Sex in Development, New York, Hoeber, 1940

Lane SL: The sexual abuse cycle, in Juvenile Sexual Offending. Edited by Ryan GD, Lane SL. Lexington, MA, Lexington Books, 1991, pp 103–142

Lane SL, Zamora P: A method for treating the adolescent sex offender, in Violent Juvenile Offenders: An Anthology. Edited by Mathias RA, Demuro P, Allinson R. San Francisco, CA, National Council on Crimes and Delinquency, 1984, pp 347–363

Longo RE, Groth AN: Juvenile sexual offenses and the histories of adult rapists and child molesters. International Journal of Offender Therapy and Comparative Criminology 27:150–155, 1983

Marshall WL, Barbaree HE, Eccles A: Early onset and deviant sexuality in child molesters. Journal of Interpersonal Violence 6:323–336, 1991

Matson JL, Esveldt-Dawson K, Kazdin A: Evaluating social skills with youngsters. J Clin Child Psychol 12:174–180, 1983

McGraw RK, Pegg-McNab J: Rorschach comparisons of male juvenile sex offenders and nonsex offenders. J Pers Assess 53:546–553, 1989

Melella JT, Travin S, Cullen K: Legal and ethical issues in the use of antiandrogens in treating sex offenders. Bull Am Acad Psychiatry Law 17:223–232, 1989

Metzner JL: The adolescent sex offender: an overview. The Colorado Lawyer 16:1844–1851, 1987

Moos RH, Moos B: Revised Family Environment Scale. Palo Alto, CA, Consulting Psychologists Press, 1981

Murphy WD, Krisak J, Stalgaitis S, et al: The use of penile tumescence measures with incarcerated rapists: further validity issues. Arch Sex Behav 13:545–554, 1984

Murray H: Manual for the Thematic Apperception Test. Cambridge, MA, Harvard University Press, 1943

National Center on Child Abuse and Neglect: Study of national incidence of child abuse and neglect (DHHS Publ No 20-01099). Washington, DC, U.S. Government Printing Office, 1987

National Task Force on Juvenile Sexual Offending: Preliminary report on juvenile sexual offending, 1988. Juvenile and Family Court Journal 39:1–67, 1988

Otey EM, Ryan GD (eds): Adolescent sex offenders: issues and research and treatment (DHHS Publ No ADM-85-1396). Rockville, MD, U.S. Department of Health and Human Services, 1985

Perilstein RD, Lipper S, Friedman LJ: Three cases of paraphilias responsive to fluoxetine treatment. J Clin Psychiatry 52:169–170, 1991

Peters D, Wyatt GE, Finkelhor D: Prevalence, in A Sourcebook on Child Sexual Abuse. Edited by Finkelhor D. Newbury Park, CA, Sage, 1986, pp 15–59

Pino CJ, Simmons N, Slowski MJ: Children's Version of the Family Environment Scale. East Aurora, NY, Slosson, 1984

Prentky RA, Knight RA, Straus H, et al: Developmental antecedents of sexual aggression. Journal of Development and Psychopathology 1:153–169, 1989

Reynolds CR, Richmond BO: Revised Children's Manifest Anxiety Scale (RCMAS). Los Angeles, CA, Western Psychological Services, 1985

Rorschach H: Psychodiagnostics. New York, Grune & Stratton, 1942

Ross J: Starting a juvenile sexual offender program, II. The New England Adolescent Perpetrator Network Newsletter 1:1–5, 1986

Ryan GD: Juvenile sex offenders: defining the population, in Juvenile Sexual Offending: Causes, Consequences and Corrections. Edited by Ryan GD, Lane SL. Lexington, MA, Lexington Books, 1991a, pp 3–8

Ryan GD: Perpetration prevention: primary and secondary, in Juvenile Sexual Offending: Causes, Consequences and Corrections. Edited by Ryan GD, Lane SL. Lexington, MA, Lexington Books, 1991b, pp 393–407

Ryan GD, Lane S, Davis J, et al: Juvenile sex offenders: development and correction. Child Abuse Negl 11:385–395, 1987

Ryan GD, Metzner JL, Krugman RD: When the abuser is a child, in Understanding and Managing Child Sexual Abuse. Edited by Oates KR. Sydney, Australia, Harcourt Brace Jovanovich, 1990, 258–274

Salter AC: Prevalence, in Treating Child Sex Offenders and Victims: A Practical Guide. Newbury Park, CA, Sage, 1988, pp 16–24

Saunders EB, Awad GA: Assessment, management, and treatment planning for male adolescent sexual offenders. Am J Orthopsychiatry 58:571–579, 1988

Shoor M, Speed MH, Bartelt C: Syndrome of the adolescent child molester. Am J Psychiatry 122:783–789, 1966

Showers J, Farber E, Joseph J, et al: Sexual victimization of boys: a three-year survey. Health Value: Achieving High-Level Wellness 7:15–18, 1983

Smith WR, Monastersky C, Deisher RM: MMPI-based personality types among juvenile sex offenders. J Clin Psychol 43:422–430, 1987

Stevenson HC, Wimberley R: Assessment of treatment impact of sexually aggressive youth. Journal of Offender Counseling, Services and Rehabilitation 15:55–68, 1990

Stevenson HC, Castillo E, Sefarbi R: Treatment of denial in adolescent sex offenders and their families. Journal of Offender Counseling, Services and Rehabilitation 14:37–50, 1990

Strong K, Tate J, Wehman B, et al: Sexual Assault Facts and Effects. Cumberland, WI, Human Growth & Development, 1986

Swanson CK, Garwick GB: Treatment for low-functioning sex offenders: group therapy and interagency coordination. Ment Retard 28:155–161, 1990

Tarter RE, Hegedus AM, Alterman AI, et al: Cognitive capacities of juvenile violent and nonviolent, and sexual offenders. J Nerv Ment Dis 171:564–567, 1983

Terman LM: Psychological Factors and Marital Happiness. New York, McGraw-Hill, 1938

Thomas J: The adolescent sex offender's family in treatment, in Juvenile Sexual Offending: Causes, Consequences and Corrections. Edited by Ryan GD, Lane SL. Lexington, MA, Lexington Books, 1991, pp 333–376

Travin S, Cullen K, Melella JT: The use and abuse of erection measurements: a forensic perspective. Bull Am Acad Psychiatry Law 16:235–250, 1988

Wasserman J, Kappel S: Adolescent Sex Offenders in Vermont. Burlington, VT, Vermont Department of Health, 1985

Wechsler D: Manual for the Wechsler Intelligence Scale for Children–Revised. New York, Psychological Corporation, 1974

Weinrott MR, Saylor M: Self-report of crimes committed by sex offenders. Journal of Interpersonal Violence 6:286–300, 1991

Wenet G, Clark T: Juvenile Sexual Offender Decision Criteria. Seattle, WA, Juvenile Sexual Offender Program, University of Washington Adolescent Clinic, 1984

Yochelson S, Samenow S: The Criminal Personality. New York, Jason Aronson, 1976

Appendix: Commentary

Metzner and Ryan have written a very useful review of the literature regarding adolescent sex offenders. In their review, they skillfully discuss clinical application related to assessment and treatment of adolescent offenders.

An area of increasing concern involves children under the age of 12 who sexually abuse other children. There is very little information on the origins of this behavior. A classification system for problematic sexual behavior in children has been proposed that includes three categories: 1) precocious sexual behavior, 2) inappropriate sexual behavior, and 3) coercive sexual behavior. *Precocious sexual behavior* refers to oral-genital contact or attempts at intercourse and similar behaviors between preadolescents in which there is no evidence of force or coercion. These behaviors may occur following exposure to sexually explicit material (e.g., cable television, videotapes, movies), from observation of adults who are indiscreet when children are around, or following sexual molestation of the child. *Inappropriate sexual behavior* refers to persistent and/or public masturbation, excessive preoccupation with sexual matters, and highly sexualized play or verbalizations. Finally, *coercive sexual behavior* refers to sexual acts in which force is used and/or threats are employed to induce cooperation from the other child, or in which there is a significant disparity in the children's ages or sizes (L. Berliner, O. Manaois, and C. Monastersky, "Child Sexual Behavior Disturbance: An Assessment and Treatment Model" [unpublished manuscript], 1986[1]).

Although previous sexual abuse of the child may play a part in the emergence of behavior in any of the three categories, it appears that a significant number of children who engage in these behaviors have not been abused. In addition, data exist that suggest that patterns of sexually aggressive behavior in some individuals emerge in the preadolescent years (Division of Children, Youth and Family Services 1987). These behaviors may subsequently become ingrained during adolescence and the young adult years, resulting in a chronic adult offender. To obtain more information about the etiology of this behavior and effective treatment for such behavior, the National Center on Child Abuse and Neglect has funded two projects: one at the University of Oklahoma Health Sciences Center in Oklahoma City, Oklahoma,[2] and the other at the Center for Prevention and Treatment of

---

[1] Available from Harborview Medical Center, 325 Ninth Avenue, 2A-07, Seattle, WA 98104.

[2] Barbara Bonner, Director; C. Eugene Walker (University of Oklahoma, Oklahoma City) and Lucy Berliner (Sexual Assault Center, Harborview Medical Center, University of Washington, Seattle, Co-Investigators.

Sexual Abuse in Waterbury, Vermont.[3] The purpose of these projects is to develop a typology regarding children with sexual behavior problems and to compare the effectiveness of various treatment approaches.

Few standardized evaluation instruments exist for use with children who engage in inappropriate sexual behavior. In the University of Oklahoma program, the child completes an evaluation battery consisting of the Revised Children's Manifest Anxiety Scale (Reynolds and Richmond 1985); the Rorschach inkblot test (Exner 1986; Rorschach 1942); the Children's Version of the Family Environment Scale (Pino et al. 1984); the Child Assessment Schedule (Hodges et al. 1982); the Kaufman Brief Intelligence Test (Kaufman and Kaufman 1990); the Pictorial Scale of Perceived Competence and Social Acceptance for Young Children (Harter 1982; Harter and Pike 1983, 1984) or the Self-Perception Profile for Children (Harter 1985); the Draw-a-Person test (Hibbard and Hartman 1990); and the Posttraumatic Stress Disorder (PTSD) Symptom Scale (Dancu et al. 1991). In addition, the parents complete an extensive demographic form and a battery consisting of the Child Sexual Behavior Inventory (Friedrich et al. 1992), the Parenting Stress Index (Abidin 1983), the Revised Family Environment Scale (Moos and Moos 1981), the Brief Symptom Inventory (Derogatis 1977; Derogatis and Melisaratos 1983), the Child Behavior Checklist (Achenbach and Edelbrock 1983), the Index of Parental Attitudes (Hudson 1982), and the Goal Attainment Scale (Kiresuk and Sherman 1968). The Goal Attainment Scale focuses on positive and negative behaviors that the parents would like to see increase or decrease in their child during treatment.

It is hoped that this database will provide information to develop a typology of children who are involved in sexually inappropriate behavior. Data from both of these projects should be available in the near future. Treatment procedures used in the projects have been developed from earlier work by Berliner and Rawlings (L. Berliner and L. Rawlings, "A Treatment Manual: Children With Sexual Behavior Problems" [unpublished manuscript], 1991), Cunningham and MacFarlane (1991), Friedrich (1990), Friedrich and Luecke (1988), and Johnson and Berry (1989). Outcome data on treatment of these children will be available a year or two following the typology.

E. Eugene Walker, Ph.D.
Karen Longest, M.A.
Oklahoma University Health Sciences Center
Oklahoma City, Oklahoma

[3] William Pithers and Alison Stickrod Gray, Directors.

Section II

Treatment and Prevention

Chapter 8

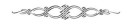

Individual Psychotherapy

Efrain Bleiberg, M.D.

Augustt Aichhorn's (1935) bold proposal to apply psychoanalytic principles to the treatment of delinquent youth gave rise to a radical notion: that it is possible to create a context of human relationships in which wayward, hateful, impulsive youngsters can be understood, cared for, and, perhaps, helped to resume their thwarted development.

Aichhorn's conception was rooted in the basic premises of psychoanalytic theory: an appreciation of the power and significance of unconscious motivation, an awareness of the double-edged potential of the transference (both as a source of resistance and as an opportunity to achieve freedom from repetition of the past), and a belief in the centrality of early development and early relationships in shaping psychic experience.

By the early 1950s, Aichhorn's seminal work had inspired a number of important contributions to the psychoanalytic understanding of delinquency. Redl and Wineman (1951, 1957) described the failure of ego controls underlying the difficulties of "children who hate." Johnson and Szurek (1952) examined adolescents' enactments of their parents' unconscious delinquent tendencies. Winnicott (1958) interpreted the antisocial tendency as an effort to test and secure relationships. Such contributions promised to pave the way for even more significant advances and stirred up hope and therapeutic enthusiasm. Yet, over the next three decades, enthusiasm gave way to

147

widespread disillusionment with the effectiveness of psychoanalytically oriented approaches in general, and of psychotherapy in particular, for youth with conduct disorder (CD).

Such a waning of therapeutic enthusiasm can hardly be surprising. Working with youngsters with CD presents a unique challenge to the clinician's skill, sensitivity, and compassion. Like perhaps no other group of patients, these children test the treatment team's cohesiveness and capacity to use countertransference reactions therapeutically. Aggressive, manipulative, and apparently unconstrained by guilt, children with CD are far more likely to elicit feelings of anger, hopelessness, and helplessness than of compassion, empathy, and concern. Furthermore, their seeming lack of suffering or of serious psychiatric impairment strains their treaters' ability to justify to third-party payers and utilization review personnel the necessity for a tortuous, lengthy, and often unsuccessful treatment. Last, but not least, these youngsters' difficulties expose the limits of the dominant psychoanalytic paradigms of ego psychology and the structural model, the focus on psychosexual development and the vicissitudes of hypothetical drives and psychic energies, and developmental notions primarily derived from analytic reconstruction.

This theoretical model—the basis of Aichhorn's and Redl's formulations—provided a new conceptual lens to investigate human behavior. By the early 1970s, however, it had become evident that this lens left out critical dimensions of human functioning better addressed by competing paradigms:

1. **Sociocultural models** (e.g., Cloward and Ohlm 1960; Merton 1957; Rutter and Giller 1983) that identify the significance of socioeconomic class; ethnicity; family size; access to social, medical, and psychiatric services; child-rearing and socializing practices; and modes of exposure to alcohol and drugs
2. **Family interaction models** (Patterson 1982; Rutter and Giller 1983) that emphasize the importance of parental violence and physical abuse; severe marital discord; and parental inadequacies in providing structure, supervision, and emotional involvement
3. **Neurobiological models** that stress genetic influences (Christiansen 1977), neuropsychiatric vulnerabilities (Lewis 1983; Lewis et al. 1979), attentional deficits and learning disabilities (Cantwell 1981), and depression (Kovacs et al. 1984)

These and other studies made abundantly clear that "CD" is a diagnostic label encompassing an array of biopsychosocial vulnerabilities, intermixed in various combinations, rather than a homogeneous condition. Attempts to subdivide these youngsters in ways that help make sense of this heterogeneity offer the potential to provide a firmer base from which to conceptualize psychotherapeutic approaches.

Subjective Experience and Personality Configurations

The subtyping of CD remains controversial. Rutter and Giller (1983), after reviewing the literature, concluded that the most meaningful distinction was along the lines of socialized versus undersocialized dimensions. According to these authors, the capacity to form enduring affectionate bonds and to experience concern for others is a psychological dimension associated with a less dysfunctional family background and a more benign outcome. (Interestingly, Rutter and Giller [1983] also questioned whether the significant differentiation is between degrees or types of personality disturbance rather than between syndromes of CD.)

Important contributions in this direction were made by Marohn et al. (1979) and Offer et al. (1979), who conducted a factor analysis study. Offer et al. divided their sample of juvenile delinquents at the Illinois State Psychiatric Institute into four psychological subtypes: 1) impulsive, 2) narcissistic, 3) borderline, and 4) depressive. What follows is my elaboration of Offer et al.'s (1979) classification of subtypes of CD, which illustrates several distorted patterns of organizing and structuring subjective experience and provides a guide for a psychotherapeutic process to ameliorate such experiential distortions. Needless to say, these four subtypes represent modal types in a clinical continuum; in most instances, youngsters with CD present different degrees of overlap, or combinations, of these subtypes.

Impulsive Conduct Disorder

Offer et al. (1979) described the impulsive subtype as represented by a socially insensitive youngster who shows more violent and nonviolent antisocial behavior than youngsters representative of the other subtypes, yet who possesses some awareness of his or her need for help. The delinquent behavior springs from a propensity for immediate discharge of affect into action. Shapiro (1965) described the impulsive "style" of these individuals' subjective lives. The central feature of this style is distortion of the experience of intention.

In nonimpulsive individuals, impulses, wishes, and whims initiate a complex process, usually carried out smoothly and automatically outside conscious awareness. First, the impulse's expression is inhibited. Subsequently, the impulse commands or fails to command attention, then gains or loses significance as it is balanced against and integrated into the person's more enduring aims, values, and motivational constellations. These stabilizing psychological systems are based on the person's mental representations of the self in relation to others. In other words, the nonimpulsive individual "asks" himself or herself: "How does this wish of the moment fit with what is going on now in my life; with my goals, ideals, and relationships; with who I am and with what I wish to become?"

Such processing allows for a momentary impulse to be suppressed, delayed in its expression, repressed (when found to be too discordant and threatening to the person's self-concept), displaced or modified into more acceptable pursuits, or given access to action and smoothly woven into the fabric of the self. This very processing transforms the whim or urge of the moment into a more sustained and active experience of decision. By virtue of this silent process of integration, individuals develop a sense of agency and ownership of their behavior. The capacity to experience guilt is one of the corollaries of assuming ownership over one's motives and impulses.

In the case of impulsive children and adults, the wishes, needs, and impulses are translated directly into action, thereby short-circuiting the mediating process. Because these individuals rush into action, their own wishes cannot evolve into sustained intentions anchored in a sense of stability and self-continuity. In fact, their chronic inability to integrate wishes, needs, and motives disrupts their capacity to develop a cohesive and continuous sense of self and others. Their low tolerance for frustration stems from an inability to connect or integrate momentary wishes with general goals and interests or to form enduring representations of self and others.

Impulsive individuals believe their actions "happen" to them rather than occur by their choice, and thus they experience little guilt or sense of responsibility. The world appears as a disconnected set of temptations and frustrations: possibilities for immediate gain and satisfaction or obstacles to gratification. Their experience of other people and relationships is equally fragmentary and shallow, resulting in an inner life that is barren and undifferentiated. As Marohn (1991) pointed out, many of these youngsters have "little awareness of an inner psychological world, cannot name affects or differentiate one affect from another, and often confuse thought, feeling, and deed" (p. 150). Their concrete, egocentric mode of experience interferes with planning, abstraction, and generalization and forms the basis for their well-known difficulty in learning from experience.

It is beyond the scope of this chapter to review in detail the many factors involved in the pathogenesis of the impulsive subtype. One pathogenic route, however, deserves to be highlighted. A chaotic, impulse-ridden environment is a salient feature in the background of many impulsive youngsters, often coupled with attention-deficit hyperactivity disorder and/or other learning disabilities, particularly dyslexia.

Narcissistic Conduct Disorder

Offer et al. (1979) pointed out that narcissistic delinquents see themselves as well adjusted rather than as delinquent, whereas clinicians perceive them as resistant, cunning, manipulative, and superficial. The subjective world of narcissistic youngsters is dominated by three main features, all involving their desperately rigid efforts at control: 1) striving for omnipotence, 2) dissociating from and disowning self experiences, and 3) projecting onto others the rejected aspects of their sense of self and attempting to evoke in others responses that match their intrapsychic representational models.

First, these youngsters engage in an ongoing, rigid, ever-desperate effort to organize and maintain their sense of self around an illusory, arbitrary experience of power, control, or perfection. This sense of omnipotence, not necessarily based on any real achievements or competence, replaces the normal process of narcissistic regulation (Bleiberg 1988, 1989a). Less-narcissistic children regulate their self-esteem and achieve a sense of mastery and control by modeling their *actual self*—conscious and unconscious representations of one's own characteristics and aptitudes—after their *ideal self* (Joffe and Sandler 1967)—mental representations built from memories, fantasies, and models provided by others and associated with safety, satisfaction, and an optimal ability to adapt. The ideal self becomes a blueprint—a model to attempt to match. When the actual self approximates the ideal self, children experience the sense of narcissistic well-being that is generally described as self-esteem, and which typically results in greater competence. In effect, the ideal self guides the child in reversing states of helplessness and passivity to achieve mastery. In narcissistic youngsters, the ideal self no longer functions as a road map, but serves instead as an illusory basis for the sense of self.

Next, narcissistic youngsters rigidly and desperately disown and dissociate from self experiences that fail to measure up to their ideals of omnipotence, control, or perfection. They deny pain, helplessness, sadness, and vulnerability as "not me." Some chronically abused children may even develop an impressive numbness to physical injury. This persistent, tenaciously maintained discontinuity of subjective experience—the chronic dissociation of some self experiences—is one of the hallmarks of a developing personality disorder.

Last, but not least, children and youth with narcissistic CD make a sustained effort to force other people to match their intrapsychic reality. They project onto others their own rejected, dissociated self experiences of weakness, pain, and vulnerability. Those features now belong to others rather than to the self. Thus, they do not experience other people, including the significant adults in their life, as helpful and reliable protectors, limit setters, sources of support, or models of identification; instead, they hold others in contempt or perceive them as worthless, inept weaklings—tools to be manipulated or objects from whom to extract admiration and confirmation of their own power. The narcissistic youngster's insistence that the interpersonal world match and support a rigidly held configuration of intrapsychic representations—and his or her desperate maneuvers to force other people to match that internal model—is another hallmark of a developing personality disorder.

Yet no matter how much confirmation of their power they receive, these persons are perennially haunted by the specter of narcissistic vulnerability—experienced as shame—and by their suspicion of impending attack. If their shortcomings are revealed, if their illusions of omnipotence are punctured, they expect to be painfully humiliated and viciously destroyed. Thus, they feel a need to control and intimidate, fully anticipating from others the same ruthlessness and lack of empathy.

This subtype of CD appears most commonly among children who are innately endowed with skills and resourcefulness (in particular, precocious language skills, unusual social prowess, and the ability to elicit responses from others) and a set of life circumstances that promotes a closure of dependency, disavowal of vulnerability, and reliance on self-nurturing capacities. Abuse and neglect within a chaotic, violent, drug-abusing environment create an especially fertile soil for this particular distortion in development. Typically, a more specific set of forces promotes the grandiosity of these children. These resourceful, sometimes charming youngsters are often recruited to serve critical, even life-saving, functions for a parent or an entire family.

Borderline Conduct Disorder

Offer et al. (1979) described the borderline subtype as represented by an emotionally empty, depleted youngster, sometimes an outcast but at other times needy and clinging. Borderline youngsters are moody, irritable, and explosive. They are constantly being swept along by the feelings of the moment and so are prone to affective storms—episodes of uncontrolled emotion without an apparent precipitant. Their sense of self and others constantly changes kaleidoscopically. One moment they feel elated and expansive, blissfully connected in perfect love and harmony to a temporarily idealized partner; the next, they plunge into bitter feelings of disappointment and rage, coupled with self-loathing and despair. This abruptly shifting, chaotic sense of self and others is the central feature of the borderline youngster's subjective experience.

To maintain even a semblance of a sense of well-being, of continuity of their sense of self, borderline youngsters require a constant stream of "supplies" to "hold" them and protect them against their own emotional whirlwinds: another person's love and attention, sex, drugs, or food. When such supplies are not forthcoming, they panic, become enraged or transiently psychotic, or experience an inner sense of emptiness. Their delinquent behavior is often associated not only with their desperate efforts to secure those essential supplies, but also with secondary difficulties that arise from drug abuse and their dependency for support and protection on other delinquents—frequently those suffering from the narcissistic subtype of CD.

Rinsley (1980) postulated that specific patterns of mother-child interaction are the central pathogenic factor in borderline disorders. In his view, the mothers of future borderline individuals take pride in and find gratification in their children's dependency. These mothers reward passive-dependent, clinging behavior while withdrawing or otherwise punishing their children for actively exploring or striving for autonomy. Such mothers are attuned to states of helplessness and proximity-seeking behavior, which they validate and respond to, but give subtle or overt rebuffs to children who show evidence of mastery or independence. The central message communicated to their children, said Rinsley, is that "to grow up is to face the calamitous loss or withdrawal of maternal supplies, coupled with the related injunction that to avoid such calamity, the child must remain dependent, inadequate, symbiotic" (p. 5). The overall developmental consequence is thus an inhibition of separation and individuation. Other investigators (Klein 1977; Stone et al. 1981), however, suggest that borderline patients suffer from an underlying problem of affective dysregulation and that a genetic linkage exists between borderline personality and mood disorders.

More recently, Gunderson and Zanarini (1989) pointed out that although studies have indeed shown a uniformly elevated prevalence of mood disorders in the relatives of borderline patients, the link is neither uniform nor specific. As Gunderson and Zanarini conclude, the genetic contribution to borderline personality disorder is more likely a broad predisposition to psychopathology rather than an increased probability of acquiring a specific disorder. In some youngsters, the genetic factor may consist of a vulnerability to mood disorders, while in others it may involve problems with impulse control. In both cases, this genetic contribution interacts with a broad range of developmental problems, including early parental loss, sexual abuse, and parental discouragement of separation and autonomy. Sexual abuse and traumatic overstimulation have increasingly been recognized as important pathogenic factors, given the powerful propensity of such traumatic experiences to induce dissociative states. As previously noted, the fragmentation of inner experience is a subjective hallmark of borderline disorders. This tendency to fragmentation, initially mediated either by genetic vulnerability and/or trauma, eventually may be actively—albeit unconsciously—produced for defensive purposes in the well-described phenomenon of splitting (O. F. Kernberg 1975).

Depressive Conduct Disorder

In Offer et al.'s (1979) view, the depressed—or "depressed borderline"—youngster with CD shows initiative in school, is liked by clinicians, and tries to engage therapeutically with treaters. These youngsters possess a strongly internalized value system and a considerable amount of guilt and depression from which delinquent behavior serves as a relief, but they also show "an anaclitic need for objects to which they cling and for which they hunger" (Offer et al. 1979, p. 52).

Numerous studies (Kovacs et al. 1984; Puig-Antich 1982) have documented the coexistence of CD and depression in children. Depressed children are often irritable and aggressive. They carry an image of themselves as unworthy and incompetent, while they experience others as unavailable. Studies of so-called attributional style (Seligman and Peterson 1986) show that depressed children—like depressed adults—attribute failures and other "bad" events to global, stable, internal causes, but they associate good events with specific, unstable, and external sources.

Although they feel depleted and deprived, these depressed children with CD typically reject or sabotage any offers of help, support, or nurturance, no matter how desperately they claim to need them. The salient features of their subjective experience include anticipating failure and frustration, feeling utterly helpless in the face of misery, and organizing their sense of self and others around the premise that they are bad and that others are indifferent or withholding. Feeling victimized is a critical component of these children's sense of identity.

Genetic studies (Weissman et al. 1987) lend qualified support to the role of genetic transmission in the etiology of depressive disorders in children. Although a biologically based proneness to irritability and aggression probably plays a part in the link of depression and CD, this association also prompts us to look at other factors. Freud (1916/1963) described the "criminal from a sense of guilt" (p. 332). People, said Freud, can engage in criminal behavior to provoke punishments, thereby appeasing their unconscious feelings of guilt while confirming their badness. Children, who have less well-structured self-critical functions, are more likely to externalize their internal needs for punishment. Freud described how children who committed theft, fraud, and arson became quiet and contented only after being punished.

Self-victimization, however, serves other purposes besides validating one's conviction of badness. Inflicting pain on oneself and causing misery to others can effectively ensure responsiveness from otherwise indifferent or exhausted caretakers. Although depressed parents may ignore quiet children, they will usually be forced to respond to angry, defiant, or self-destructive ones. Thus, "conduct problems" may become the currency of relatedness every bit as much as they represent a protest against neglect, an unconscious search for punishment, or an expression of a biologically based predisposition to mischief.

Self-defeating behavior acquires other meanings over time. In addition to provoking punishment from others, self-inflicted pain helps children to actively produce the very misery they expect will befall them. Thus, paradoxically, self-victimization can induce a secret sense of activity, control, and power and in so doing reverse traumatic states of passivity and helplessness. In the same way, in the case of borderline youngsters, the active use of splitting can counter the passivity and helplessness associated with a traumatically evoked sense of fragmentation.

Furthermore, the "victims" can derive narcissistic gratification from their suffering. They can claim entitlement to special treatment: the world owes them something because they belong to the long-suffering, morally superior breed of the martyrs.

Psychotherapeutic Approaches: A Representational Mismatch

Faced with the amazing, intimidating, and deflating challenge of how best to treat youngsters with CD, therapists have often despaired of finding basic principles to guide their interventions. An important recent contribution by P. F. Kernberg and Chazan (1991) describes in detail a "trio of therapies"— individual supportive-expressive play psychotherapy, parent training, and play group psychotherapy—specifically for elementary school–aged children with mild to moderate CD.

Kernberg and Chazan (1991) indicate that their approaches are intended for children who demonstrate a capacity for social bonding as manifested by at least two of the following criteria: forming and sustaining peer-group friendships for at least 6 months, extending themselves on others' behalf, experiencing at least a minimal sense of guilt, exhibiting loyalty toward companions, and showing concern for the welfare of others.

The three therapeutic modalities described by P. F. Kernberg and Chazan (1991) can be used separately or in combination. The treatment approach presented in this chapter is based on the premise that the treatment of youngsters with CD should always integrate individual and family approaches—both conceptually and clinically.

Developmental research (Stern 1985; Sameroff and Emde 1989) has clearly demonstrated that the efforts to build and maintain sustaining connections with others constitute a central motivational system and a critical organizer of psychological experience. Research also documents the powerful, innate bias toward mastery, control, integration, and perceptual-experiential coherence (Emde 1989). As Stern (1985) puts it, the human brain is biased to put together what goes together in reality, and to respond with distress and anxiety when such experiential coherence is disrupted.

These two motivational systems join forces in the organization and structuring of children's internal representational models (Bowlby 1973). As internal representational models of the self in relation with others are generated, they serve to guide active, intentional behavior. Internal representational models also organize future interactions and become increasingly resistant to change (Sroufe 1989). In both normality and psychopathology, the need for experiential coherence mandates a "match" between the individual's internal representational model and the interpersonal world around him or her. In fact, children with CD are rigid and desperate in their insistence on inducing interpersonal responses that support and validate their intrapsychic organization.

A perverse cycle typically evolves in which youngsters evoke interpersonal dysfunction that in turn reinforces their intrapsychic pathology. To put it differently, these children exemplify the pertinence of a transactional perspective (Minuchin and Fishman 1981): a child shapes, modifies, and reinforces his or her family's dysfunction every bit as much as the family's dysfunction shapes, modifies, and reinforces the child's individual psychopathology. Interactions aimed at the child's subjective experience (i.e., individual psychotherapy) necessarily have an impact on the family's relational patterns, whereas approaches designed to modify patterns of family interaction inevitably modify the child's developmental context and intrapsychic organization. Thus, much greater therapeutic leverage can be achieved by carefully coordinating individual psychotherapeutic approaches with family treatment.

Patterson (1982) delineates specific approaches to help parents consistently set limits and effectively promote prosocial behavior in their delinquent children. P. F. Kernberg and Chazan (1991) advocate a similar approach in a four-phase program of parental guidance. In the first phase, the parents' management techniques are assessed and agreement is reached on how to modify these techniques. During the second phase, parents are taught general principles of development and modification of behavioral problems. The third phase focuses on specific approaches for parents to apply with their children. The fourth phase helps parents learn how to monitor their children's behavior at home to provide input to the therapist. Structural-strategic (Minuchin and Fishman 1981) family therapists emphasize the importance of interventions and assignments designed to establish clear generational boundaries and extricate symptomatic children from the roles they play within the family—often precisely through their disruptive behavior. For example, disruptive behavior can detour one parent's hostility onto the child instead of onto the other parent, or it can serve as a stimulus to keep parents engaged with each other, preventing marital dissolution.

From a developmental perspective, these various approaches all foster an interpersonal context that can function as a "holding environment" (Winnicott 1965). A holding environment is a human system that communicates to children, "We, the adults, are strong and competent, capable of nurturing you and caring for your needs, soothing and comforting you when you are distressed. We will hold you and prevent you from feeling that you are about to collapse, but we will also contain your destructive and maladaptive behavior."

From a therapeutic-intrapsychic vantage point, the process of creating a holding environment introduces what Horowitz (1985) called a representational mismatch, that is, an interpersonal reality that contradicts rather than supports the child's intrapsychic representational model. Thus, narcissistic children find that a holding environment implicitly challenges their claim to omnipotence and their insistence that others are worthless, weak, and incompetent. Borderline youngsters are prevented from engaging in their usual maladaptive maneuvers—around sex, drugs, or food—from which they derive a momentary sense of well-being, self-cohesion, and connection with others. Impulsive children are precluded from automatically translating impulses into action, challenging a view of the world as a disconnected series of temptations or obstacles to gratification. Depressed children's self-defeating and self-victimizing behaviors are thwarted, along with their insistence that caretakers are unreliable, indifferent, and mean.

A review of the clinical literature (Bleiberg 1987, 1989b; Marohn et al. 1980; Masterson 1988; Patterson 1982; Rinsley 1989) reveals that although authors conceptualize their interventions differently, they all agree that the treatment of children with CD cannot take place without first establishing effective limits for impulsive, manipulative, and destructive behavior.

From a clinical standpoint, the crucial considerations in deciding between an inpatient or a residential setting, on the one hand, or an outpatient or a community-based plan, on the other, are 1) the capacity of the youngsters' parents to establish and maintain a clear and consistent holding environment; 2) the extent of the youngsters' need for containment, support, and structure; and 3) the availability of community resources and services to support the family's containment. Clinical experience has long suggested the necessity of maintaining a holding environment that can withstand youngsters' storms of rage and that can limit their efforts to corrupt real therapeutic engagement.

Faced with a parental effort to set limits and provide structure (i.e., a representational mismatch), children with CD react blatantly or subtly to sabotage adult competence. In so doing, they attempt to re-create an interpersonal context characterized by the caretaker's ineptitude, inconsistency, and unreliability and by adult reliance on the children's power and manipulation, instead of one in which children can count on adult protection.

Pseudocompliance and pseudoinsights are frequent maneuvers these children use to preserve the status quo. Their seductive efforts to sexualize relationships with clinicians or to become "good buddies" with them can render treaters ineffective. On the other hand, such children can also be openly defiant, threatening, assaultive, contemptuous, or bent on instigating chaos in the family, the school, or the hospital.

A consistent holding environment is a prerequisite to achieving the initial goals of treatment, which include 1) challenging the youngster's pathological defenses enough to induce therapeutically useful anxiety; 2) establishing the adults, both parents and treaters, as reliable protectors and limit setters; and 3) promoting the child's capacity to share some aspects of self-experience with the treaters.

Whether the treatment is conducted in an inpatient or outpatient setting, the specific elements of each therapeutic holding environment should be based on the developmental needs of the children. Those with prominent narcissistic features require a therapeutic context that, while implicitly challenging their omnipotence and curtailing their efforts to derail treatment, avoids unnecessary exacerbation of their sense of vulnerability. Borderline and impulsive children need an environment that provides structure, support, and self-regulation. Stimulants or mood-stabilizing medications and special educational programs can also be important elements in creating a holding environment for these youngsters. Group therapy provides a controlled opportunity for these—and for narcissistic—children to be challenged by peers.

Yet perhaps the most critical factor in determining therapeutic success is the alliance established between parents and treaters. Following diagnostic assessment, patients can be excluded from the first one or two sessions while the treaters share the diagnostic formulation and treatment plan with the parents. Simply excluding the child from these early planning sessions conveys a powerful message that the adults will be in charge and begins the process of creating a mismatch between the child's expectations and external reality.

Beginning Phase of Individual Therapy: Self–Other Relatedness and the Therapeutic Alliance

Redl and Wineman (1951) succinctly posed the dilemma facing treaters in the beginning phase of psychotherapy with youngsters with CD. "What to do until the ego comes?," they wondered. In the treatment model proposed in this chapter, individual psychotherapists attempt to create a context in which a therapeutic alliance can emerge—that is, a context that promotes the development in the patients of the notion that a collaborative activity with the treaters is possible, safe, and potentially helpful. Clinical experience suggests that a minimum of one—and preferably two—sessions per week is necessary for a therapeutic relationship to develop. Narcissistic children with CD, however, often need three or more sessions per week to break through their narcissistic defenses. Achieving such a sense of collaboration is, of course, easier said than done. A therapist typically contends with an opening phase in which the patient's behavior is marked by ruthless tyranny, aloofness, suspiciousness, demands for control of the sessions, or attempts to reduce the therapist's role to that of captive audience for an elaborate show. Older school-age and adolescent narcissistic patients often present themselves as "hotshots" filled with bravado and pretentious self-sufficiency, bent on demeaning the therapist. On the other hand, they may appear grateful and seemingly compliant, brimming with intellectual insights or seductively communicating to the therapist that they find him or her exceptionally sensitive, brilliant, and attractive. Borderline youngsters can fall madly in love with their therapist and are eager to declare their good fortune in having found the perfect person to love—and be loved by. Impulsive children play aggressively and destructively, but those who have experienced significant trauma or who are depressed often display a narrow range of verbal and emotional involvement and concrete, repetitive, joyless play themes. These initial gambits provide a window into the subjective experience and characteristic defensive maneuvers of these children.

Robert, a 15-year-old hospitalized adolescent with a mixture of borderline and narcissistic features, began therapy with a superficial eagerness to solve his problems. This therapeutic zeal soon gave way to rather flamboyant expressions of contempt for the hospital, the hospital's treatment team, and me. He had expected that a famous clinic would provide him with a therapist perfectly suited to treat him—"a perfect match." He had some hope (on first meeting me) that I was such a match, as he noticed that I, like him, have blue eyes and blond hair. He was quickly disappointed, however, especially when he heard my obviously foreign accent. He could not understand why he had been subjected to the ignominy of having a "spic" (his reference to my Hispanic accent) for a therapist. I commented that he seemed to experience my accent as a put-down—a flaw he would be embarrassed to be associated with.

"Not bad for a spic," he replied, quickly turning to his doubts about whether "spics" could understand the concerns of someone of obvious Nordic descent, such as he. At that point I mentioned that, if I heard him right, he seemed to be saying that if we were not identical—not only in our looks but in our backgrounds as well—I would not be able to understand him and appreciate him. "Not bad for a spic," was again his response. Yet I could detect some budding relatedness in his mocking compliment.

Such relatedness, of course, was only tentative. He could confide then, nonetheless, his concerns that if he trusted me, I would find a way to sabotage his plans to "behave appropriately" and maintain a "positive attitude." Such behavior would, he was sure, convince the clinical staff and his parents that he was ready to return to his beloved home state, instead of enduring the disgrace of rotting in dreadful Kansas. This comment, of course, betrayed Robert's own questions about how effectively manipulation and pretense could serve to solve his problems. Not picking up on this issue, I commented instead that I appreciated his concern about what would happen to him—again, what would happen if I "could hear him right"—if he trusted me, even a bit. Would it help him or would it hinder him?

This clinical vignette illustrates how initial interventions should focus on clarifying the patient's subjective experience ("Let me see if I understand what you are saying . . . am I hearing you right?"), with the primary goal of helping the patient find an area of subjective experience that can be safely shared, either verbally or in play. The therapist should avoid prematurely interpreting the patient's envy, sadness, vulnerability, or rage, as well as the related defenses of grandiosity, dissociation, denial, and projective identification. In other words, the therapeutic intent is to facilitate the establishment of a beachhead, an area of self–other relatedness.

Prematurely confronting the patient's defenses before this beachhead is established only exacerbates the need for distance, control, or devaluation of the therapist and the therapy.

Elliot, an 11-year-old boy with a narcissistic CD, responded to my premature inquiry into his feelings of pain and sadness by frantically denying any dysphoric experiences. He proceeded to launch into a tirade that explained how "any idiot knows that babies only learn to feel pain when their mothers get all hysterical" after they injure themselves. Without such "hysteria," he claimed, babies would never learn to feel pain. He, fortunately, had been forced to rely on his own resources by his parents' self-absorption, so he had been spared the need to learn to feel vulnerable. Instead, his task was to monitor his mother's mood and to keep her amused and buoyant. Disappointment, particularly regarding the failings of an unavailable husband, threw this chronically depressed woman into a suicidal despair from which only Elliot could rescue her.

Bent on convincing me of both his power and his lack of familiarity with either pain or vulnerability, Elliot began to lose his grip on reality. His tirade became increasingly desperate as he insisted on demonstrating the power of his mind over ordinary matter. Before long, he was telling me how once he had wished to fly so badly that he had been able to defy the laws of gravity. Then he grew anxious, keenly aware that maintaining an illusion of omnipotence was requiring him to treat reality in an ever more arbitrary fashion.

Helping Elliot at this juncture presented me with a dilemma. To acknowledge my mistake in addressing his vulnerability before he was ready would only add the insult of implying that he was not tough enough to deal with the injury of exposure. I offered him a compromise: I asked, "Are you saying that when you really put your mind to something, no matter how impossible it may seem, you can accomplish it?" He agreed, but only after first dismissing my formulation ("No, that's not it.") A moment later, however, he replied, "What I really mean is that when you really put your mind to it, you can accomplish just about anything. You can even learn to fly in an airplane." Elliot was thus able to save face, regain his grip on reality, maintain his sense of omnipotence unchallenged, and use my help without having to acknowledge it.

Interventions that help these youngsters save face can pave the way for a therapeutic alliance. That is, therapists help their patients to maintain a sense of control even when confronted with the blow of the family's or inpatient staff's growing capacity to provide a holding environment. Such face-saving help facilitates the patients' ability to accept their representational mismatch and the implicit "humiliation" of therapy itself. As the case of Elliot illustrates, such tasks involve a delicate balance between fostering more adaptive solutions to life's demands, maintaining a semblance of control, and keeping anxiety and shame within manageable limits. Therapists, for example, can discuss how youngsters might respond more adaptively to their parents'—or the inpatient staff's—limits on manipulative or provocative behavior or to the enraging, anxiety-provoking prohibition on using drugs and alcohol.

Not only the patients' reactions require careful attention, however. Perhaps the greatest therapeutic obstacle is the therapist's countertransference. Therapists often experience dread of the sessions, concern about being fooled by the patient, and wishes to show who "really is in charge"; feelings of worthlessness, helplessness, and defeat; irritation and urges to reject these patients; and boredom or indifference. O. F. Kernberg (1975, 1977) has pointed out the usefulness of countertransference reactions as invaluable clues to the patient's rejected self-experiences being projected onto the therapist. Kohut's (1971) contributions enhanced therapists' awareness of the necessity of paying minute attention to children's feelings of disappointment in their therapists. Kohut's stress on empathy highlights the importance of respecting patients' needs to feel powerful and in control without prematurely interpreting warded-off feelings of envy or vulnerability.

Middle Phase: Expanding the Range of Relatedness and the Interpretation of Defenses

Children's readiness to enter the middle phase of therapy is signaled by two indicators: the obvious appearance of anxiety and the beginning of a therapeutic alliance. Anxiety is generated largely by the representational mismatch created by the holding environment—whether as a result of the parent's greater competence or of the inpatient milieu's limits. To some degree, however, anxiety can also be traced to children's own wishes for closeness with their therapists and the dawning conviction (fraught with uncertainty and fears of being subjugated, destroyed, or humiliated) that hope and help can be derived from therapeutic relationships. Only rarely can these youngsters openly acknowledge their attachment to their therapists. More commonly, children demonstrate some embryonic collaboration in the form of sharing experiences with the therapist or in using their treaters to find face-saving solutions to the adults' "conspiracy" to deprive them of their usual coping mechanisms.

The presence of some form of collaborative relationship allows therapists to gently encourage their patients to consider an expansion in the range of "shareable" experiences: narcissistic youngsters are invited to share their experiences of vulnerability, depression, pain, helplessness, and dependency. Borderline and impulsive children are introduced to the notion of a continuity of the self and relationships. Depressed patients are encouraged to look at the restrictions in their play and emotional ranges.

> Jimmy, a 10-year-old narcissistic boy, created a play theme in which his father was the president of the United States. This pathetic father-president, however, could barely function without Jimmy's guidance. Jimmy instructed the therapist to play the role of the father and relished ordering him around, barking directives for the country. The therapist began to point out the child's desire to share in the power of an exalted, yet secretly diminished, ruler. If he could share in such power maybe he would not have to feel little, vulnerable, or envious of anyone else.

Only at this point can therapists attempt to systematically confront children's characteristic defenses and begin the exploration of the motives and functions of those defenses. However, as children face their vulnerability, pain, and depression, they are filled with stark panic. Jimmy, for example, became extremely anxious when the therapist pointed out his defensive need to cover up fears of helplessness and vulnerability.

Not surprisingly, a heightened reliance on old defensive mechanisms becomes apparent—that is, attempting to control, devalue, intimidate, manipulate, or seduce the therapist; rejecting help; running away; abusing drugs; and intensifying antisocial behavior outside the sessions or attempting to pit parents and therapists against one another.

> Joe, a 13-year-old borderline narcissistic boy, had been subjected to brutal physical and sexual abuse by an alcoholic father while his mother pursued her theatrical career. Almost in spite of himself, he began to feel more comfortable with me, even to look forward to the sessions. Yet, desires for closeness were almost unbearable for him. Thus, he began to carefully look for "mistakes" on my part—for example, my interrupting him or "invading" his space while walking. Discovering such mistakes would then trigger hateful barrages. He told me of his plans to run away from the hospital and find out my house's location ("I have good sources, you know") so that he could set it on fire after raping my wife and murdering my children with intravenous injections of cocaine. He would spare my life, but only to ensure that I would suffer the devastation of the loss of everything I hold dear.

Joe's tirade spoke volumes of what closeness meant to him: a painful, destructive invasion of his house-fortress, a rape, a painful penetration of his body and bloodstream that could evoke burning, devastating feelings leading to total collapse; the envy of my possessions and my relationships and the associated rage at his own deprivation and abuse; the wish to eliminate all possible rivals for my love but also the desire to leave me as deprived, lonely, and needy as him.

Obviously, such outbursts can evoke rather intense countertransferential responses in treaters. Interestingly, while attempting to weather the storm of Joe's vindictive rage, I felt neither threatened nor cut off from him. I wondered if he wished to provoke me yet remain connected to me, all the while denying attachment. He did not love me, he seemed to be telling me; in fact, he hated me. I was a pedantic, know-it-all, rich shrink who could not possibly understand someone hardened by a life in the mean streets of the big city.

Sensing his desire to maintain a relationship while overtly disowning it, I commented on the meanness and cruelty of his imagery. Where did that come from? He looked at me with a mix of contempt and amusement and proceeded to describe, in a wildly exaggerated fashion, the toughness of his neighborhood and its brutal gang wars. He was sure that my wimpy, nerdy self had been shielded from such roughness.

Together with contempt and devaluation, I sensed an inviting, playful teasingness in Joe's account of his gang escapades. In effect, he had grown up in the far more sedate environment of an upper-middle-class community in New England. His interest and knowledge of gangs had mostly been acquired through extensive reading on the subject. Prior to his outburst, he had brought to the sessions magazines and tapes glorifying gangs.

I picked up (perhaps with more hope than conviction) on the implied teasing and replied with an even more fantastic account of my own heroic battles as a gang kingpin—a secret identity hidden behind my deceptively mild appearance.

He seemed to enjoy this gambit, and over the next few sessions we engaged in a good deal of increasingly more good-natured bantering. Only after we reestablished our relationship at a distance he could more readily tolerate did I bring back to his attention the rage he had experienced and the abuse he had inflicted upon me.

This vignette illustrates how these youngsters often require a transitional area of relatedness akin to Winnicott's (1953) transitional experience. In this transitional, as-if area (often jointly created by patient and therapist) between fantasy and reality, patients can both own and disown their rejected feelings and experiences while testing out the therapist's attunement, respect, and responsiveness to the vulnerable aspects of their selves.

Younger narcissistic patients often introduce, as a transitional relationship, a play theme involving an imaginary twin. The twin typically embodies the "weak," dependent, sad, helpless experiences these children find unbearable. Another version of the transitional experience, common to all children with CD, consists of somatic complaints. These complaints offer a way of requesting help without acknowledging it and of reconnecting with feelings of pain and inadequacy while keeping open the possibility of disowning such feelings.

Borderline youngsters fight mightily to prevent disruptions of their transitional space. They create play themes so vivid and absorbing that they—and, at times, their therapists—can no longer tell the difference between fantasy and reality. It is in their play themes that these youngsters come to life—and in which they adamantly refuse to allow reality to intrude and question the arbitrariness they need to impose on their life and relationships.

> Cory, a Taiwanese-born 8-year-old girl who was adopted as a baby by a Caucasian family from the Midwest, was referred for therapy when she began to react to threats of separation from her adoptive mother by exhibiting dramatic disruptions in her reality contact as well as raging outbursts, stealing, and disruptive behavior in school. Facing the possibility of separation—such as when her adoptive mother visited her own mother in a nearby town for a few days—also prompted Cory to take refuge in an elaborate fantasy about her biological mother, whom she "knew" was an Oriental princess.
>
> The fantasy was extraordinarily vivid for Cory and animated her lashing out at the world in which reality failed to appreciate her entitlement to royal prerogatives. Yet, even without reality's assistance, a dream or a bad thought typically sufficed to disrupt the idyllic fantasy. In her dreams and play, the Oriental princess would be replaced by a witch, a vicious vixen whose features combined Oriental and Caucasian traits. This woman would taunt Cory and try to drag her to a bottomless pit, leaving the child with no choice but to strangle the witch in self-defense. Cory herself changed. Without the love and protection of the princess, she would become a "Chinese bitch." These play themes were soon incorporated into her therapy.

As this vignette illustrates, the transitional sphere of the play's theme provides the illusion of a perfect, magical union with the therapist. At the same time, the split-off, threatening aspects of both the patient's self and the world of reality are kept safely apart.

Tooley's (1973) "Playing It Right" is a beautiful account of how the therapist can more closely attempt to align borderline children's play and fantasy with reality's constraints. Gradually, children are nudged to introduce small modifications in their play to better encompass the complexities, limitations, conflicts, and frustrations of reality. The transitional space of play and fantasy becomes a stage on which to try out new identifications, to practice imagined solutions to life's dilemmas, to explore new ways of being in the world and relating to others, and to test behavior that promises greater mastery, more effective coping, and increased pleasure and adaptation. In particular, play offers borderline children the magic of anonymity in which to attempt to bring together split-off representations of the self and others. In the safe haven of the transitional sphere of relatedness, therapists can safely confront children with systematic explorations of the youngsters' pathological defenses and the motives for such defenses. In particular, they can examine, as in Cory's case, the advantages of splitting—that is, of keeping the hated and hateful image of the witch carefully disconnected from the memory of the loving and lovely princess. Thus, in a transitional space, children can be invited to consider that a whole region of their experience stands unlived, so to speak—never owned or shared.

Therapists' acknowledgment of the utter terror children feel as they enter into rejected, dissociated, denied aspects of their lives and relationships can prevent therapeutic stalemates and limit regression. Therapists should always point out the many advantages of *not* changing—in effect, the price children would have to pay if they were to give up their maladaptive, but often life-saving, defenses. Ultimately, therapists present to their patients, implicitly or explicitly, a therapeutic "bargain": by relinquishing their pathological defenses and the illusion of control and safety, they make way for the far more exposed and laborious process of attempting to achieve real mastery and meaningful relationships.

Such a "bargain" is unlikely to prove appealing unless a number of factors are operant in the child's interpersonal world. Thus, it is essential for the psychotherapist to maintain close and ongoing contact with the hospital or residential treatment staff and the family therapist. Such meetings provide invaluable information to both psychotherapist and staff regarding the child's subjective experience, the realities of his or her life, and the ways that milieu, family treatment, and psychotherapy can be effectively aligned. Family treatment must address the powerful coalitions often apparent between one of the parents and the symptomatic child. It is particularly imperative to extricate these children from their roles as saviors, confidants, or special partners of one of the parents (typically the other-sex parent). At the same time, opportunities should be provided to foster the relationship between the child and the same-sex parent while promoting the ability of that same-sex parent to function as a model to the child (a relationship that requires the other parent's sanction).

The family therapist gives the individual psychotherapist access to a vantage point from which to assess the consequences to the family of the patient's relinquishment of symptoms and the anxieties that the child's changes may trigger in the family. Bringing the parents into the treatment serves to address a major source of the child's resistance to treatment: an overwhelming anxiety that his or her growth and change will shatter the family and cause the parents to hurt each other, divorce, commit suicide, or abandon the child.

Educational programs and activities and occupational therapy provide opportunities to promote real mastery and competence, thereby lessening children's needs to rely on illusory solutions. Yet, teachers and other therapists need to sensitively approach children's fears of exposing their limitations and the gaps in their knowledge. Cognitive approaches are useful in the individual sessions to increase children's ability to anticipate, process, and plan. Group therapy sessions serve to promote adaptive ways of relating to peers and provide new sources of support and identification.

Interventions that change children's interpersonal contexts help bring to the fore material usefully pursued in individual psychotherapy. Themes of dependency, safety, autonomy, envy, rage, and vulnerability become available for exploration, often mixed with items of oedipal competition, fears of bodily integrity, and unconscious guilt over destructive wishes. Just as important as attunement to feelings of real pain and vulnerability is therapists' sharing in the real joy, renewed hope, and genuine pride children experience as a result of their growth, increased competence, and comfort with their feelings.

Termination Phase: Mourning and Resuming Development

The harbingers of termination are found both within and without the therapy process. Naturally, a sustained amelioration of symptomatic behavior is a hopeful sign. The achievement of nondelinquent peer relationships and interests is perhaps more significant than the simple absence of overt antisocial activities. Changes in family interaction and school functioning are particularly important. Children's growing ability to use their parents—and/or other nondelinquent adults—as sources of protection and comfort and as models of identification bodes the end of the psychotherapeutic process. When children can approach parents and teachers for help in solving problems in reality, the beginning of termination is in view.

Within the therapeutic process itself, therapists recognize other clues of impending termination: children's open acknowledgment of missing their therapists during interruptions and vacations; youngsters' expressions of gratitude for help received; patients' spontaneously bringing to the sessions their sense of how they utilize outside the sessions something they learned in therapy; and—perhaps the most sensitive clue—patients' bringing to the sessions their sense of loss regarding missed or botched opportunities and life's unfairness.

The final stage of psychotherapy offers a chance to test children's readiness to relinquish pathological defenses. Beginning to discuss a termination date with patients and parents fuels anxiety and often brings about a reactivation of symptoms in the patient and of dysfunctional interaction patterns in the parents.

Jill, a 10-year-old girl in residential treatment, began attending public school. This move meant clearly that discharge from the residential treatment center and termination of psychotherapy were looming. This narcissistic girl proceeded—as was characteristic of her before beginning treatment—to alienate her classmates with her petulance and manipulativeness, her tall tales about extraordinary accomplishments, and her demands to be the center of everyone's attention. Along with this return of old patterns, Jill attempted to present in therapy a rosy picture of her adaptation to the world outside the residential treatment center. She was liked by her peers, she said, was eagerly sought out as a playmate, and could count two or three girls as her best friends.

Only a school report brought home the true picture of the girl's struggles. Confronted with the discrepancy, Jill could speak of her fears of disappointing me, the staff in the residence, and her parents. She wondered if her progress was completely contingent upon the therapy and the staff's support, and worried about whether she could sustain it without such a protective envelope. She was skeptical as to whether her parents and I would really appreciate her if she was anything less than a perfect, smashing success. Could she be loved if she was just a regular girl? Only after much work did another dimension of the girl's regression emerge: her difficulties in dealing with the sadness and loss associated with termination.

Mourning the anticipated loss of the therapy and the therapist is an essential task of the termination phase. Just as important is the opportunity to work through children's disappointments: with their own shortcomings, with the adults who never measured up to their expectations, with everything they could not achieve in therapy, and with the therapists' limitations.

Regardless of apparent regressions and symptomatic reactivations, the termination phase requires a relaxation of supervision and the provision of expanded responsibilities and increased privileges to the youngster. Naturally, such a stance is not without risk. The following vignette illustrates the vicissitudes that can be encountered during termination.

Adam, a 12-year-old boy, had found himself in the state's custody after repeated desertions by his mother. His unremitting destructiveness and defiance landed him in a residential treatment center. There he explained to his therapist, in the metaphor of his play, the reasons for his hatred: the therapist, who was the leader of the "Irams"—this vignette occurred at the time of the Teheran embassy hostage crisis—had kidnapped the mother of "Billy." Billy naturally was bent on revenge and fully intended to rob all the banks in the world and kill people until his mother was released.

Much work went into turning this play theme slowly around until it could encompass the possibilities of maternal abandonment, rage at his mother, and the notion that Billy's badness, greed, and neediness had damaged his mother and driven her away.

As discharge to a group home was becoming a realistic possibility, Adam ran away. He returned, however, on his own, a few days later. He had traveled more than 100 miles and had located his mother (a feat that had eluded the investigative powers of child protective services). Having found her, he said, he had made peace with this distraught and rather limited woman. Soberly, Adam told his mother that "he knew what she had done," and no matter what happened between them, he still loved her and would go on with his life.

Anna Freud herself could not have stated more eloquently the criteria for termination: the child's experience of reinstatement in the path of growth and development.

Conclusion

This sketchy review fails to do justice to the complexities that are part and parcel of the psychotherapeutic treatment of youngsters with CD. Systematic evaluation of the effectiveness of this and other treatment modalities is sorely needed before more definitive statements can be made regarding what interventions, in what timing or sequence, predict positive outcomes in children with specific forms of CD.

Developmental research continues to expand the boundaries of our understanding of how subjective experience is organized and structured. Family therapists' growing appreciation of individual differences is building new bridges between family and individual psychotherapy. These advances promise to dramatically enhance our conceptual sophistication and clinical effectiveness.

For now, clinical experience suggests that individual psychotherapy can play a pivotal role in helping children with conduct disorder break the grips that anxiety, anger, vulnerability, and loneliness have fastened on their lives.

References

Aichhorn A: Wayward Youth. New York, Viking, 1935

Bleiberg E: Stages in the treatment of narcissistic children and adolescents. Bull Menninger Clin 51:296–313, 1987

Bleiberg E: Developmental pathogenesis of narcissistic disorders in children. Bull Menninger Clin 52:3–15, 1988

Bleiberg E: Adolescence, sense of self and narcissistic vulnerability. Bull Menninger Clin 52:211–228, 1989a

Bleiberg E: Stages of residential treatment: application of a developmental model. Residential Treatment for Children and Youth 6(4):7–28, 1989b

Bowlby J: Attachment and Loss, Vol 2: Separation. New York, Basic Books, 1973

Cantwell DP: Hyperactivity and antisocial behavior revisited: a critical review of the literature, in Vulnerabilities to Delinquency. Edited by Lewis D. New York, Spectrum, 1981, pp 21–38

Christiansen KO: A review of studies of criminality among twins, in Biosocial Bases of Criminal Behavior. Edited by Mednick S, Christiansen KO. New York, Gardner Press, 1977, pp 89–108

Cloward RA, Ohlm LE: Delinquency and Opportunity. Chicago, IL, Free Press, 1960

Emde R: The infant's relationship experience, in Relationship Disturbances In Early Childhood. Edited by Sameroff A, Emde R. New York, Basic Books, 1989, pp 33–51

Freud S: Some character-types met with in psycho-analytic work (1916), in The Standard Edition of the Complete Psychological Works of Sigmund Freud, Vol 14. Edited by Strachey J. London, Hogarth Press, 1963, pp 309–333

Gunderson JG, Zanarini MC: Pathogenesis of borderline personality, in American Psychiatric Press Review of Psychiatry, Vol 8. Edited by Tasman A, Hales RE, Frances AJ. Washington, DC, American Psychiatric Press, 1989, pp 25–48

Horowitz M: Introduction to Psychodynamics. New York, Basic Books, 1985

Joffe WG, Sandler J: Some conceptual problems involved in the consideration of disorders of narcissism. Journal of Child Psychotherapy 2:56–66, 1967

Johnson AM, Szurek SA: The genesis of antisocial acting out in children and adults. Psychoanal Q 21:323–343, 1952

Kernberg OF: Factors in the treatment of narcissistic personalities. J Am Psychoanal Assoc 22:243–254, 1975

Kernberg OF: Borderline Conditions and Pathological Narcissism. New York, Jason Aronson, 1977

Kernberg PF, Chazan SE: Children With Conduct Disorders: A Psychotherapy Manual. New York, Basic Books, 1991

Klein DF: Psychopharmacological treatment and delineation of borderline disorders, in Borderline Personality Disorders. Edited by Hartocollis P. New York, International Universities Press, 1977, pp 365–383

Kohut H: The Analysis of the Self. New York, International Universities Press, 1971

Kovacs M, Feinberg TL, Crouse-Novak MA, et al: Depressive disorders in childhood. Arch Gen Psychiatry 41:229–237, 1984

Lewis DO: Neuropsychiatric vulnerabilities and violent juvenile delinquency. Psychiatr Clin North Am 6:707–714, 1983

Lewis DO, Shanok SS, Balla DA: Perinatal difficulties, head and face trauma, and child abuse in the medical histories of seriously delinquent children. Am J Psychiatry 136:419–23, 1979

Marohn RC: Psychotherapy of adolescents with behavioral disorders, in Adolescent Psychotherapy. Edited by Slomowitz M. Washington, DC, American Psychiatric Press, 1991, pp 145–161

Marohn RC, Offer D, Ostrov E, et al: Four psychodynamic types of hospitalized juvenile delinquents. Adolesc Psychiatry 7:466–483, 1979

Marohn RC, Dalle-Molle D, McCarter E, et al: Juvenile Delinquents: Psychodynamic Assessment and Hospital Treatment. New York, Brunner/Mazel, 1980

Masterson J: Psychotherapy of the Disorders of the Self. New York, Brunner/Mazel, 1988

Merton RK: Social Theory and Social Structure. New York, Free Press, 1957

Minuchin S, Fishman HC: Family Therapy Techniques. Cambridge, MA, Harvard University Press, 1981

Offer D, Marohn RC, Ostrov E: The Psychological World of the Juvenile Delinquent. New York, Basic Books, 1979

Patterson GR: Coercive Family Processes. Eugene, OR, Castalia, 1982

Puig-Antich J: Major depression and conduct disorder in prepuberty. Journal of the American Academy of Child Psychiatry 21:118–128, 1982

Redl F, Wineman D: Children Who Hate. Glencoe, IL, Free Press, 1951

Redl F, Wineman D: The Aggressive Child. Glencoe, IL, Free Press, 1957

Rinsley DB: The developmental etiology of borderline and narcissistic disorders. Bull Menninger Clin 44:127–134, 1980

Rinsley DB: Developmental Pathogenesis and Treatment of Borderline and Narcissistic Disorders. New York, Jason Aronson, 1989

Rutter MP, Giller H: Juvenile Delinquency: Trends and Perspectives. New York, Penguin, 1983

Sameroff A, Emde R: Relationship Disturbances in Early Childhood. New York, Basic Books, 1989

Seligman MEP, Peterson C: A learned helplessness perspective on childhood depression: theory and research, in Depression in Young People: Developmental and Clinical Perspectives. Edited by Rutter M, Izard CE, Read PB. New York, Guilford, 1986, pp 223–249

Shapiro D: Neurotic Styles. New York, Basic Books, 1965

Sroufe A: Relationships, self and individual adaptation, in Relationship Disturbances in Early Childhood. Edited by Sameroff A, Emde R. New York, Basic Books, 1989, pp 70–96

Stern DN: The Interpersonal World of the Infant: A View From Psychoanalysis and Developmental Psychology. New York, Basic Books, 1985

Stone MH, Kahn E, Flye B: Psychiatrically ill relations of borderline patients: a family study. Psychiatr Q 53:71–84, 1981

Tooley K: Playing it right: a technique for the treatment of borderline children. Journal of the American Academy of Child Psychiatry 12:615–631, 1973

Weissman MM, Gammon GD, John K, et al: Children of depressed parents: increased psychopathology and early onset of major depression. Arch Gen Psychiatry 44:847–853, 1987

Winnicott DW: Transitional objects and transitional phenomena. Int J Psychoanal 34(2):89–97, 1953

Winnicott DW: The antisocial tendency, in Collected Papers. New York, Basic Books, 1958, pp 306–315

Winnicott DW: The Maturational Processes and the Facilitating Environment. New York, International Universities Press, 1965

Chapter 9

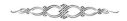

Manual-Based Psychotherapy

Gregory G. Wilkins, Ph.D.
G. Pirooz Sholevar, M.D.

lthough substantial strides have been made in the conceptualization and assessment of conduct and other disruptive behavior disorders, the translation of empirical findings into treatment-relevant approaches continues to be deficient for many reasons. Treatment interventions are often described in anecdotal and ambiguous terms, without adequately specifying the nature of the intervention, the intensity, the process variables, and the duration. Because of shifting conceptual boundaries, problems of comorbidity, and changes in diagnostic practices, target populations are often tenuously defined—a condition that makes assessment of treatment interventions difficult. The search for effective treatment modalities is particularly important for children with conduct disorder (CD) because these children are among those most commonly referred by parents and teachers for professional intervention (Breen and Altepeter 1990; Herbert 1978; Kazdin 1985; Safer and Allen 1976; Wells and Forehand 1985). Children with CD manifest a variety of oppositional, noncompliant, disruptive, and aggressive behaviors. Equally important, they fail to behave in a manner consistent with established societal norms and situation-specific rules, exhibit irritating and aversive interpersonal behaviors, and, with older age, increasingly manifest serious delinquent actions.

Against the background of the urgent need to develop treatment-relevant interventions for children with disruptive behavior disorders, the manual developed by Paulina F. Kernberg and Saralea E. Chazan with their collaborators from Cornell Medical College—"Children With Conduct Disorders: A

Psychotherapy Manual" (1991)—assumes a unique position. The intent of this manual is to advance teaching and research in psychotherapy with children by discussing the treatment needs of children with CD and describing suggested interventions. Kernberg and Chazan's text outlines three distinct, but highly integrated, treatment approaches for children with CD: individual supportive-expressive play psychotherapy (SEPP), parent training, and play group psychotherapy (PGP). In this chapter we summarize these treatment approaches, as well as relevant issues, as concisely as possible, necessarily excluding the richness of the detailed clinical material presented in the text. Effective use of these techniques requires a thorough perusal of the text in addition to successful completion of a training curriculum, including ongoing supervision.

Candidates for these psychotherapeutic interventions include children with oppositional defiant disorders and those with mild to moderate conduct disorder. Children with a primary diagnosis of attention-deficit hyperactivity disorder (ADHD) are generally excluded from SEPP and PGP as a result of their extreme attentional fluctuations, heightened overactivity, and demonstrated failure to benefit from insight-oriented treatment approaches (Barkley 1990).

Although a number of prerequisite conditions should be met for the use of SEPP, parent training, and PGP, particular consideration is given to the child's capacity to establish a therapeutic alliance and to experience guilt or remorse with regard to antisocial behaviors. Children with CD exhibit diverse behavioral and interpersonal problems of varying complexity and determination. Nonetheless, these children share a characteristic impulsiveness and a subsequent tendency to express themselves through actions rather than words. Accordingly, P. F. Kernberg and Chazan's treatment approaches emphasize defining psychotherapeutic interventions that enable action-oriented behaviors to be transformed—or at least moderated—into the language of subjective experience. The three approaches described in the manual use concepts based on ego psychology and object relations theory and emphasize the development of representational thought and the use of play.

Over the last decade, many attempts from diverse theoretical and empirical perspectives have been made to formulate a clinical description for assessing and diagnosing CD (Bemporad and Schwab 1986; Hinshaw 1987; Kazdin 1985; Quay 1986). In developing their manual-based treatment approaches for children with CD, P. F. Kernberg and Chazan relied heavily on the distinction between two subtypes of CD: socialized aggressive and undersocialized aggressive (Wells and Forehand 1985). According to this perspective, children with the socialized aggressive subtype demonstrate "a capacity for peer relationships, social attachments, guilt, shame, and remorse"; those with the undersocialized aggressive form of CD manifest "overt antisocial behavior and an inability to understand rules or the feelings of others" (P. F. Kernberg and Chazan 1991, p. 2). The treatment approaches described in the manual were intended to be used with children who exhibit a capacity for social bonding. With the importance attached to social bonding, assessment of the dimension of socialization and social competence revolves around such criteria as sustaining peer-group relations for at least 6 months, extending oneself for others, experiencing at least a minimal sense of guilt, exhibiting loyalty to friends, and evidencing a concern for the welfare of others.

In conceptualizing CD, a predominant psychoanalytic model based on ego psychology and object relations theory is used (Freud 1965; Hartmann 1958; O. F. Kernberg 1977; Spitz 1957, 1958; Winnicott 1965, 1971). According to these theoretical perspectives, the major difficulties of children with CD result from distortions based on structural deficiencies within their internal worlds. These distortions ultimately progress to major developmental impairments that are most evident in the areas of attention, impulse regulation, social judgment, cognitive functioning, language, and tolerance for anxiety, stress, and frustration. Although a psychoanalytic model is principally employed in P. F. Kernberg and Chazan's manual, other theoretical approaches are integrated into the treatment: attachment theory (Bowlby 1973, 1980), temperament theory (Thomas et al. 1968), and learning theory (Patterson 1982; Wells and Forehand 1981). It is stressed that only through the complementary use of these four theoretical perspectives can an adequate understanding of CD in children be attained.

Objectives of a Psychotherapy Manual

The primary objective of a psychotherapy manual is to describe the most representative and commonly used techniques in the practice of a particular psychotherapeutic approach with a reasonably well-defined patient population exhibiting a certain disorder. The development of a manual was stimulated by "small revolutions in psychotherapy research about 20 years ago which demanded that an official 'manual' be devised for each psychotherapy so that methods and theories could effectively be implemented and compared" (Luborsky 1984, p. 15). A wide range of manuals were developed, particularly in behavioral, cognitive, and family therapies. The first groundbreaking work in the area of psychoanalytic psychotherapy was Lester Luborsky's *Principles of Psychoanalytic Psychotherapy: A Manual for Supportive-Expressive Treatment* (1984).

The development of manuals for child psychotherapy followed the above initiatives. In this area, three manuals are particularly representative of these initiatives to delineate treatment approaches and their parameters. The first—a manual for individual and group psychotherapy for children with CD—was developed by P. F. Kernberg and S. E. Chazan and their colleagues at Cornell

Medical College (P. F. Kernberg and Chazan 1991); this is the manual summarized in this chapter. Two other child psychotherapy manuals are currently under development: one on psychoanalytic psychotherapy with neurotic children by a group from the Anna Freud Clinic in Hempstead, England (Luborsky and DeRubeis 1984), and one on prevention of emotional disorders in children of depressed parents—"Prevention of Emotional Disorders in Children of Depressed Parents: A Manual" (manuscript in preparation)—by William Beardslee at Harvard Medical College (Beardslee 1990).

In addition to serving as helpful training tools for therapists, teachers, and supervisors, manuals for child psychotherapy can be profitably used by experienced therapists to improve their skills and to serve as a reference for supervision. The scales for measuring therapist compliance with the treatment techniques can be used to judge when—and to what extent—a therapist is able to practice the therapy in conformity with the manual, and thus has fulfilled the goals of the training.

Just as important, such manuals are expected to delineate the principles to be followed by therapists in understanding patients' motives and intentionalities. This process is expected to unearth *core conflictual relationship themes* (CCRTs)—a concept considered to be the cornerstone of the supportive-expressive treatment described by Luborsky (1984). Furthermore, a manual for psychotherapy should provide guidelines for evaluating and strengthening the supportive therapeutic relationship, be useful for both short-term and open-ended psychotherapy, and be applicable with a broad range of patients, including patients who are hospitalized and treated by many different professionals—for example, hospital staff, doctor, and primary psychotherapist.

The purpose of a manual for psychotherapy, as outlined by Luborsky (1984), is to provide therapists with the essential principles regarding a definitive description of the techniques of a particular form of psychotherapy, a detailed guide for practicing the techniques, and a measure of the degree to which the therapist has mastered the techniques and conforms to them in his or her practice. Such a manual should be written with a special empathy for the therapist's tasks. In this way, it can help the therapist to understand the patient's communications and the process by which inferences may be drawn from those communications. The format for a psychotherapy manual should satisfy the following criteria:

1. The treatment recommendations should be as complete as the type of treatment permits and should state the techniques that are integral to the treatment.
2. The treatment principles and the operations to be performed by the therapist must be clearly explained. This is best accomplished by presenting concise descriptions and providing examples.

3. A set of scales should be included for measuring the degree to which the therapist has mastered the main treatment techniques.

Multiple Dimensions of Treatment

The multiple dimensions of treatment with children with CD include the use of SEPP, parent training, and PGP. These treatment approaches are conceptualized and described separately; however, at the therapist's discretion and depending on the child's treatment needs, any combination of the interventions may be used concurrently. In fact, this is frequently done, particularly with regard to parent training. These treatment approaches share a number of similarities. In all three approaches, treatment issues are divided into beginning, middle, and ending phases. Recommendations are provided regarding the use of play in each stage of SEPP, and phase-specific treatment tasks are delineated in parent training and PGP. As we discuss in greater detail later in this chapter, the types of therapist verbal interventions used in SEPP, parent training, and PGP are critical and are described by treatment phase. Such a formulation of well-defined treatment interventions affords researchers a means of assessing outcomes of child psychotherapy.

Common Concepts and Techniques

An emphasis on social relationships, play, and verbal interventions by the therapist is shared by SEPP, parent training, and PGP. Because children with CD have significant disturbances in interpersonal relationships, all three treatment approaches stress interventions aimed at improving social cognition and the experience of the child within various social contexts, including family, school, and peer relations. On the other hand, "play provides a context within which the relationship between the child patient and therapist unfolds. Children with CD frequently demonstrate an impaired capacity to play, for interacting and sharing with others, or for problem-solving" (P. F. Kernberg and Chazan 1991, p. 10). The objective is for play to become transformed from a vehicle for discharging aggression and impulses to one for achieving constructive self-expression. Play follows an orderly transition throughout the course of treatment, from gross motor play to structured games and, finally, to a form of creative fantasy. With appropriate play activities, the therapist facilitates the child's social awareness and expression of feeling from within a protective setting.

A fundamental focus of these approaches is the therapist's verbal interventions with the child. Such a focus is considered to be of paramount importance with children with CD, because they need to enhance their capacity to tolerate affects through verbal channels as a substitute for habituated actions, often of an impulsive nature. A hierarchical model of therapist verbal interventions is used in which ascending categories subsume the characteristics of categories under them. These categories are as follows:

1. **Ordinary social interactions.** The aim of these interventions is to engage the child in neutral, everyday social behaviors and exchanges that increase the child's comfort and diminish his or her level of apprehension. Content includes conventional expressions of greeting and politeness. (Examples: "Thank you." "Good-bye, Jacob.")

2. **Treatment-related statements.** The aim of this type of intervention is the specification of treatment parameters, which, as a therapeutic alliance is established, attenuates a child's anxiety through orientation and anticipation. Content encompasses statements regarding the structure of the treatment sessions, the role of the therapist, the behavioral limits within treatment sessions, and the process of psychotherapy. (Examples: "We will meet at this time every Thursday for the next several weeks." "You are not permitted to destroy any object in the office.")

3. **Requests for factual information.** The aim of these interventions is to elicit objective information, thereby facilitating the process of psychotherapy and communication with the child. (Examples: "Did you first feel that way after your mother went on vacation?" "Was that when you were in the third or fourth grade?")

4. **Supportive interventions.** Slightly at variance with interventions requesting factual information, the aim of supportive interventions is to strengthen a child's sense of mastery and self-esteem through educative and empathic remarks. Content may range from providing objective information to teaching new skills. (Examples: "You did that well even though you thought you couldn't do it." "I'm glad that you noticed that Jerry felt sad about losing his pet." "It would take you more that an hour to walk that far.")

5. **Facilitative interventions.** These verbal interventions are directed toward enhancing the therapist-child interchange, usually by employing review statements. Ongoing attention and understanding of the child are conveyed by the therapist through these interventions. (Examples: "What are you thinking about?" "In class today, you learned the names of the first four Presidents of the United States." "Tell me the other things I do that are wrong.")

6. **Attention-directing interventions.** These verbal interventions focus the child's attention on events, feelings, and behaviors, and there is the firm implication that new construals may be achieved, often through the support of preparatory statements. Therapist statements are divided between directing attention and identifying new behavioral, affective, and cognitive patterns. Directing attention and identifying patterns are achieved through "look-at" (past and present) and "see-the-pattern"

statements. (Examples: "Have you ever noticed that your headaches never happen after school?" "If you pick up the chair again, I'll have to restrain you." "Last week, you were sad about losing your friend.")

7. **Interpretative interventions.** The primary aim of these interventions is to enable the child to view the interrelatedness between behaviors, emotions, and ideas of which he or she is aware and assumptions and beliefs of which he or she is not aware. Content includes the interpretation of defenses and motives, both of which provide information to the child about unrecognized determinants of behavior. (Examples: "You expect me to hit you, because actually you are angry at me and would like to hit me." "You're afraid that your angry thoughts may become real." "You wish that you could be king of the world, because then you would be the boss of everybody and no one could do anything that would hurt you.")

In addition to this hierarchy of therapist verbal interventions (described in more detail later in this chapter), therapist statements can be categorized in terms of *mode*:

1. *Direct* interventions refer to the child's behaviors, thoughts, feelings, and descriptions (e.g., "You look angry today").
2. *Therapist-related* interventions concern the child's perceptions of the therapist (e.g., "You're feeling frustrated with me today because I disagreed with you").
3. *Indirect* interventions relate to the child's behavior, affects, and thoughts by using fantasy, role playing, or play (e.g., "The rabbit doesn't like to be alone").
4. Other interventions consist of the therapist's verbalizations of his or her own feelings, thoughts, and behaviors. The primary purpose of such interventions is to introduce the child to another person's perspective.

Supportive-Expressive Play Psychotherapy (SEPP)

Luborsky (1984) originated the concept of a "supportive-expressive" parameter for conceptualizing types of psychoanalytic psychotherapy. "The ego functions targeted for intervention include impulse control; tolerance for frustration, anxiety, or depression; capacity for anticipation and reflective thought; and sublimation and communication through play or language. The expressive component refers to the therapist's efforts to address the patient's unconscious conflicts and maladaptive coping mechanisms, so as to render them conscious and therefore within ego control" (P. F. Kernberg and Chazan 1991, p. 23). Play is included in this treatment approach because it is deemed an essential part of individual supportive-expressive psychotherapy with children.

Initial assessment procedures by a multidisciplinary team ensure that appropriate candidates, as previously specified, are selected for SEPP. Clinical assessment of CD must incorporate multiple sources of information, focus primarily upon the child's behaviors across multiple contexts, and be directly tied to subsequent treatment interventions. In addition to obtaining information about a child's behavioral difficulties through a review of historical data and parental interview, other instruments such as the Child Behavior Checklist (Achenbach 1978; Achenbach and Edelbrock 1983), the Conners Teacher and Parent Rating Scales (Conners 1969, 1989), and standard intellectual, educational, and neuropsychological assessments may prove useful in understanding the severity and determinants of a child's behavioral problems.

When other criteria have been met, SEPP is particularly useful for a child who exhibits an impaired capacity to play and who has substantial difficulty in relating with parents and peers in a rewarding manner. The use of play is accorded a central place in the implementation of SEPP. P. F. Kernberg and Chazan conceptualize the play of children with CD as being primarily aggressive and destructive. The aggressive use of play often serves the defensive functions of blocking feelings of rejection and devaluation from a child's awareness. Play is not used in a reciprocal manner, but instead is used to control others and situations to tolerable levels. For this reason, the therapist's task is to encourage the process of sublimatory play activity. "The therapist must be attuned to the changing levels of play, from sensorimotor efforts to establish contact (ball playing, dart games), to symbolic play (war games), which increasingly serve the purpose of communication, to structured games with consensually shared rules, to role-playing in creative fantasy play" (P. F. Kernberg and Chazan 1991, p. 30).

SEPP proceeds predictably through initial, middle, and ending phases. All phases share the three common goals of reducing behavioral difficulties, improving social adaptation, and consolidating healthy self-esteem. Each phase also has specific goals. The initial phase is concerned with establishing a therapeutic alliance in a structured and safe environment that permits a child to express his or her concerns. In the middle phase, the goal is to increase the child's repertoire of social coping strategies, to improve communication skills, and to become more aware of behavior and its meanings, both within and outside the treatment sessions. The objective of the ending phase is to increase the child's appropriate behavioral regulation and autonomous strivings, as well as to consolidate overall treatment gains.

Because the therapist's verbal interventions assume much significance in P. F. Kernberg and Chazan's text, we next trace the predominant types of verbal interventions through the initial, middle, and ending phases of the treatment. Throughout SEPP, one objective is for the child to experience himself or herself as an active agent, capable of reflection and of making decisions. Every effort is made to strengthen the child's impulse control by transforming action into words and play, and to enhance social competence by developing the child's awareness of his or her behaviors and the perspectives of others through therapist-child interactions.

Initial Phase

In the initial phase of SEPP, communication—relying upon the *indirect mode*—is achieved predominantly through metaphor and play. Because they fail to perceive the therapist as a separate individual, children anticipate that their personal understanding of events exists within their own perspective. To build a therapeutic alliance and to foster self-esteem and feelings of competence, the therapist uses verbal interventions that consist largely of ones involving *ordinary social behavior* and *support* in the form of education, redirection, encouragement, and empathy. These interventions contribute to the child's understanding of his or her identity. The therapist is attentive to the child and facilitates the therapeutic dialogue by encouraging the child's communications. The therapist also abstracts—usually in the form of review statements—the substance of the child's communications, both verbal and nonverbal. This process enables consensual validation between the therapist and child to be approximated so that the child's experiences of the world become shared. Subsequent to these interventions, a shift is made toward enhancing the child's awareness as the therapist's interventions convey the potential of new meanings and interconnections among events, behaviors, and ideas.

Five types of verbal interventions are characteristic of the initial phase of SEPP: ordinary social interactions, treatment-related statements, requests for factual information, supportive interventions, and facilitative interventions.

In the beginning phase, play is an avenue of assisting the child to increase his or her level of comfort with therapy and with the therapist. Such play usually consists of games and activities of a gross motor nature, such as dart games and basketball. Often, the therapist offers suggestions with regard to playing a game with definite rules. The child gradually becomes capable of moving into more creative and symbolic fantasy play. It should be clear that, at this and subsequent phases, the therapist assumes the role of participant-observer.

Middle Phase

In the middle phase of SEPP, children use words to a greater extent in communicating with their therapists, and *direct* interventions become increasingly prevalent. Sequences and patterns of experience can be related more directly to the children by the therapist, and children are more able to recognize these patterns as logical. "The children's awareness of their patterns of behaving and thinking gives them a new perspective, and they begin to experience themselves as the agent of circumstances, not their victim. Furthermore, they now know that they can influence their surroundings by autonomously choosing alternative adaptive responses" (P. F. Kernberg and Chazan 1991, p. 35). It is evident that, in the middle phase of treatment, the therapist and the child interact either within the metaphor of play or directly through verbal exchanges. A significant milestone of progress is reached when the child's communications indicate that he or she has formed a therapeutic alliance with the therapist.

Several changes in the pattern of verbal interventions occur during the middle phase of SEPP. Whereas verbal interventions regarding *ordinary social behavior* remain essentially unchanged, statements related to *treatment* are expected to decrease significantly as the child becomes more familiar with treatment parameters. Requests for *factual information,* with respect to biographical aspects of the child's life, decrease and are substituted with inquiries concerning current situational and interpersonal happenings involving the child's experiences outside treatment. *Supportive* interventions continue as from the initial phase of treatment, although their content shifts as treatment themes expand. *Facilitative* interventions, particularly in the form of review statements, increase in frequency during the middle phase. Such interventions convey the therapist's interest in the child and facilitate the child's willingness to talk about himself or herself. Preparatory to later interpretations, *attention-directing* communications are the most characteristic intervention of the middle phase. Interventions of this type are designed to prepare the child for subsequent interpretations by enhancing the child's capacity for critical self-observation and interest in learning that his or her thoughts, actions, and emotions have potential meaning of which he or she may not be aware.

Ending Phase

During the final stage of SEPP treatment, several significant changes occur in the focus of the therapist's verbal interventions. Interventions related to *ordinary social behavior* remain unchanged, and statements and questions related to *treatment* increasingly become focused on the implications of treatment termination. Requests for *factual information* continue, although with diminished frequency, and are related more to current interpersonal events and stressors. *Supportive* interventions continue to be of considerable importance as they are centrally employed to reassure the child that his or her behavioral improvements should remain relatively stable after treatment concludes. Themes of mastery, competence, and self-esteem continue to be focal to educating the child regarding the level and the vicissitudes of his or her improved functioning. *Facilitative* interventions remain largely unchanged with again the prominent use of review statements. *Attention-directing* and *interpretative* interventions become focused on the child's impending separation from the therapist and its potential impact on his or her behavior.

Interpretations are provided more in a therapist-related mode and specifically address the termination of treatment.

Parent Training

Research has amply substantiated the benefits of educating parents regarding the principles underlying behavior change (Foreman and Atkinson 1977; Kazdin 1985, 1987; Patterson et al. 1975). Parents are able to apply the principles they have learned, and they derive much satisfaction from seeing substantial behavioral changes—in the form of greater compliance and lessened social disruptiveness—in their child.

Initial Phase

In the initial phase of parent training, the therapist supplies parents with "a theoretical framework within which to understand their child's behavior and to provide a basis for meaningful dialogue with their therapist" (P. F. Kernberg and Chazan 1991, p. 132). Parents are given two guidelines— "Basic Principles" and "Building and Maintaining a Secure Parent-Child Relationship"—that explain the principles and the underlying rationale of the treatment approach. These guidelines, together with the professional assistance of a skilled clinician, educate parents with regard to behavioral interventions with children with CD.

The Basic Principles guideline discusses the ways in which a child's basic relationship with his or her parents establishes a prototype for relationships with others. Attachment, separation, and individuation as concepts (Mahler et al. 1975) assume importance in parents' attunement to their child's feelings as well as in their capacity to respond in ways that are appropriate to the child's developmental level. Several developmental concepts that contribute to an understanding of ways in which an insecure parent-child relationship might develop are discussed vis-à-vis children with CD. These concepts include temperamental traits (e.g., activity level, distractibility, persistence, adaptability, approach/withdrawal, intensity, regularity, sensory threshold, mood) (Thomas et al. 1968), problematic phases in child development (e.g., "the terrible twos" and preschoolers entering grade school), temperamental mismatches between parent and child, and the dimension of the good-enough parent (Winnicott 1965).

The Building and Maintaining a Secure Parent-Child Relationship guideline elaborates on the role that a secure relationship between parent and child plays in the child's development of a sense of boundary organization and role regulations. Secure relationships grow by providing warmth, acceptance, and empathic support; establishing firmness, strength, and objectivity; and maintaining structure, regulation, and organization. The guideline includes a description of each of these components, a summarization of efficient strategies for rewarding children, and an explication of the damaging effects of negative, rejecting, and punitive responses.

Middle Phase

In the middle phase of parent training, the therapist expands his or her repertoire of verbal interventions to include ones that focus on the parents' actions and experiences. Greater effort is made to direct the attention of parents to their child's behaviors and the determinants of those behaviors, from both psychoanalytic and behavioral perspectives. The therapist integrates what the parents have related or implemented in terms of behavioral interventions. Role playing may be used to clarify required interventions. As part of their training, parents are introduced to the practice of maintaining a behavioral log for their child. In this log, they are requested to record detailed information, including the date and time that a behavioral event occurred, a description of the event, their response to the event, and the consequences of specific interventions.

Systematic training is provided to parents concerning ways of improving parental interpersonal skills, including focusing and attunement, self-reflection and problem solving, and effective limit setting. Focusing enables parents to direct their attention to their child in ways that facilitate an adequate understanding of the child's needs, conflicts, and behaviors. Because parents are not necessarily adept at attending to their child's relevant verbalizations, behaviors, and affects (Stern 1985), P. F. Kernberg and Chazan include a number of clinical vignettes that illustrate exercises in parental attunement and empathic understanding so that these eventually become acquired skills.

Effective limit setting circumscribes a number of dimensions, all aimed at lessening "coercive interchanges" (Patterson 1982):

1. **Rewarding and ignoring.** Rewards should follow specific behaviors that have been evaluated as positive. Parents are taught to administer three kinds of rewards: physical and affectionate rewards, unlabeled verbal rewards, and labeled verbal statements that specify the behavior the parent is reinforcing (Forehand and McMahon 1981). Counterbalancing the use of positive parental attention is the use of withdrawal of attention or ignoring.
2. **Giving commands.** Research has demonstrated the critical role that parental commands have in influencing the level of a child's compliance (Peed et al. 1977; Roberts et al. 1978). The command-training segment of parent training corresponds to the training described by Forehand and McMahon (1981). Essentially, it is stressed that optimal commands should be specific and direct, be provided individually, and allow a sufficient interval for the child to comply.

3. **The time-out procedure.** Time-out procedures are universally incorporated into a clinician's armamentarium of behavioral interventions. They are defined as any therapeutic interruption of the focus of a child's interaction. P. F. Kernberg and Chazan describe two important characteristics of time-out procedures. First, although the child's activity is interrupted, allowance is made for the child to pursue an alternative activity or a silent project. Second, a time-out procedure should be initiated as immediately following the noncompliance as possible, and verbal exchanges regarding appropriate behaviors and consequences should follow the time-out procedure.

4. **The quiet-time procedure.** In addition to the time-out procedure, regular time should be allocated for the child to settle down and achieve a degree of comfort in solitary activities (Winnicott 1965).

5. **The playtime procedure.** Because children with CD are so habitually involved in negative interactions with their parents, scheduled quality time should be shared frequently between parent and child. With regard to the level of parent involvement, playtime activities may range from passive observations to joint participation, depending on the activities.

Ending Phase

Parent training is discontinued when an amelioration of the child's symptoms has been achieved, and when it appears that the child's gains have been maximized. As termination becomes imminent, the therapist reduces the activity level and the scope of interventions. Specific criteria for termination include the improvement and maintenance of target behaviors, the recognized effectiveness of strategies for achieving behavioral change, and an enhancement of attachment between parent and child. The latter criterion is critical in that it supports the child's efforts toward psychological separation or individuation. Sessions are usually tapered in intensity and frequency, gradually restructuring the therapist's role to one of a consultant. This termination timetable takes into account the extremity and enduring nature of CD behaviors as well as the intense difficulties with personal attachment experienced by the parents of these children.

Play Group Psychotherapy (PGP)

PGP refers to the methodology and approach to group treatment for children with CD. This approach is heavily influenced by Scheidlinger's (1982) conceptualization of group psychotherapy (also see Chapter 12). Given the difficulty that socialized children with CD have with verbal expression, play becomes a modality for nonverbal expression of impulses, feelings, and thoughts. PGP is intended for a subgroup of children who meet the criteria for SEPP. Additional treatment considerations include primary difficulties in peer relations; limited effectiveness of and progress in individual psychotherapy; extreme negative reactions to authority figures that preclude the establishment of a therapeutic alliance; the need for a more forceful, directed focus on social interactions; and serious deficiencies in social skills, including participation with peers in game activities. Exclusionary criteria include marked deviance from other children and the manifestation of symptoms (e.g., acute suicidal ideation and gestures) that demand prompt management through individual attention. In the PGP model of group psychotherapy, there are two co-therapists and the group is composed of same-sex peers; concurrent parent groups are also conducted so that supplemental support and direction may be provided to the work occurring in the children's group.

In PGP, therapeutic effects, with regard to a reduction of CD behaviors, are achieved by providing structure, fostering group cohesiveness, and encouraging socialization. Each child selects, with the therapist, treatment objectives that are required on the basis of individual history and treatment need. Characteristically, these objectives involve relevant aspects of immature social adaptation, unsocialized behaviors, and damaged self-esteem. Toward this end, play materials are selected by the group therapists to optimize opportunities for socialization and communication experiences. Finally, categories of therapist verbal interventions replicate, with appropriate variances, the schema outlined for SEPP, including the four modes of communication. Given the importance attached to therapist verbal interventions with respect to treatment outcome, these interventions are traced through the beginning, middle, and ending stages of PGP.

Initial Phase

Before beginning PGP, each child meets individually with one of the group therapists for a general orientation and brief description of group activities. The child is told that a general treatment objective is to learn more effective ways of making friends and relating to peers, and individual treatment goals are developed with the child's participation. For PGP to be effective, "the therapists must convey their authority to set limits and establish norms of the group and yet remain flexible enough to adapt the norms for the specific group of children with whom they are working" (P. F. Kernberg and Chazan 1991, p. 207). Play continues to be a critical part of treatment. In the beginning, activities are designed so that a dynamic transition—from individual projects to pair play to activities involving the entire group—unfolds naturally over the course of treatment.

During the initial phase of PGP, therapist verbal interventions are directed toward reducing the children's anxiety and uncertainty about being members of a group. While attempting to enhance the children's effectiveness and level of adaptation in social relatedness, the therapist continues to focus verbal interventions on *ordinary social interactions* as well as on *supportive and facilitative* statements. Supportive statements are largely restricted to direct communications about peer relationships. As in SEPP, the therapist's verbal interventions are designed to introduce and elaborate on another person's perspective, an area of marked deficiency in children with CD (Barkley 1990; Breen and Altepeter 1990). These verbal interventions facilitate peer interaction, model social skills in supportive and educational ways, and use role playing at critical treatment junctures.

In PGP, the group therapists emphasize the use of words as opposed to actions by providing clarifications and review statements. From a careful analysis of PGP transcripts included in the manual, it is clear that the verbal interventions of the initial phase frequently consist of specific requests for *factual information,* "see-the-pattern" statements used in discussing angry and hurt feelings among group members, encouragement for the children to evaluate critically their own feelings and attitudes, constructive suggestions of ways in which social interactions might be improved, and discussions of such developmentally central issues as fairness and perceptions of rules.

Middle Phase

The middle phase of PGP is characterized by major themes of dependency issues and authority concerns, and the development of prosocial skills continues to be a primary focus. Many opportunities are provided for the group members to practice adaptive ways of expressing aggression. The children are encouraged "to recognize the beginning of aggressive feelings before they turn into impulsive actions, to modulate aggressive feelings by giving oneself time to react, and to channel aggression into words or appropriate competitive activities" (P. F. Kernberg and Chazan 1991, p. 233). As the group sessions progress, play activities become less structured, allowing imaginative activities to unfold.

Because of the group's greater cohesiveness at this phase, the children are more receptive to the comments of the therapists. Although statements related to the *treatment* decrease in number, rules about behavioral expectations within the group need to be periodically restated, and group planning for subsequent sessions is encouraged. As in the middle phase of SEPP, therapist verbal interventions regarding requests for *factual information* shift to information related to recent events and those evoked by the group process. Children are encouraged to discuss critical happenings in their lives outside the group as a way of reinforcing their ties to the outside world. In an attempt to educate children in new ways to handle aggression, decrease impulsivity, and improve their repertoire of social skills, therapists use *supportive* interventions in a variety of contexts. In this phase, *facilitative* interventions, largely in the form of review statements, increase as the children need to have their progress—or lack of same—reflected by the therapists.

The social awareness of group members is also expected to increase during the middle stage of PGP, and verbal interventions related to *directing attention* enable the children to attend to events in greater detail and to focus their attention on themselves and others. This process is achieved through preparatory and "see-the-pattern" statements (in both the past and the present). Finally, *interpretations*—"clarifications and confrontations about how the children are reacting toward their peers and toward adults and how they perceive others' behavior and their own intentions"—are critical during this period. Such interventions help the children become "aware of their defenses, affects, and motives" (P. F. Kernberg and Chazan 1991, p. 238). Interpretations are often used to encourage children to look at their interactions and infer possible motivations for these interactions; this process usually entails viewing another person's perspective.

Ending Phase

As the group progresses toward termination, increased individuation and group cohesiveness become evident. Children advance in their social awareness, their ability to observe critically, and their capacity to channel impulses, affects, and aggression into self-expressive modes—all of which constitute significant gains for children with CD. A number of specific issues are relevant to PGP, and specific opportunities for handling these issues are provided, particularly in the middle and ending phases of PGP. These special issues are as follows:

1. **Fighting.** Fighting among children is conceptualized and interpreted with respect to both group dynamics and individual psychopathology. When fighting occurs, the children are afterward engaged in active discussions related to the aggressive behavior that has taken place and the implications of that behavior for the children involved. The therapist must focus the group on alternative ways of handling aggressive impulses and of preventing their expression in unsocialized forms.
2. **Scapegoating.** When scapegoating occurs, the therapist should stop the action and clarify the process as a group defensive posture. Children need to understand that the scapegoated child serves the needs of the group.
3. **Refusal to attend sessions.** Resistance to treatment is frequently encountered with children with CD. Whenever a child is absent from the group frequently, possible reasons for the absence should be discussed by the group. This discussion should occur with the group member present so that group members may express their reflections and feelings directly.
4. **Introducing new members.** Ideally, new members are introduced to the group in pairs to lessen the pressure placed upon a child who already lacks critical social skills. Whenever new members are to be introduced to the group, a minimum of 2 weeks' notice is given so as to attenuate anxieties aroused by changes in the group's composition.

5. **Removal of members.** Any child unable to abide by minimal rules of coexistence is considered for removal after a trial of 4–6 weeks. Removal of a member usually occurs on the basis of unremitting antisocial behavior that cannot be adequately contained, managed, or moderated within the group. Children within the group are integrally involved because such an intervention arouses guilt about expelling a member as well as fears of being extruded. If the removal of a child is necessary, alternative provisions for treatment are made for the child in conjunction with his or her parents.

6. **Ending the year of treatment.** The ending of PGP is dealt with explicitly, both by making an announcement about the last session and by marking the event on the calendar for all the children to see. Individual meetings with the children and their parents are planned at the conclusion of the group to summarize individual progress and to review future treatment needs. The termination of the group allows each child—and the group as a whole—to experience separation and to express feelings of attachment. With the active participation of the children, therapists should review the group's progress and the achievements of group members throughout the year. The children are encouraged to demonstrate, through words and play, their positive and negative feelings about their experiences within the group.

During the ending phase of PGP, the same kinds of therapist verbal interventions continue to be used as had been throughout the initial and middle phases. Of the categories of verbal interventions employed, however, *attention-directing remarks* and *interpretations* are primary, buttressed by secondary use of *supportive* and *facilitative statements.* "Interpretations and 'look-at' statements are useful to clarify and share feelings of rivalry, defeat, and envy among those who have improved versus those who remain behind, as well as overall feelings of loss for the group that is coming to a close" (P. F. Kernberg and Chazan 1991, p. 280).

Some of the children who participated in PGP will be sufficiently improved to terminate treatment. In addition to substantial gains in the acquisition of social skills, these children will have progressed in modulating their aggression and impulses within more acceptable social parameters, and they will have consolidated a healthier self-esteem. Their conflicts with authority figures will have been moderated, and their capacity for self-awareness and for appreciation of another person's perspective will have improved.

Conclusion

The need for treatment-relevant interventions for children and adolescents with CD has been amply demonstrated in both the research and the literature of current psychotherapy practice. P. F. Kernberg and Chazan's (1991) manual-based psychotherapy for SEPP, parent training, and PGP directly addresses this need. These three approaches constitute a formal curriculum, supported with individual supervision, for the integrated treatment of children with CD.

Because children with CD suffer from behavioral impulsiveness and a tendency to express themselves through actions rather than words, the three treatments formulated by P. F. Kernberg and Chazan share a heavy emphasis on the therapist's verbal interventions. By means of such interventions, therapists seek to enhance the capacity of these children to express affects through verbal channels as a substitute for impulsive actions. Another objective common to SEPP, parent training, and PGP is to improve the child's functioning by promoting the acquisition of social skills, the expression of aggression and impulses within more acceptable social parameters, and the consolidation of healthier self-esteem.

A final contribution of manual-based treatment approaches deserves note: By their systematic and rigorous specification of all aspects of a particular treatment, these approaches afford defined avenues for formal outcome studies of the efficacy of various interventions.

References

Achenbach TM: The child behavior profile, I: boys aged 6 through 11. J Consult Clin Psychol 46:478–488, 1978

Achenbach TM, Edelbrock CS: Manual for the Child Behavior Checklist and Revised Child Behavior Profile. Burlington, University of Vermont, Department of Psychiatry, 1983

Barkley RA: Attention Deficit Hyperactivity Disorder: A Handbook for Diagnosis and Treatment. New York, Guilford, 1990

Beardslee W: Development of a preventive intervention for families in which parents have serious affective disorders, in Depression and Families: Impact and Treatment. Edited by Keitner GI. Washington, DC, American Psychiatric Press, 1990, pp 103–120

Bemporad JR, Schwab ME: The DSM-III and clinical child psychiatry, in Contemporary Directions in Psychopathology: Toward the DSM-IV. Edited by Millon T, Klerman GL. New York, Guilford, 1986, pp 135–150

Bowlby J: Attachment and Loss, Vol 2: Separation. New York, Basic Books, 1973

Bowlby J: Attachment and Loss, Vol 3: Loss, Sadness and Depression. New York, Basic Books, 1980

Breen MJ, Altepeter TS: Disruptive Behavior Disorders in Children: Treatment-Focused Assessment. New York, Guilford, 1990

Conners CK: A teacher rating scale for use in drug studies with children. Am J Psychiatry 126:152–156, 1969

Conners CK: Conners' Rating Scales Manual: Instruments for Use With Children and Adolescents. North Tonawanda, NY, Multi-Health Systems, 1989

Forehand R, Atkinson BM: Generality of treatment effects with parents as therapists: a review of assessment and implementation procedures. Behavior Therapy 8:575–593, 1977

Forehand R, McMahon RJ: Helping the Noncompliant Child: A Clinician's Guide to Parent Training. New York, Guilford, 1981

Freud A: Normality and Pathology in Childhood. New York, International Universities Press, 1965

Hartmann H: Ego Psychology and the Problem of Adaptation. New York, International Universities Press, 1958

Herbert M: Conduct Disorders of Childhood and Adolescence: A Behavioral Approach to Assessment and Treatment. New York, Wiley, 1978

Hinshaw SP: On the distinction between attentional deficits\hyperactivity and conduct problems\aggression in child psychopathology. Psychol Bull 101:443–463, 1987

Kazdin AE: Treatment of Antisocial Behavior in Children and Adolescents. Homewood, IL, Dorsey Press, 1985

Kazdin AE: Treatment of antisocial behavior in children: current status and future directions. Psychol Bull 102:187–203, 1987

Kernberg OF: Object Relations Theory and Clinical Psychoanalysis. New York, Jason Aronson, 1977

Kernberg PF, Chazan SE: Children With Conduct Disorders: A Psychotherapy Manual. New York, Basic Books, 1991

Luborsky L: Principles of Psychoanalytic Psychotherapy: A Manual for Supportive-Expressive Treatment. New York, Basic Books, 1984

Luborsky L, DeRubeis RJ: The use of psychotherapy treatment manuals: a small revolution in psychotherapy research style. Clinical Psychology Review 4:5–14, 1984

Mahler M, Pine F, Bergman A: The Psychological Birth of the Human Infant. New York, Basic Books, 1975

Patterson GR: Coercive Family Processes. Eugene, OR, Castalia, 1982

Patterson GR, Reid JB, Jones RR, et al: A Social Learning Approach to Family Intervention. Eugene, OR, Castalia, 1975

Peed S, Roberts M, Forehand R: Evaluation of the effectiveness of a standardized parent training program in altering the interactions of mothers and their noncompliant children. Behav Modif 1:323–350, 1977

Quay HC: A critical analysis of the DSM-III as a taxonomy of psychopathology in childhood and adolescence, in Contemporary Directions in Psychopathology: Toward the DSM-IV. Edited by Millon T, Klerman GL. New York, Guilford, 1986, pp 151–165

Roberts MW, McMahon RJ, Forehand R, et al: The effect of parental instruction-giving on child compliance. Behavior Therapy 9:793–798, 1978

Safer DJ, Allen D: Hyperactive Children. Baltimore, MD, University Park Press, 1976

Scheidlinger S: Focus on Group Psychotherapy: Clinical Essays. New York, International Universities Press, 1982

Spitz R: No and Yes. New York, International Universities Press, 1957

Spitz R: On the Genesis of Superego Components: The Psychoanalytic Study of the Child. New York, International Universities Press, 1958, pp 375–404

Stern DN: The Interpersonal World of the Infant: A View From Psychoanalysis and Developmental Psychology. New York, Basic Books, 1985

Thomas A, Chess S, Birch HG: Temperament and Behavior Disorders in Children. New York, New York University Press, 1968

Wells KC, Forehand R: Child behavior problems in the home, in Handbook of Clinical Behavior Therapy. Edited by Turner SM, Calhoun K, Adams HE. New York, Wiley, 1981, pp 527–567

Wells KC, Forehand R: Conduct and oppositional disorders, in Handbook of Clinical Behavior Therapy With Children. Edited by Bornstein PH, Kazdin AE. Homewood, IL, Dorsey Press, 1985, pp 218–265

Winnicott DW: The Maturational Processes and the Facilitating Environment. New York, International Universities Press, 1965

Winnicott DW: Playing and Reality. New York, Basic Books, 1971

Chapter 10

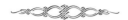

Family Interventions

G. Pirooz Sholevar, M.D.

T he interpersonal dimension of conduct disorder (CD) in children and adolescents has been broadly recognized. CD tends to occur extensively in families characterized by a high level of disagreement and tension between parents (Rutter and Giller 1983), and it is this discord, not the presence of a divorce or separation in the family, that creates the risk factor (Hetherington et al. 1979). Family interventions with youth with CD have been a significant focus of inquiry beginning with the pioneering work of Minuchin et al. (1967), Patterson (1982), and other investigators. Progress in this area has continued with the contributions of the school of functional family therapy (Alexander and Parsons 1982), Reiss and his colleagues (Reiss 1981, 1982; Reiss and Olivieri 1983), and psychodynamic family therapy (Ackerman 1958; Friedman et al. 1971; Sholevar 1991; Sholevar and Schwoeri, in press; Sonne 1981). Family intervention for CD assumes further significance based on two additional factors: 1) the high prevalence of these disorders—CDs are estimated to account for up to 50% of clinically referred youth, or 5% of the youth population in general (Rutter et al. 1970, 1975); and 2) this population's heavy use of mental health and psychiatric services, residential treatment centers, court-affiliated facilities, and correctional institutions. In addition to the high costs associated with such lengthy and extensive interventions, the treatment can be frequently rendered ineffective by the continued negative effect of families on the youngsters following their physical separation.

The purpose of this chapter is to review the disturbances in family relationships and interpersonal interactions of children with CD reported by different investigators and to describe the range of intervention options available for such families. A separate chapter in this volume (Chapter 11) is devoted to the ground-breaking work of Patterson and parent management training programs because of the extensiveness of the findings by this productive group.

Early History

The role of parental psychopathology in the genesis of antisocial behavior in the children was first described by Johnson and Szurek (1952). These authors discussed moral deficiencies and "superego lacunae" in antisocial children corresponding to psychopathic tendencies in the parents that were transmitted to their offspring in the course of their development. The collusive relationship between these parents and their children resulted in active maintenance of the children's antisocial tendencies by the parents, who acted as enablers at the time of antisocial crises.

A more systematic study of antisocial tendencies was undertaken by the Multiple Impact Therapy (MIT) group (MacGregor 1967) in Galveston, Texas. In this investigation, a team of mental health professionals met intensively with family and family subgroups over a 2-day period. Four patient groups described by the investigators included two groups each of "rebels" and "autocrats." The rebels showed traits closely resembling those defined in DSM-III-R (American Psychiatric Association 1987) for CD. These patients exhibited a preadolescent level of functioning during their adolescence, exemplified by behaviors such as running away, sexual promiscuity, and legal difficulties; demanded the privileges of adults and were highly ambivalent but fascinated by authority figures; and manifested great interest in their membership and status with groups and gangs. The autocrats displayed qualities similar to those defined in DSM-III-R for oppositional defiant disorder. They were characterized by temper tantrums and oppositional and defiant behavior at home; seemed oblivious and "blind" to the authority of parents and teachers; and reacted strongly when frustrated, frequently exhibiting explosive behavior.

Family relationships of rebels.   The homes of rebels were highly organized and had a definite institutional flavor. Both husband and wife were extremely competent in their activities, inside and outside of the home, but their enjoyment of each other was very limited. There were no projects shared between the couples. There seemed to be a tacit agreement between the husband and wife not to invade each other's privacy or domain. Both parents generally worked and were highly involved in the community. The adolescent was also involved in the community and with a peer group but was isolated from the family at home. The problems were generally acted out by the adolescent in the school to allow the father to remain uninvolved at home. The problematic behavior appeared to have the flavor of acting out the wishes of the parent of the same sex. There seemed to be a crush on the parent of the other sex. At home there was the lack of differentiation between genders and between youth and old age. The fathers appeared cooperative and "good" but pompous in the family sessions. Most mothers had career training but felt inferior to the fathers. Some of them had physical or fertility problems early in the marriage. At home, the mothers were aggressive figures, whereas the fathers exhibited passive-aggressive behavior. Outside the home, the fathers were aggressive whereas the mothers behaved in a passive-aggressive fashion. The adolescent behaved in an unpredictable and emotionally unstable manner. The communication system in the family did not allow for the direct processing of information, and the family members learned about each other through indirect routes.

Family relationships of autocrats.   The family relationships of autocrats revealed emotional distance between the father and the mother. The mother was "consumed" with the adolescent and his problems, and the adolescent's actions seemed to be an attempt to gain autonomy from this close mother-child bond. The peer relationships were poor due to the explosiveness and poor frustration tolerance of the autocrat. The autocrats wanted to be involved with other children only on their own terms. They were more interested in manipulating adults than in spending time with peers. They greatly enjoyed feelings of omnipotence and were afraid of limits being put on them.

The home spirit was low, echoing the gray and depressed mood of the fathers. The mothers did not seem to have any adult interests, were preoccupied with their children, and neglected their husbands. The mothers were the aggressive figures in the home. They married beneath themselves, were disappointed in their husbands, and exploited their children for their own needs. Fathers were passive at home but aggressive outside the family. As husbands, they ignored their wives' needs and frequently were absent from the home in the early stages of the family life.

Although both rebels and autocrats responded relatively well to treatment, the therapeutic rate of success for rebels (64%) was somewhat inferior to the positive therapeutic results achieved with autocrats (75%).

Family Characteristics

The parents and families of children with CD have been described as exhibiting a number of dysfunctional characteristics. The family members of children with CD are more likely to suffer from various psychiatric disorders than are those of children in the general population (Rutter et al. 1970). Antisocial behavior and alcoholism, particularly of the father, are two of the more consistently reported parental characteristics of youth with CD (Robins 1966;

Rutter and Giller 1983; West 1982). Parental disciplinary practices and attitudes have been especially well studied. Parents of youth with CD tend to be harsh in their attitudes and disciplinary practices with their children (Farrington 1978; Glueck and Glueck 1968; McCord et al. 1961; Nye 1958). Child abuse tends to be more common in families of children with CD than in families in the general population or in families of other children referred to child guidance clinics (Behar and Stewart 1982; Lewis et al. 1979). Erratic, inconsistent, and lax disciplinary practices by one or both parents are also characteristic of families of children with CD: one parent may be severely punitive while the other may be lax in disciplinary practices (Glueck and Glueck 1950; McCord et al. 1959). Parents of antisocial children are more likely to issue frequent commands to their children, to reward deviant behavior directly through attention and compliance, and to ignore or provide adverse consequences for prosocial behavior. Lax parental supervision, as another aspect of the parent-child interaction, has been frequently reported in youth with CD (Glueck and Glueck 1968; Goldstein 1984; Robins 1966). Parents of children with CD are less likely to monitor their children's whereabouts, to make arrangements for childcare when they are temporarily away from the home, and to provide rules in the home about where the children can go (Wilson 1980).

Parents of children with CD show less acceptance of their children; provide less warmth, affection, and emotional support; and report less attachment (Loeber and Dishion 1983; McCord et al. 1959; West and Farrington 1973) than parents of youth without CD. Unhappy marital relations, interpersonal conflict, and aggression characterize the parental relationships of delinquent and antisocial children (Hetherington and Martin 1979; Rutter and Giller 1983). Early marriage of the parents, lack of parental interest in the child's school performance, and lack of family participation in activities have also been reported (Glueck and Glueck 1968; Wadsworth 1979).

Different family characteristics are reported in families of children with different subtypes of CD. Children with aggressive symptoms have been found to exhibit significantly more aversive and coercive behaviors in their interactions at home and are less compliant with their parents' requests than are children who steal (Patterson 1982; Reid and Hendricks 1973). The parents of "stealers" show greater emotional distance in relation to their children (lack of responding, less disapproval, fewer commands) than do the parents of "aggressors."

The Cambridge-Somerville Youth Study (McCord et al. 1959) attempted to examine the roots of delinquency in the general population. The mass of data gathered in a 30-year follow-up of the group of children in this study demonstrated a link between the disciplinary patterns in the homes of the children and their subsequent conduct problems. The study reported that if the quarrelsome, neglectful, and lax disciplinary practices of parents were coupled with withdrawal of love as a punitive measure, only 14% of the children became delinquent. The next lowest rate of delinquency (21%) was found in the settings in which consistently punitive disciplinary methods were maintained. When a more loving kind of discipline was employed, the rate rose to 27%, possibly because of the confusion created by the affect.

Boyle and Offord (1990) compared the parental divorce rate in a group of children with CD with that in a control group. Within the 5 years of study, they found a higher divorce rate in the parents of children with CD than in those of the control group.

Contemporary Family Approaches

Structural Family Therapy

The contributions of Minuchin and his colleagues to the understanding of CD and delinquency in boys first emerged in the book *Families of the Slums* (1967), in which they described families of a group of delinquent boys in Wiltwyck School in New York City and elaborated on a variety of functional and structural family characteristics. The families of these boys seemed to be functionally organized around the mother, who maintained a tight coalition with the children, excluding the physically or emotionally absent father. The interactions between the mother and the children served the function of underlining the significance of the mother, who felt very unsure of her own value and identity. The children were used as a group of interchangeable objects—essentially soulless creatures who were expected to submit totally to maternal demands in order to make the mother feel effective and valuable. Minuchin labeled these families "mother-centered" because the whole family was expected to function in a way that promoted the importance of the mother. Once the children were out of the mother's sight, their behavior was considered unimportant because it no longer reflected upon her competence. Therefore, a major functional deficiency reported was the lack of a code of rules and values by which the children could be guided regardless of the presence or absence of the mother. In the presence of the mother, they were expected to fully comply with the maternal expectations without asking for explanations. However, because they lacked an internal code of rules and values, the children were at a total loss as to how to behave in the mother's absence.

The father in such families was generally left out of the close coalition between the mother and the children because he was seen as a competitor for the maternal position. The mother also exhibited little capacity to relate to another adult on an equal and cooperative basis. The frequent outcome of this type of family structure was the gradual drifting of the father away from the family unit, resulting in separation and divorce. The father maintained little contact with the children after his departure from the family.

Minuchin described delinquency occurring in both enmeshed and disengaged families—the two major family types described in structural family therapy. In enmeshed families, the delinquency was the result of lack of individuation. The overly reactive quality of interpersonal interactions made the children prone to much mischief and misbehavior both outside and inside the family. In disengaged families, the weakness of parental executive power resulted in the parentification of one of the older children, who in turn acted as a bully toward the younger children due to the lack of parental involvement and supervision. Later on, this bullying behavior extended to others outside the family when the child acted in an aggressive and destructive way toward the peer group or joined a peer group with the same characteristics.

Minuchin has emphasized the low level of cooperative behavior and poor role differentiation in families of delinquent youth.

Parent Management Training

Patterson and his colleagues have studied delinquent children and their families over the past 20 years. Their recent work has focused on observing and coding family interactions in home situations.

The work of Patterson et al. has been described in a large number of publications, particularly in Patterson's comprehensive book *Coercive Family Processes* (1982). Patterson's approach is based on social learning theory. It recognizes the high prevalence of aggressive behavior in such families. Because of the high prevalence of aggressive behaviors, the youngster is likely to exhibit aggression disproportionally to the situation. The mother will then react to the child's behavior by excessively aggressive and punitive behavior. The child persists and accelerates his or her aggressive behavior. The parent backs away and withdraws the punishment. This aggregation of behaviors—called the "coercive trap" by Patterson—tends to teach the child over a period of time that persistence and acceleration of aggressive behavior is rewarding.

The goal of parent management training is to institute planned and effective disciplinary and management practices with parents while simultaneously rewarding the child's prosocial behavior. The extensive application of parent management training with a large number of families with children who have CD over the last 20 years has resulted in the following findings:

1. Parent management training is superior to alternative interventions or no treatment with aggressive youth.
2. The result of parent management training is generalizable to other situations: children exhibit behavioral improvement in school and other environments.

3. The effective treatment of CD reduces both the likelihood that younger siblings will develop similar disorders and the risk of parental (maternal) depression.

The work of Patterson et al. has also enhanced our understanding of the connection between CD and depression, both in children and in their mothers (caregivers). Although in the short term depression can act as a coercive mechanism by inhibiting aggression or forcing compliance in other family members, in the long term it results in further aggressive behavior. According to this model, mothers may react to CD in their children by exhibiting short-lived depression, succumbing to chronic depression, or resisting depression. The major behavioral link is irritability in the mother, who can overreact to as well as provoke the behavior of the child. Therefore, irritable behavior in the mother may instigate as well as maintain the coercive family interactions.

Chapter 11 of this volume contains a complete description of parent management training.

Functional Family Therapy

Functional family therapy (FFT) was developed by Alexander and his co-workers (Alexander and Parsons 1982; Barton and Alexander 1981). This model emphasizes the functional value of the child's aggressive behavior in maintaining family operations and structure. FFT is an integrative approach that relies on systems theory and behaviorism. More recently, a cognitive perspective that emphasizes the attributional–information-processing component of change has been added to the FFT model. Clinical problems are conceptualized from the standpoint of the functions they serve in the family as a system, as well as for different family members. The therapist assumes that the problem behavior in the child represents the only way that some interpersonal functions, such as support and distancing, can be achieved among family members. The problematic behaviors and interactions within the family are considered a direct means of fulfilling these functions. Therefore, the goal of treatment is to alter interaction and communication patterns in such a way as to enhance adaptive functioning.

The therapeutic strategies in FFT draw from the extensive behavioral family relational research studies describing specific maladaptive parent-child interactions. For example, research underlying functional family therapy has found that families of delinquents show higher rates of defensiveness in their communication, both in parent-child and in parent-parent interactions, and lower rates of mutual support. Such families use high rates of system-disintegrating and defensive communications. In contrast, more adaptive families use more system-integrating or supportive communications. The goal of treatment is to improve communication within the family and to enhance supportive interactions and reciprocity among family members.

The FFT approach particularly concentrates on two types of family interactions: supportive and defensive. Supportiveness is exhibited by listening to the views of other family members, attempting to understand their perspectives on different situations, and making compromises in one's own position to accommodate the other family members' viewpoints. Compared with families of nondelinquents, families of youth with CD show a lower rate of mutual support (Alexander 1973). Improving supportive communication is a functional goal of treatment and has been correlated with a lower rate of recidivism of delinquent behavior in the youth.

In terms of treatment methodology, FFT encourages family members to examine the relational function that conduct problems serve within the family. The therapist points out the interdependencies among family members in their day-to-day functioning, with specific reference to the presenting problems. This alternative way of viewing the problem results in more constructive modes of family interaction and problem solving. Reframing and positive attribution are also used as important tools for cognitive structuring.

The goal of treatment is to enhance support, positive reinforcement, and reciprocity among family members as well as to establish clear interpersonal communication and negotiation to solve problems. The family is provided with a manual that describes behavioral principles (e.g., reinforcement and extinction) in order to help them become familiar with the concepts used in treatment. The family is then asked to identify the behavioral changes expected from different members. These expectations are incorporated into a reinforcement system at home that aims to enhance adaptive behavior in exchange for privileges. The interventions focus heavily on in-session behaviors where the family communication can be altered directly. The therapist can also help provide social reinforcement for clarification of problems and solutions.

In terms of treatment outcome, the impact of FFT has been measured in a study of status and index offenses in male and female adolescents: runaway behavior, truancy, unmanageability, and theft. FFT was compared with attention-placebo intervention and no treatment. After eight treatment sessions, FFT was found to have led to greater and more equitable discussions among family members and to an increase in frequency and duration of spontaneous speech. The changes were superior to those demonstrated with the placebo and the no-treatment conditions. Furthermore, Alexander and Parsons (1973) compared FFT with client-centered family groups, psychodynamically oriented family therapy, and no treatment. Their results suggested greater improvement in family interactions and lower recidivism rates of juvenile offenses lasting up to 18 months after treatment. The follow-up data obtained $2\frac{1}{2}$ years later indicated that siblings of the adolescents who received FFT showed significantly lower rates of referral to juvenile courts. Therefore, the study suggests beneficial effect of FFT on the index adolescents as well as their siblings.

Behavioral Family Therapy

Behavioral family therapists emphasize that aggression is a fairly stable characteristic in youth with CD and that aggressive behavior makes a significant contribution to family patterns. The problems are made worse by poor parental management skills. The extensive findings of behavioral groups have been summarized succinctly by Tolan and Mitchell (1989):

1. There is a high level of parental conflict around the transmission of values and the disciplining of the children.
2. There is a lack of hierarchical differentiation between parents and children, leading to confusion in family conversations and decision making. This lack of differentiation results in children exhibiting an inappropriately significant role in family decisions, with the parental role reduced to one of complaining.
3. There is a low level of positive mood and a predominance of aversive and oppressive affect in the family.
4. Effective communications are frequently mislabeled as aggressive.
5. One or a few family members dominate family communications and refuse to negotiate or compromise.

In terms of treatment course, a number of principles are emphasized by behavioral family therapists. Progress in treatment is slow and can take from 6 to 9 months of weekly sessions. The general aggressive tendency of these youngsters is an important contribution to the problem and should be addressed consistently. In addition to altering problematic behaviors exhibited by the child with CD, treatment should enhance prosocial behavior. Treatment should support a functional parent-child hierarchy and parental authority. The influence of deviant and normative peer groups should be addressed. Families should be assisted in recognizing the availability of social resources and in making use of them.

Psychodynamic Family Therapy

Psychodynamic family therapy emphasizes the importance of parent-to-child transmission of motivational forces for delinquent and antisocial tendencies. The ground-breaking work of Johnson and Szurek (1952) provided an early description of the transmission of poorly integrated parental antisocial tendencies to children. The transmission of such parental tendencies results in a poorly integrated internal system of conscience or superego that contains many lacunae and allows the child's delinquent behavior. Johnson and Szurek's concepts were further elaborated in the extensive work of Stierlin (1974), who described the *delegate* mode of family interaction, wherein the child's engagement in delinquent activities is correlated with the parents' desire to have the child act as an agent for their own unacceptable tendencies and actions. Stierlin further expanded his model by including the role of *ego activities*. According to this concept, the parents may refrain from participating in an activity because their egos or superegos are unwilling or unable to process such actions. Here, the child is assigned a role to act as the scout or agent of the parents to explore the activities in which the parents are unable to participate directly. However, the parents are keenly attentive to the exploits of their children and derive vicarious gratification from them. In the delegate mode of interaction, the child is sent out on a long leash and returns periodically to have the parents share his or her experiences and pleasures. The delegation process is one manifestation of an unresolved separation-individuation process between the child and the parents. The other two manifestations of the failure of this process are the "binding" mode of interaction, reflecting excessive undifferentiation and closeness between the child and one parent, and the "rejecting" mode, representing parental neglect of the child.

The more contemporary psychodynamic family approach to CD (Sholevar and Schwoeri, in press) emphasizes the mediating role of developmental failures, resulting in continued and shared family conflicts as well as shared family defenses for the containment of such conflicts. The model addresses both the conflictual modes of the relationship based on past conflicts transplanted to the present, and the "deficit" model, representing the lack of ego development and the corresponding behavioral and skill deficits resulting from this lack (Karasu 1992). The particular issues and patterns targeted in the therapeutic inquiry and resolution are historically based conflicts in the areas of

1. Neglect and abandonment.
2. Sexual and physical abuse.
3. Parental failure to create an adequate "holding environment" for the child in infancy, early childhood, and subsequent years.
4. Internalization of a family image (Sonne 1981) centered around parental conflict, uncooperation, and lack of reciprocity. Identification with parental defensiveness and uncooperation can interfere with a child's capacity for compliance and reciprocity in relationships.

The pathogenic effects of abusive, exploitative, and neglectful child-rearing practices can lead to repression of such memories and of their attendant affects, as well as to a propensity to view everyday interpersonal interactions as abusive. Parents who endured such childhoods can readily become involved in the "coercive family processes" described by Patterson (1982). The behavioral manifestations of such dynamically active conflicts are being irritable, provoking others, and being easily provoked by the actions of others. Remembering, reconstructing, and working through such memories can result in a reduction and resolution of irritability and provocativeness.

In some cases, clarifying communicational systems in the family, establishing a more adequate family structure, reducing defensiveness, and enhancing supportiveness may still result in little improvement in the child's symptomatic behavior. In such situations, the lack of therapeutic effectiveness may be related to the absence or failure of an emotional "holding environment" (Winnicott 1965), both in the present and extending backward to the child's infancy. Psychodynamic family therapy enhances those "holding" qualities in the family and corrects the ill effects of such past deficits.

Failure of "Coordination"

Reiss (1982) examined the three parameters of configuration, coordination, and closure in the families of patients with conduct and personality disorders as compared with those of schizophrenic patients. Such parameters are established by means of a card-sorting procedure (Reiss 1982), in which family members perform a neutral task that requires them to interact with one another. The parameters of configuration, coordination, and closure represent different family dimensions, or *paradigms*—that is, the ways in which family members define and organize their experiences (Reiss 1982; Reiss and Olivieri 1983; Olivieri and Reiss 1984). *Configuration* refers to the ability of family members to recognize the different patterns and the underlying rules; this ability remains unimpaired in families with CD. *Coordination* refers to the ability of family members to cooperate in order to achieve joint results. Coordination remains the weakest of the three parameters in families of youth with CD. *Closure* refers to the family's ability to adapt, change, and remain flexible.

With high configuration, the family views the world as ordered and itself as capable of mastery; with low configuration, the family sees the world as disordered and itself as helpless and threatened.

With high coordination, the family sees itself as a cohesive entity—a united group; with low coordination, the family is unable to discuss or reconcile different views and thus appears less integrated as a group and less able to problem-solve.

Early closure refers to the family's inability to change despite the need to do so. A family with delayed closure is one that sees the world as offering new and interesting experiences and itself as evolving and changing.

Reiss refers to families with delinquent children as "environment distance sensitive." These families are viewed as isolated from one another emotionally, with independent motives and perspectives in their interactions.

The model proposed by Reiss appears to have significant face validity. It is supportive of the findings of family therapists who have emphasized the lack of adaptive relatedness and growth promotion in children. It is also supportive of individual schools of psychotherapy for CD (Kernberg 1991; also see Chapter 8 of this volume) that have emphasized the narcissistic orientation and pattern of development in children and adolescents with CD.

Family Therapy and Acute Hospitalization

Hospitalization and Chronic Family Dysfunction

The hospitalization of children with CD frequently occurs at the height of the negative escalation between the parents and children. The child is hospitalized after repetitive fights with the parents, often because of school nonattendance or failure to complete school assignments. Through hospitalization, the parents may hope to enlist the assistance of the hospital to make the child comply with school attendance. After a few days of compliance with hospital procedures (or of absolute refusal to comply), the child may be discharged home without any change in his or her actual behavioral pattern. It would be helpful to investigate the likelihood of hospitalization's being effective in enabling a child to return to school following discharge. In cases in which the pattern of oppositional and rebellious behavior against parental expectation is severe and extreme, it seems unlikely that hospitalization will result in school attendance. The only possible exception to this pattern is if a dramatic shift in family dynamics has occurred whereby the family has become able to effectively address issues avoided for many years. If the school attendance problem is a chronic one and no resolution of significant emotional issues occurs in treatment, the likelihood of rapid change is low. The task may be better viewed as searching for ways to "manage" and "rehabilitate" a chronic and disabling symptom. Here, the parents and the child can be assisted to recognize that neither side possesses sufficient leverage to win the situation and be encouraged to forge a compromise. The compromise may be that the adolescent gets a job and contributes to paying for his or her own expenses in exchange for room and board and some access to the family car. In terms of children younger than the age of 14, a boarding school may be a more viable alternative, particularly if an intermediate outpatient family treatment course has proven ineffective. A small dose of humility can help the therapist to recognize that lack of improvement through family therapy is frequently a commentary on the severity of family dysfunction and the relative weakness of family rehabilitative forces, rather than directly reflective of the competence and skills of the family therapist or the efficacy of a particular family therapy approach.

Hospitalization and Children of Divorce

An emerging new phenomenon is the interface between hospitalization of children with CD and parental divorce. Divorce is significantly higher in parents of children with CD than in the general population. While the parents are still married, each parent tends to blame the child's problems on the shortcomings of the other parent and to overestimate his or her own ability to contain the child's behavior. In reality, a divorce often intensifies the conflict between the child and one parent and creates a pattern of rapid negative escalation, resulting in extreme behaviors such as suicidal threats on the part of the child and depression in the parent at the height of an escalated crisis. At one point, the child and one parent—usually the parent who was overinvolved before the divorce—reach an impasse. As the result of years of blaming the other parent as inadequate and as having caused the child's difficulties, the custodial parent cannot consider the option of sending the child to the noncustodial parent. Therefore, hospitalization is called upon to mediate the situation. The frequent outcome is that the child enters the hospital following a crisis with the custodial parent and is discharged to the house of the noncustodial parent following the hospital course. Although there are no definite statistics available for this phenomenon, probably somewhere between 10% and 20% of hospitalized CD children of divorced parents end up returning to the second parent following the hospitalization course. Here, the hospital seems to serve the function of introducing and opening an alternative residential custody option. Hospitalization can be made more efficient if hospital staff recognize their limited and specific role at this point rather than attempting to pursue a more ambitious course.

This phenomenon of "child switching" or "child keeping" has also occurred historically in nondivorcing families but with less frequency. In such circumstances, the nuclear and extended families have arranged to shift the children back and forth at the time of crisis in order to diffuse the tension.

Family Intervention in
Residential Treatment Centers

Family intervention in a residential treatment center should be guided by two variables: 1) the state of disintegration of the family unit, and 2) the level of availability of the family as a potential care provider or participant in psychiatric treatment. Based on assessment of these variables, families of patients in residential treatment centers can be divided into the following four groups: 1) available families, 2) potentially available families, 3) partially available families, and 4) totally unavailable families.

Available Families

The available family is forced to institutionalize the child following family confrontations at the height of negatively escalated interactions. However, the family and child are strongly bonded and dependent on one another to the point that they cannot "live with or without each other." Such families are available for home visits and participation in family sessions. The communication in available families is generally a covert attempt to force others into excessive concessions, which, although frequently granted, are followed by feelings of resentment and disappointment and coercive maneuvers. The therapeutic task is to enhance these families' leadership, power sharing, problem solving, and negotiation capabilities in an effort to enable them to form appropriate compromises. An underlying self-punishing or masochistic attitude in one or both parents may also require attention.

The major challenge in working with available families is to prevent premature interruption of treatment by the family after only a short stay in the residential treatment center. Such interruptions are primarily precipitated by collusive family maneuvers, dependency issues, feelings of loss, and the inability of the family and the child to tolerate separation. This danger should be addressed at the time of admission and remedial measures taken by establishing objective and clear goals before discharge from the treatment center.

Potentially Available Families

The potentially available family has lost its immediate ability to care for the child because of a loss of functional capacity in the nuclear or extended family. A history of divorce, remarriage, physical or psychiatric illness, or death should alert the treatment team to such limitations in family resources.

The therapeutic task is to recognize the limitations in the functional and caretaking capacity of these families and protect them from any unrealistic and premature demands. Furthermore, the functional capacity of the family should be increased by resolving conflict between the nuclear and extended families, improving the functional and economic capacity of the parents, and activating the parents' social networks.

A therapeutic goal for a family with this diminished level of functioning is to remain available as a support system to the child or adolescent while his or her ego capacity is increased and his or her dangerous and provocative behavior is modified through the residential treatment.

Partially Available Families

The partially available family only incompletely supports the child through erratic phone calls, occasional visits, or irregular attendance in treatment sessions. Its members cancel family sessions frequently and are defensive and unproductive when they attend. A major clinical finding in such families is the extreme nature of parental incapacity in managing life tasks. Severe personality disorders, long-standing covert depression, substance abuse, and unemployment or underemployment are common findings. Another important clinical finding is social isolation, lack of contact with extended family members, and very constricted and low-functioning social networks.

The primary therapeutic task is to prevent such families and their children from misleading one another into unrealistic expectations of reunion, particularly in the foreseeable future. Parental promises of family reunion here are usually countered by blaming the child for being unmanageable and therefore unsuitable to return home.

A realistic treatment strategy is to maintain the family's connection with the child psychologically while making realistic living plans for the child following discharge from the residential treatment center. The family can continue to remain as a resource to the group home or foster family following the child's discharge from the residential treatment center.

Totally Unavailable Families

The totally unavailable family is characterized by loss of contact with the child many years before his or her admission to a residential treatment center. The family of Shawn, described in Chapter 16, characterizes this type of family. There is usually a distorted and unrealistic expectation of a potential reunion between the family and the child. Such distorted fantasies should be discussed both immediately and continuously throughout residential treatment. It would be helpful if the families could be located early in the course of residential treatment and be made to verify—either in person or by telephone—their inability to take care of the child. This strategy would help resolve some of the child's dormant conflicts and facilitate his or her future adaptation to other living possibilities. Other innovative tactics with such families may include bringing them in for an extended family session with the specific goal of resolving some of the distortions of the past and enhancing the child's future adaptation.

Summary and Conclusions

Low levels of parental skills and cooperation are the prominent roots of arrested socialization, and a lack of appreciation for intimate and gratifying human relationships is evident in children with CD. The relational problems are further exaggerated by the child's observation of chronic parental discord and internalization of a family image constructed around intrafamilial conflict and isolation. Skill deficits in parental and marital communication and problem solving and conflicts in these relationships play significant roles in producing family dysfunction. The low level of parental differentiation and identity formation plays a fundamental role in family dysfunction by interfering with the development of an adequate self-image, self-esteem, and internal codes of behavior in the child. The transmission of parental antisocial tendencies to their children is facilitated by the low level of differentiation between parent and child.

Family treatment should focus on enhancing cooperation 1) between parents and children and 2) between parents as coparents and as a couple. Enhancing parent management skills can undermine the use of coercive, punitive, and impulsive interactions in the families. The higher divorce rate in parents of children with CD should be addressed with parents directly and early in treatment with the hope of mobilizing the rehabilitative and cooperative marital forces.

Future Direction

In the future, family studies should address and incorporate the expanding knowledge of biological and psychological characteristics of children with CD and the possible impact of such characteristics in undermining family development and integrity. Such investigations should include the following:

— The role of sustained and intense aggression in some children on family functioning and development
— The possible role of diminished response to punishment and excessive search for gratification in children with CD
— The role of the child with CD in promoting marital and family discord and divorce
— The role of neurotransmitters (serotonin) in the production of irritability, provocativeness, coercive family processes, and subsequent depression in the caregiver or the child
— Effective models of intervention with children with CD in hospitals and residential treatment centers

References

Ackerman N: The Psychodynamics of Family Life. New York, Basic Books, 1958
Alexander JF: Defense and supportive communications in normal and deviant families. J Consult Clin Psychol 40:223–231, 1973

Alexander JF, Parsons BV: Short-term behavioral intervention with delinquent families: impact on family process and recidivism. J Abnorm Psychol 81:219–225, 1973

Alexander JF, Parsons BV: Functional Family Therapy. Monterey, CA, Brooks/Cole, 1982

American Psychiatric Association: Diagnostic and Statistical Manual of Mental Disorders, 3rd Edition, Revised. Washington, DC, American Psychiatric Association, 1987

Barton C, Alexander JF: Functional family therapy, in Handbook of Family Therapy. Edited by Gurman AS, Kniskern DP. New York, Brunner/Mazel, 1981, pp 403–443

Behar D, Stewart MA: Aggressive conduct disorder of children. Acta Psychiatr Scand 65:210–220, 1982

Boyle MH, Offord DR: Primary prevention of conduct disorder: issues and prospects. J Am Acad Child Adolesc Psychiatry 29:227–233, 1990

Farrington DP: The family background of aggressive youths, in Aggressive and Antisocial Behavior in Childhood and Adolescence. Edited by Hersov LA, Berger M, Shaffer D. Oxford, UK, Pergamon, 1978, pp 73–93

Friedman A, Sonne J, Speck R, et al: Therapy With Families of Sexually Acting-Out Girls. New York, Springer, 1971

Glueck S, Glueck E: Unravelling Juvenile Delinquency, Cambridge, MA, Harvard University Press, 1950

Glueck S, Glueck E: Delinquents and Nondelinquents in Perspective. Cambridge, MA, Harvard University Press, 1968

Goldstein HS: Parental composition, supervision and conduct problems in youths 12 to 17 years old. Journal of the American Academy of Child Psychiatry 23:679–684, 1984

Hetherington EM, Martin B: Family interaction, in Psychopathological Disorders of Childhood, 2nd Edition. Edited by Quay HC, Werry JS. New York, Wiley, 1979, pp 247–302

Hetherington EM, Cox M, Cox R: Family interaction and the social, emotional and cognitive development of children following divorce, in The Family: Setting Priorities. Edited by Vaughn V, Brazelton T. New York, Science & Medicine, 1979

Johnson AM, Szurek SA: The genesis of antisocial acting out in children and adults. Psychoanal Q 21:323–343, 1952

Karasu B: Developmentalist metatheory of depression and psychotherapy. Am J Psychother 46:37–57, 1992

Kernberg OF: Conduct Disorders in Children and Adolescents. New York, Basic Books, 1991

Lewis DO, Shanok SS, Pincus JH, et al: Violent juvenile delinquents: psychiatric, neurological, psychological, and abuse factors. Journal of the American Academy of Child Psychiatry 18:307–319, 1979

Loeber R, Dishion TJ: Early predictors of male delinquency: a review. Psychol Bull 94:68–99, 1983

MacGregor R: Progress in multiple impact therapy, in Expanding Theory and Practice in Family Therapy. Edited by Ackerman NW, Beatman FL, Sherman SN. New York, Family Service Association of America, 1967

McCord W, McCord J, Zola IK: Origins of Crime. New York, Columbia University Press, 1959

McCord W, McCord J, Howard A: Familial Correlates of aggression in nondelinquent male children. Journal of Abnormal and Social Psychology 62:79–93, 1961

Minuchin S, Montaluo B, Guerney B, et al: Families of the Slums: An Exploration of Their Structure and Treatment. New York, Basic Books, 1967

Nye FI: Families and Family Therapy, Cambridge, MA, Harvard University Press, 1958

Olivieri M, Reiss D: Family concepts and their measurement are seldom what they seem. Fam Process 23:33–48, 1984

Patterson GR: Coercive Family Process. Eugene, OR, Castalia, 1982

Reid JB, Hendicks AFCJ: Preliminary analysis of the effectiveness of direct home intervention for the treatment of predelinquent boys who steal, in Behavior Change: Methodology, Concepts and Practice. Edited by Hamerlynck LA, Handy LC, Mash EJ. Champaign, IL, Research Press, 1973, pp 20–219

Reiss D: The Family's Construction of Reality. Cambridge, MA, Harvard University Press, 1981

Reiss D: The working family. Am J Psychiatry 139:1412–1420, 1982

Reiss D, Olivieri M: Sensory experience and family process. Fam Process 22:289–308, 1983

Robins LN: Deviant Children Grown Up: A Sociological and Psychiatric Study of Sociopathic Personality. Baltimore, MD, Williams & Wilkins, 1966

Rutter MP, Giller H: Juvenile Delinquency: Trends and Perspectives. New York, Penguin, 1983

Rutter MP, Tizard J, Whitmore K (eds): Education, Health and Behavior. London, Longman, 1970

Rutter MP, Cox A, Tupling C, et al: Attainment and adjustment in two geographical areas, I: the prevalence of psychiatric disorder. Br J Psychiatry 126:493–509, 1975

Sholevar GP: The family interview, in Textbook of Child and Adolescent Psychiatry. Edited by Wiener JM. Washington, DC, American Psychiatric Press, 1991, pp 84–91

Sholevar GP, Schwoeri L: Psychodynamic family therapy, in Textbook of Family and Marital Therapy. Edited by Sholevar GP. Washington, DC, American Psychiatric Press (in press)

Sonne J: Transference considerations in marriage and marital therapy, in The Handbook of Marriage and Marital Therapy. Edited by Sholevar GP. New York, Spectrum Medical & Scientific Books, 1981, pp 103–130

Stierlin H: Separating Parents and Adolescents: A Perspective on Running Away, Schizophrenia and Waywardness. New York, Quadrangle, 1974

Tolan PH, Mitchell ME: Families and the therapy of antisocial and delinquent behavior. Journal of Psychotherapy and the Family 6:29–48, 1989

Wadsworth M: Roots of Delinquency: Infancy, Adolescence and Crime. New York, Barnes & Noble, 1979

West DJ: Delinquency: Its Roots, Careers and Prospects. Cambridge, MA, Harvard University Press, 1982

West DJ, Farrington DP: Who Becomes Delinquent? London, Heinemann, 1973

Wilson H: Parental supervision: a neglected aspect of delinquency. British Journal of Criminology 20:215–221, 1980
Winnicott D: The Maturational Process and the Facilitating Environment. New York, International University Press, 1965

Chapter 11

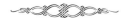

Parent Management Training

Karen C. Wells, Ph.D.

The practice of child therapy began more than 100 years ago and first took the form of direct intervention for children exhibiting behavioral, emotional, and cognitive disturbances. Contact with parents of child patients was often avoided, based in large part on the theories of Freud, who took the position that because of the family's pathological influence, the patient must be isolated from his or her family if improvement was to occur. In addition, Freud adopted the position that it is not factual events, but the patient's subjective perceptions, opinions, and fantasies about those events, that is of primary therapeutic importance. Therefore, observing and intervening in overt family interactions was considered unimportant and potentially counterproductive (Wells 1988).

Unfortunately, even though prodigious research efforts by many investigators over the last 25 years have documented the *direct controlling influence* of family interactions on child adjustment and maladjustment (Maccoby and Martin 1983; Parke and Slaby 1983; Wahler and Dumas 1987), the dominating influence of Freud has resulted in slow acceptance, in some quarters of the psychiatric community, of approaches that involve intervention with the parents and/or family as a vehicle for treating the child. It is the purpose of this chapter to provide a brief overview of empirically driven theoretical work on the relationship of parent and family variables to conduct disorder (CD) in children, and to present a therapy model—parent management training (PMT)—that arises out of that body of work. There is now considerable evidence attesting to both the efficacy and the limitations of this model, and that work will be presented as well. An aim of this review is to inform or update practitioners as to advances in the fields of theory and treatment of child CD so that treatment possibilities for this population can be expanded. In this regard, PMT is presented not as an alternative to traditional individual child therapy, but as an important component in the treatment armamentarium of those offering services to this difficult child population.

The emergence of contemporary PMT as a viable, theoretically sound, and empirically validated approach to the treatment of child CD can be traced to the 1950s and 1960s, when two reviews appeared noting the relative ineffectiveness of traditional forms of psychotherapy with children (Levitt 1957, 1963). Although Levitt's conclusions were subsequently criticized on several grounds (Barret et al. 1978), his work had an impact on a number of young researchers beginning their careers at that time. For example, in his book *Coercive Family Processes,* Patterson (1982) relates that at the time the Levitt reviews appeared, he (Patterson) was a trainee learning the fundamental child treatment techniques of that day (intensive, individual analytic therapy and nondirective play therapy). Patterson noticed, however, that not only he, but also even the most highly trained therapists, failed to effect permanent, objective changes in most aggressive child disorders. The Levitt reviews reinforced the idea that these experiences were not unique.

Observations of this sort led Patterson, Wahler, and other contemporaries and colleagues to conduct work advancing theory development and treatment progress in the area of child CD (Patterson 1982, 1986; Patterson et al. 1989; Wahler and Dumas 1989). This work led inexorably to examinations of parent and family influences in the development and maintenance of child aggressive behavior, as well as to therapeutic approaches that incorporate attention to family factors. PMT as a therapy model has arisen out of this work.

PMT is based on the central assumption that child aggression is acquired and maintained through social learning processes in the family. Social learning theory also posits temperamental characteristics in the child and psycho logical attributes of the parents as components contributing to the etiology of child aggression (Patterson 1982). However, the theory places primary emphasis on complex microscopic and macroscopic learning processes that occur in the context of family interactions. What is the evidence for the controlling function of these processes?

The first wave of research addressing this question looked at the behavioral characteristics and patterns that differentiate aggressive children from nonreferred children. This literature is substantial and has been reviewed in detail by Patterson (1982), McMahon and Wells (1989), Wells and Forehand (1981, 1985), and Wells (1984). To summarize, when children referred to clinics for problems of aggression are observed in the home by trained observers using reliable complex behavioral coding systems, they have been shown—not unpredictably—to engage in higher rates of aversive behaviors, such as negative commands, disapproval, humiliating statements, noncompliance, negativity, physical aggression, and yelling, than their nonreferred counterparts. Furthermore, these behaviors are displayed in the context of interactions with other people and often occur in "bursts." What characterizes the aggressive child is the frequency and duration of these chains or bursts of aversive social interactions. Aggressive children display more frequent chains and ones of longer duration. Furthermore, their aversive behaviors are not random but contingent: the aversive behaviors are used contingently to produce a reliable impact on another family member (i.e., to control his or her behavior).

These same studies have shown that the parents of aggressive children also display a number of behavioral characteristics that differentiate them from the parents of nonaggressive children. The parents of aggressive children exhibit a significantly higher rate of aversive behavior directed toward their children. Their commands are poorly formulated and poorly delivered. A significantly higher proportion of their commands are delivered in a threatening, angry, or nagging way. They criticize their children more frequently and supply more negative and ineffective consequences to deviant as well as nondeviant behavior. These parents also provide significantly lower rates of positive attention and rewards for their children's prosocial behavior, and confront deviant behavior with effective consequences less frequently than do parents of nonaggressive children (Forehand et al. 1975; Patterson 1982).

The most interesting findings from this research are that aversive parent and child behaviors do not occur in isolation from one another, but rather take place in tight, reciprocal control processes during moment-to-moment interactions. Aggressive children and their parents tend to respond to one another in mutually reinforcing and escalating chains of aversive interaction, thereby accounting for the "burst" phenomenon noted in behavioral observations.

In summarizing the results of studies such as these, Patterson (1982) has called attention to an essential theme: The parents of aggressive children cannot or do not punish well. Instead of applying effective consequences to aggressive behavior, they engage in other behaviors—such as scolding, threatening (with no follow-through), nagging, and repeating commands—that do not effectively confront the child's behavior. Patterson and Reid have referred to this ineffective parent behavior as "nattering" or "irritable aggression"; that is, negative verbal interchanges that are not backed up by effective consequences. In one of his most important findings, Patterson (1982) showed that this irritable parental behavior has a paradoxical effect in that it actually serves to *escalate* the child's aggressive behavior. Thus, it has an effect exactly the opposite of that intended by the parent. After repeated interactions of this type, the child learns that nattering signifies irritation with no intention to follow through.

Lest the above analysis sound too much like an indictment of parents, it is essential to point out that the process of coercion among family members is a reciprocal-influence process in which aggressive behavior on the part of both parent and child is escalated and maintained by the behavior of the other member of the interacting dyad. In addition, Patterson (1982) reviews evidence that the propensity to behave aggressively on the part of both parent and child is also affected by the temperaments and psychological states of children and parents. Temperamentally difficult children, he asserts, require greater skill to deal with and, therefore, are more likely to elicit irritable reactions in even the most well-meaning parents.

There are currently two theories that attempt to explain the reinforcement processes inherent in these coercive interchanges. In his theoretical model, called "coercion theory," Patterson gives central status to negative reinforcement processes in moment-to-moment interactions. The key assumption is that some of children's coercive behaviors function to terminate aversive intrusions by other family members. Patterson's (1982) analyses show that family members in families of aggressive children are more likely than their counterparts in families of nonaggressive children to deliver aversive events to the child. When a child's coercive responses (e.g., yelling, hitting, humiliating) cause the attacker to terminate his or her intrusion, negative reinforcement occurs. In addition, because aversive intrusions produce negative autonomic arousal, the child's coercive behavior is further negatively reinforced by the reduction of arousal accompanying termination of the attack. The combined reinforcement effects of removing the aversive intrusion and reducing arousal produce coercive behaviors that are highly resistant to extinction.

Wahler and his colleague Dumas (Dumas 1984; Dumas and Wahler 1985; Wahler and Dumas 1986) have offered an alternative theoretical explanation for the reinforcement effects inherent in coercive bursts of family interaction. Variously labeled the "predictability hypothesis" or the "inconsistency theory," their explanation focuses on the larger context of parent-child interactions. They have shown that mothers of aggressive children are more indiscriminate in their use of aversive behavior toward their children, thereby providing an unpredictable environment for the child (Dumas and Wahler 1985). Reviewing laboratory work showing that unpredictable environments are inherently aversive, Wahler and Dumas postulate that the child's coercive behavior is negatively reinforced because it produces a *predictable* response from the parent regardless of the valence of that response (i.e., positive or negative). The predictable—albeit negative—response is reinforcing because it temporarily removes the unpredictable contextual background. This process would account for the puzzling clinical observation that some aggressive children seem to "seek out" negative attention from their parents.

Processes involving irritable, ineffective discipline are present in families of children with both overt (oppositional behavior, arguing, physical aggression) and covert (stealing, lying, truancy) forms of aggressive behavior (Patterson 1982). Interestingly, families with covertly aggressive children have lower rates of engaging in irritable aggression than do families with overtly aggressive children—that is, parents of oppositional children are more irritable in their verbal aggression than parents of antisocial children, who, in turn, display more irritability than parents of nonaggressive children (Patterson 1982, p. 252). What further distinguishes the parents of overtly and covertly aggressive children is a parenting construct variously labeled *supervision* and *monitoring* (Lobber and Dishion 1983; Patterson and Stouthamer-Loeber 1984). At a behavioral level, this construct refers to failure on the part of parents of covertly aggressive children to monitor and track both the child's whereabouts and the child's performance of basic expectations. At a more basic relational level, the construct reflects a lack of parental involvement with the child and/or poor parental bonding to the child (Patterson et al. 1989). Therefore, the picture in the families of covertly aggressive children tends to be one of distance and disengagement. When family members do talk, they also display more irritability than do nonaggressive families.

In addition to *effective discipline* and *monitoring*, Patterson and his group have also investigated the association of other macroscopic parenting constructs with aggressive child behavior. These constructs include the ability of parents to define and set clear *house rules* and to use effective *problem-solving skills* when confronted with novel situations presented by the child. Although both of these constructs show some empirical association with aggressive child behavior, the most robust predictors are *discipline* and *monitoring* (Loeber 1990; Loeber and Dishion 1983).

Several research groups have examined the impact of other family context variables on parenting behavior and child aggression. For example, parents of aggressive children experience more personal distress (depression and anxiety), more marital distress (overt marital conflict and divorce), and more extrafamilial distress (insularity and social isolation) than do parents of nonaggressive children (see Griest and Wells 1983 for a review). Each of these factors has been demonstrated to have a significant relationship to child aggression. For example, Wahler (1980) reported *daily* negative covariation between mothers' friendly contacts outside the home and maternal aversive and child oppositional behavior inside the home. On days when mothers reported high-friendship contacts, maternal aversive behavior and oppositional child behavior were consistently lower than on low-friendship days.

Forehand's research group has shown that maternal depression negatively biases mothers' perceptions of their children and also adversely affects mothers' parenting behavior (e.g., Forehand et al. 1986). The relationship of marital conflict and divorce to child aggression is well documented (Emery 1982; Hetherington et al. 1982).

The question of how these molar family context variables affect child aggression has been the subject of recent efforts by various research groups. Most authors conclude that these variables have an impact on child aggression because they disrupt parenting practices (Fauber and Long 1991). For example, in his recent expansion of coercion theory, Patterson describes a class of variables called "disrupters." Disrupters include stressors such as divorce, "daily hassles," unemployment, and medical problems. Parental substance use constitutes another subset of disrupters. Patterson's group has already collected data consistent with the model that the effects of these variables on child aggression are mediated by disruptions in parenting practices and behaviors (Patterson 1986; Patterson et al. 1989). Fauber et al. (1990) showed that the relationship between marital conflict and externalizing problems of young adolescents could in large part be explained by perturbations in parenting practices.

Wahler and Dumas (1989) have reviewed the literature on stress and attention in the context of a model linking parenting to child aggression. They propose an ecosystemic, interbehavioral analysis linking stressful context variables (e.g., marital strife, socioeconomic disadvantage, social insularity) in the larger system to disruptions in complex parental attention and monitoring functions, irritable and indiscriminate parenting behaviors, and child aggression. In the interbehavioral model, the stress-performance linkage is mediated by the construct of parental *surveillance* (attention and monitoring), which Wahler and Dumas consider a keystone component of the parent-child relationship. Parents who display deficient attention/monitoring processes are prone to develop response-response linkages that permit stimuli in one setting to influence behavior in other settings. The interbehavioral model is an interesting heuristic device because in departing from the tight stimulus-response requirement of traditional behaviorism, it opens up theoretical explanations for the observed relationships between ecosystemic variables and child aggression.

The extensive literature, which I have only briefly reviewed and summarized here, indicates that a complex set of parenting dysfunctions is directly related to child aggression. There is a growing body of evidence supporting a causal connection between dysfunctional parenting and child aggression. The social learning model posits that when child aggression is displayed early in life (i.e., in *early starters*) it is importantly affected both by child temperamental variables (impulsivity, hyperactivity) and by the transmission of poor parenting practices via poor grandparental models (Loeber 1990; Patterson 1986; Patterson et al. 1989). For *late starters*, it is likely that disrupters in the ecosystem perturb parenting and family management practices. In both early and late starters, deficient or disrupted family management and parenting practices set the stage for disturbed parental monitoring and a spiral of coercive, irritable family interactions leading to child aggression. In his expanded developmental model of child CD, Patterson (1986) has convincingly argued that this "basic training for aggression in the family" leads to the well-known concomitants of child CD—namely, low self-concept, poor peer relationships, and academic failure.

Parent management training (PMT) as a therapy model has arisen out of the empirically driven theoretical work reviewed above. It is based on the notion that because the most direct mechanism of effect on child aggression is disrupted family and parenting processes, intervention at the level of parenting practices represents an accessible and potentially effective intervention tactic (Fauber and Long 1991). In fact, in his recent comprehensive review of treatment research for childhood CD, Kazdin (1987) concluded that PMT is the most promising treatment tested to date.

A more expanded behavioral family therapy model (Wells 1985) utilizes PMT but also incorporates attention to ecosystemic variables (e.g., parental depression, marital distress) into the overall therapy program. An expanded model has been recommended to address these broader context variables, under the assumption that doing so will lead to enhanced treatment effects for systemically distressed families. However, this chapter is confined to a discussion of PMT alone.

Parent Management Training Programs

Several eminent clinician/researchers have been involved in the development and evaluation of PMT programs for aggressive children, among them Patterson and his group, Forehand and his group, Wahler and his group, K. Daniel O'Leary, Elaine Blechman, and others. This review focuses on programs developed at two major centers that have produced the most extensive research: Rex Forehand and his colleagues at the University of Georgia, and Gerald Patterson, John Reid, and their colleagues at the Oregon Social Learning Center (OSLC). Forehand's program has been used primarily with younger children, whereas Patterson's and Reid's programs have been used mostly with older children and adolescents.

It should be noted that although the various PMT programs focus on different age populations and entail different technologies, there is considerable consensus across the programs on the fundamental concepts and basic elements of intervention. As recently reviewed by Miller and Prinz (1990), these fundamentals include 1) pinpointing and accurately labeling child behavior; 2) placing emphasis on prosocial behavior and away from an exclusive focus on antisocial behavior; 3) implementing daily tracking of specific child behaviors; 4) administering social and tangible reinforcers; 5) using nonphysical, nonviolent punishment procedures; 6) communicating clearly and at developmentally appropriate levels; and 7) learning to anticipate and solve new problems. These parenting skills are taught through a directive therapy process that includes discussion, in-session modeling and role playing of skills, homework assignments, and performance feedback. In most programs, therapy is paced so that new skills are not taught until previous ones have been mastered.

Another commonality across programs is the emphasis placed on *non-compliance* and its prosocial opposite, compliance, as essential targets for intervention. This focus on treatment of noncompliance is grounded in a number of studies showing that noncompliance is the keystone behavior in both overt and covert dimensions of aggressive behavior (Loeber and Schmaling 1985). The term *keystone* means that constituent members of a particular behavioral class covary together, such that when one behavior in the class changes, other behaviors in the same class reliably change with it. Thus, in a number of treatment studies, the modification of noncompliance led indirectly to decreases in other nontargeted aggressive behaviors (Patterson 1982; Russo et al. 1981; Wells et al. 1980a).

In addition, a number of developmentalists have shown that noncompliance, and the behaviors associated with it (e.g., arguing, whining), are developmental precursors of later, more antisocial forms of aggressive behavior (C. Edelbrock, "Conduct Problems in Childhood and Adolescence: Developmental Patterns and Progressions" (unpublished manuscript), August 1985; Patterson 1986). As mentioned earlier, Patterson's model also suggests that noncompliance plays a role in later academic and peer relationship problems. The implication is that early intervention at the level of behavioral noncompliance may interrupt the developmental unfolding of more serious forms of aggressive behavior in addition to forestalling social and academic failure. For all of these reasons, PMT programs attach central importance to the treatment of noncompliance.

Hanf-Forehand Parent Training Program

Rex Forehand and his colleagues developed a line of research based on a treatment program developed by Connie Hanf for use with $2\frac{1}{2}$- to 8-year-old children. This program has been explicated in detail by Forehand and McMahon (1981). Briefly, the program is divided into two phases.

In Phase I, parents learn a specific set of skills for improving their child's prosocial behaviors. To accomplish this, parents learn to be more effective reinforcing agents for their children by increasing the frequency and range of social rewards. They learn to attend to and describe the child's appropriate, prosocial behavior as well as to reduce their use of commands, questions, and criticisms directed to the child (i.e., nattering). After training in attending and describing, parents learn to use verbal and physical rewards contingent upon compliance and other prosocial behaviors that the parents consider desirable. Furthermore, they learn to ignore minor inappropriate behavior. Daily homework assignments are given to the parents to spend at least one 15-minute period (each) per day attending to and rewarding appropriate behavior. Parents are also required to use these skills outside the clinic to increase at least two prosocial child behaviors. All of these skills are taught with modeling, behavior rehearsal, and feedback from the therapist.

In Phase II, parents learn to decrease noncompliance displayed by their child. First, parents are taught to give clear, direct, age-appropriate commands (instructions) to their child. If the child does not comply with the initial command, parents learn to give a warning followed by a time-out procedure if the warning does not result in compliance. The time-out procedure consists of placing the child in a chair in a corner. The child must remain in the chair for 3–10 minutes (depending on the child's age) and must be quiet for the last 15–30 seconds. The child is then returned to the uncompleted task and the initial command is restated. The procedure continues until the child eventually complies. Time-out is administered in a very straightforward and matter-of-fact manner designed to eliminate nattering and irritable verbal interchange.

Once parents learn this fundamental set of skills, additional strategies may be used to promote generalization of treatment effects outside the home and to other behaviors. For example, once parents learn to apply a time-out procedure for noncompliance, they may establish a set of "house rules" that, if violated, result in an immediate time-out (e.g., no fighting, no name calling). This procedure is especially helpful for behaviors over which parents expect children to learn self-control. Likewise, parents learn how to implement time-out procedures outside the home or—in situations in which immediate time-out is not feasible—a marked time-out procedure. As with punishment inside the home, parents are always guided to accompany any punishment plan outside the home with a positive reinforcement plan for encouraging prosocial behavior.

Empirical Evaluation

Forehand and his colleagues have conducted an extensive program of research evaluating the efficacy and the generalization of treatment effects with this model of parent training as well as identifying factors that predict or moderate treatment outcome. Some of this research is reviewed in detail by Wells and Forehand (1981, 1985).

As is often the case in the first wave of research on a treatment program, the first several studies evaluating the efficacy of this approach to parent training were pre-/postanalyses with no control group (Forehand and King 1974; Forehand et al. 1974; C. Hanf and F. Kling, "Facilitating Parent-Child Interaction: A Two-Stage Training Model" (unpublished manuscript), September 1973). Each of these studies demonstrated significant improvement from pre- to posttreatment with oppositional children.

The first true experimental evaluation of this program was conducted by Peed et al. (1977). In this study, behavioral observations were conducted by trained, reliable observers in the clinic and in the homes of oppositional children at pre- and posttreatment. A number of parent report inventories of child adjustment were also used. Subjects were randomly assigned to either an immediate treatment group or a waiting-list control group. Mothers and children in the treatment group evinced significant improvement in their respective dysfunctional behaviors, whereas families in the control group did not.

In the only study that has compared the Hanf-Forehand program with an active, viable treatment alternative, Wells and Egan (1988) recently treated 19 children meeting DSM-III (American Psychiatric Association 1980) criteria for oppositional disorder and their families with either PMT or systems family therapy (Nichols and Everett 1986). Families were randomly assigned to treatments, and measures included behavioral observations conducted in the clinic as well as several parent report inventories assessing aspects of parent adjustment empirically related to child disorders (see Griest and Wells 1983). Results of this study showed that PMT was more effective than systems family therapy in reducing the primary symptom of oppositional disorder—noncompliance with parental instructions. No differences were noted on secondary measures of parental adjustment (i.e., parental depression, anxiety; marital adjustment). Although this study suggests that PMT is more effective than systems family therapy for oppositional disorder, it says nothing about systems family therapy's efficacy for other childhood disorders—for example, anxiety or psychosomatic disorders.

The studies reviewed above show that PMT is an effective treatment approach for problems of social aggression in young children and is more effective than another frequently used treatment strategy. Its efficacy having been demonstrated, a line of research was conducted to evaluate the generalization of treatment effects obtained with PMT. *Generalization* refers to the extent to which treatment effects obtained in the clinic are maintained over time (temporal generalization); generalize to other behaviors not targeted in treatment (behavioral generalization); generalize to other situations such as the home and school (setting generalization); and generalize to other persons such as siblings or classmates (subject generalization).

Temporal generalization.   Regarding temporal generalization, Forehand and Long (1988) recently reviewed most of the published literature pertaining to maintenance of treatment effects. They evaluated 12 studies that collected long-term follow-up data from 1 to 9 years posttreatment. Of these 12 studies, 8 showed evidence of maintenance of treatment effects on all measures, 3 showed maintenance on some measures but not others, and 1 showed lack of maintenance of treatment effects at 1-year follow-up. In the latter study, as well as in one study not reviewed by Forehand and Long (1988) that failed to show maintenance of treatment effects, mothers had very low income and low educational attainment, lived in high-crime areas, and reported multiple problems besides their children's aggressive conduct (e.g., maternal depression, marital violence, chronic maternal illness) (Wahler

1980; Wahler and Dumas 1987). Wahler (1980) has referred to these mothers as "insular"—that is, mothers who are cut off from positive social contact and who experience high rates of negatively valenced social contact. Wahler and his colleagues have repeatedly demonstrated that insular mothers fail to maintain treatment-acquired gains after a parent training program. On the other hand, Baum and Forehand (1981) reported maintenance of treatment effects at $1-4\frac{1}{2}$ years on all measures. In that sample, only one of the 34 families studied was receiving welfare.

It appears from the above review that, in general, treatment effects obtained with parent training do generalize across time. Insular mothers represent a notable exception to this general statement. In discussing the insular mother's special problems in parenting, Wahler and his colleagues have noted that it is not simply low socioeconomic status that results in disrupted parenting and child behavior problems; rather, it is the process of insularity that is at least one of the more direct controlling influences.

Setting generalization. A few studies have looked at the setting generalization of the Hanf-Forehand PMT program. In the Peed et al. (1977) study previously described, generalization from the clinic to the home was examined by conducting pre- and postobservations in the clinic and home settings and conducting treatment in the clinic. Results showed that positive changes obtained in the clinic did generalize to the home, in that home improvements were noted in critical parenting skills and in target child behaviors. No changes occurred in the control group in home observational measures.

Two studies have evaluated generalization of treatment effects to school by using behavioral observations in both home and school (Breiner and Forehand 1981; Forehand et al. 1979). Both studies showed no statistically significant changes in school behavior following treatment in the clinic. Inspection of the individual data in both studies showed that some children exhibited increased levels of noncompliance at school whereas others displayed decreased levels—the two groups, in effect, canceling each other out.

These studies reveal that generalization from clinic to home does occur, probably because of similar stimulus conditions in both of these settings (i.e., parents displaying similar behaviors toward their children in the clinic and at home). However, generalization to the school, where a different set of adult caregivers interact with the child, does not necessarily occur. In fact, although some children improve, others may become worse at school, indicating that an idiosyncratic assessment of school behavior needs to occur during or following clinic treatment for home-referred behavior problems.

Behavioral generalization. One study has directly examined behavioral generalization of the Hanf-Forehand PMT program (Wells et al. 1980a). In this study, the effects of treatment for noncompliance were examined on related but untreated disruptive behaviors such as throwing tantrums, hitting, and crying by assessing changes in a code category—Other Deviant Behavior—collected during behavioral observations. Results showed that these other deviant behaviors decreased significantly from pre- to posttreatment even though they were not targeted for treatment. These data indicate that behavioral generalization does occur, at least for coercive behaviors in the same response class as noncompliance; however, this conclusion is somewhat equivocal since Patterson's research group has reported nonsignificant decreases in nontargeted deviant behaviors following their treatment program (Patterson 1974; Patterson and Reid 1973; Patterson et al. 1975). Therefore, as with generalization to school, behavioral generalization should probably be assessed on a case-by-case basis if the clinician and parents wish to see changes in other deviant behaviors. If generalization does not "spontaneously" occur, then treatment efforts need to be directed to those behaviors.

Subject generalization.   One study examined generalization of parenting skills and treatment effects to untreated siblings following treatment of a referred child (Humphreys et al. 1978). Results showed that without any prompting from the therapist, mothers did generalize positive parenting skills and siblings did improve their noncompliance following treatment of a target child. These results indicate that behavioral improvement can be seen in nontargeted children even without specific instructions to mothers to generalize the use of their skills.

Based on group outcome data from the studies reviewed in this section, a general statement can be made that whereas temporal, behavioral, and subject (sibling) generalization of the effects of PMT with the Hanf-Forehand program does occur, setting generalization does not reliably occur. However, because the results are based on group statistics, they do not predict generalization effects with 100% accuracy for every individual. For example, in Patterson's work, even though treatment effects are generally maintained (based on group statistics), up to one-third of the sample does not maintain treatment-acquired gains at follow-up, and "booster" sessions are required across posttreatment follow-up to bolster treatment effects (Patterson 1974). For these reasons, clinicians should assess the extent of generalization and provide adjunctive treatment strategies when necessary. Examples of such strategies are discussed in the next section.

Enhancing Treatment Effects

Because of the recognition that all children do not maintain treatment-acquired gains, a series of studies examined adjunctive treatment strategies designed to promote and enhance treatment effects obtained with PMT. Wells et al. (1980b) designed a self-control program that involves instructing parents in self-monitoring, self-evaluation, and self-reinforcement of parenting skills they learned during PMT. Results of an experimental evaluation of this program showed that treatment effects for children whose parents received PMT and self-control training were significantly enhanced at follow-up compared with those for children whose parents received only PMT.

Likewise, McMahon et al. (1981) showed that formal training in social learning principles during the course of therapy results in enhanced maintenance of treatment effects. In addition, parents who receive such formal training report greater satisfaction with treatment.

Miller and Prinz (1990) have recently reviewed strategies for enhancing treatment effects obtained with PMT. These strategies arise out of a broad-based model that addresses more comprehensive family context variables; they encompass what Wells has referred to as a behavioral family therapy model. The reader is referred to Griest and Wells (1983), Miller and Prinz (1990), and Wells (1985) for reviews of this expanded model.

The studies reviewed above indicate that adjunctive treatment strategies can enhance the effects of parent training. Formal training in social learning principles should probably be incorporated into all parent training therapy plans. Self-control strategies can be used when parents have difficulty generalizing skills from clinic to home.

Oregon Social Learning Center
Parent Training (Patterson and Reid)

The parent training approaches of Patterson, Reid, and their colleagues have been used with older children (up to 16 years of age). The basic treatment program can be loosely divided into three stages, with progression to each successive stage contingent upon successful completion of the preceding one.

The first phase focuses on teaching parents the language and concepts of social learning theory using programmed texts. Parents must pass a test assessing their knowledge of these concepts before passing on to the next stage of treatment.

In the second stage, parents learn to define, track, and record behavior and are asked to delineate two deviant and two prosocial behaviors of their child. The parents then record these behaviors for a 3-day period at home.

In the third phase, parents learn to develop intervention programs beginning with two or three easily tracked behaviors. A point system is set up whereby the child earns and loses points contingent upon positive and negative behavior, respectively. Points are exchanged daily for backup rewards selected by the child. In addition, parents learn to use social reinforcers, such as verbal, labeled rewards for positive behavior, and to implement a time-out procedure for negative behaviors. Thus, the child or young adolescent earns multiple reinforcers for positive behavior and multiple negative consequences for deviant behavior.

In more recent discussions of treatment procedures, Patterson has emphasized the addition of problem-solving skills training as part of basic parent training. Such training involves teaching parents how to generate solutions to problematic situations that arise, using the concepts and skills they have learned earlier, with decreasing amounts of input from the therapist. Problem-solving training is designed to assist parents in coping with children on their own as children exhibit new behaviors or as new developmental issues arise. (For a complete presentation of Patterson's treatment approach, see Patterson et al. 1975.) Table 11–1 outlines a sequence of therapy sessions employing PMT strategies based on Patterson's model.

Patterson and his colleagues conducted a number of studies early in the development of their clinical procedures that demonstrated the efficacy of this approach to PMT. Treated families showed improvements equal to or greater than 30% reduction from baseline in scored deviant behavior (home observations) following treatment (Patterson 1974; Patterson and Reid 1973; Patterson et al. 1973). Data demonstrating generalization across time and siblings were also reported (Arnold et al. 1975; Patterson 1974). In addition, children treated with this clinical program have been compared with both waiting-list control subjects (Wiltz and Patterson 1974) and attention-placebo control subjects (Walter and Gilmore 1973). In each case, PMT led to greater improvement in deviant child behavior than control conditions. However, in both of these studies, there were differences in baseline data for the experimental and control groups, suggesting possible selection bias in group assignment. In addition, the treatment time was abbreviated in both studies.

Because of these flaws, Patterson et al. (1982) conducted a third controlled study in which cases were randomly assigned to PMT or to community control conditions. In the community control group, families were referred to local mental health practitioners who employed treatments based on their own standards of care. All families submitted to a standardized assessment battery before and after treatment.

Results showed that the group receiving PMT experienced a 63% reduction in the rate of deviant child behavior in the home from the baseline level, whereas the community control group showed a 17% reduction. At termination, 70% of the PMT subjects had scores within the normal range, whereas 33% of the community control subjects had scores within this range. Both groups experienced a decrease in parent-reported problem behaviors. Differences between the groups in parent daily report data were not significant.

Because this study corrected many of the design flaws of earlier studies employing control groups, the conclusion that PMT, when applied in an open-ended, time-unlimited fashion by relatively experienced therapists, is more effective than standard treatment procedures available in the community would appear to be a valid one.

Since the early demonstrations of efficacy, research on the clinical procedures of Patterson, Reid, and their colleagues has turned to questions of replication and community dissemination, adjunctive treatment procedures

Table 11–1. Parent management training sessions

Session	Topic	Description
1	Introduction and overview	The parents are given an overview of the program. The trainer outlines the demands to be placed upon them and explains the focus of the intervention.
2	Defining and observing	Parents are trained to pinpoint, define, and observe behavior. The parents and trainer define specific problems that can be observed and develop a specific plan to begin observations.
3	Positive reinforcement	Parents are taught the concept of positive reinforcement. Factors that contribute to the effective application of reinforcement are explained, and parents rehearse how they will apply these principles in relation to the target child. Specific programs are outlined in which praise and points are to be provided for the behaviors observed during the week.
4	Review of the program and data	Observations of the previous week as well as application of the reinforcement program are reviewed. Details about the administration of praise, points, and back-up reinforcers are discussed and enacted as needed so that the trainer can identify how to improve parent performance. Changes are made in the program as needed.
5	Time-out from reinforcement	Parents learn about time-out and the factors related to its effective application. The use of time-out periods is planned for the next week for specific behaviors.
6	Shaping	Parents are trained to develop behaviors by reinforcement of successive approximations and to use prompts and fading of prompts to develop terminal behaviors.
7	Review and problem solving	The concepts discussed in all prior sessions are thoroughly reviewed. The parent is asked to apply these concepts to hypothetical situations presented within the session. Areas of weakness in understanding the concepts or their execution in practice serve as the focus.
8	Attending and ignoring	Parents learn about attending and ignoring; they then choose an undesirable behavior that they will ignore and a positive, opposite behavior to which they will attend. These procedures are practiced within the session.
9	School intervention	Plans are made to implement a home-based reinforcement program to develop school-related behaviors. Prior to this session, discussions with the teachers and parents have identified specific behaviors to focus on in class (e.g., deportment) and at home (e.g., homework completion). These behaviors are incorporated into the reinforcement system.
10	Reprimands	Parents are trained in effective use of reprimands.

(continued)

Table 11–1.   Parent management training sessions *(continued)*

Session	Topic	Description
11	Family meeting	The child and parent(s) are brought into the session. The programs are discussed along with any problems. Revisions are made as needed to correct misunderstandings or to alter facets that may not be implemented in a way that is likely to be effective.
12	Review of skills	The programs are reviewed along with all concepts about the principles. Parents are asked to develop programs for a variety of hypothetical everyday problems at home and at school. Feedback is provided regarding program options and applications.
13	Negotiating and contracting	The child and parent meet together to negotiate new behavioral programs and to place these in contractual form.
14	Low-rate behaviors	Parents are trained to deal with low-rate behaviors such as fire setting, stealing, or truancy. Specific punishment programs are planned and presented to the child as needed for behaviors characteristic of the case.
15, 16, and 17	Review, problem solving, and practice	Material from other sessions is reviewed in theory and practice. Special emphasis is given to role-playing application of individual principles as they are enacted with the trainer. Parents practice designing new programs, revising ailing programs, and responding to a complex array of situations in which principles and practices discussed in prior sessions are reviewed.

Source. Reprinted from Kazdin AE: "Conduct Disorders," in *International Handbook of Behavior Modification and Therapy, 2nd Edition.* Edited by Bellack A, Hersen A, Kazdin AE. New York, Plenum, 1982, p. 167. Used with permission.

relating to therapist clinical skills, and development of specialized approaches for different diagnostic groups.

Replication and community dissemination.   Fleischman (1981) conducted a systematic replication of the procedures developed by Patterson. Although some attempt was made to conduct the study without input from Patterson and his senior colleagues, the clinic at which the treatment was conducted was established by the research center directed by Patterson; Fleischman was a student of Patterson's; and therapists had 2–6 years of experience in parent training, presumably at Patterson's research center, prior to their work in this study. However, neither Patterson nor his senior colleagues served as supervisors of the treatment or the methods. Treatment was open-ended and conducted by experienced therapists. No control group was employed. Results of this study showed significant reductions in deviant child behavior by termination, as measured by objective home observations, parent daily reports of symptoms, parental attitudinal descriptions of the child, and parents' own counts of problematic behavior. Improvements were maintained at 1-year follow-up.

In another replication study, Fleischman and Szykula (1981) evaluated Patterson's procedures in a true community setting funded by Title XX funds. Again, therapists initially were trained by staff at Patterson's research center. Results of this study were comparable to those reported earlier from studies conducted in research facilities; that is, significant treatment effects were found for Total Aversive Behavior measured in the home by trained, objective observers, parent-collected daily behavior data, and global ratings of improvement by parents. The cost of treatment per family was $776.00 in the third year of the clinic, and referrals to the clinic were steadily increasing. Thus, it appears that the results of Patterson's research on PMT can be replicated by others. In addition, PMT procedures can be implemented effectively in clinical settings in an efficient and cost-effective manner.

Adjunctive treatment procedures. Despite the positive results obtained by Patterson and others affiliated with his research center, a number of studies conducted in the 1970s failed to show unequivocally significant treatment effects with PMT procedures (Bernal et al. 1980; Eyberg and Johnson 1974; Ferber et al. 1974). Two factors differentiated these studies from those obtaining positive results: 1) the use of a session-limited format, and 2) the use of relatively inexperienced therapists who had been taught to administer the treatment in a standardized, educative format.

These observations have prompted a line of research examining the clinical skills displayed by experienced therapists; such research may assist therapists in dealing with patient "resistance" or noncooperativeness with treatment procedures. Studies examining therapy process have shown that such resistance is systematically related both to phase of parent training therapy and to therapists' ratings of treatment outcome (Chamberlain et al. 1984). In addition, Patterson and Forgatch (1985) have shown that therapists' efforts to teach and confront are significantly related to client noncompliance. This effect was also demonstrated in an experimental study in which therapist behaviors of Teach and Confront were manipulated and increases in client resistance were systematically observed (Patterson and Forgatch 1985). These findings represent a considerable paradox for parent trainers: on the one hand, trainers are required to teach a systematic set of parent training procedures; on the other, they encounter increased noncooperativeness in trainee parents when they do so.

These studies and other observations have led Patterson and his colleagues to postulate three components of effective treatment: 1) a parent training technology to alter ineffective parent management practices, 2) therapist clinical skills for dealing with parent noncooperativeness, and 3) a therapist support system for maintaining effective therapist performance (Patterson 1985).

Although therapist clinical skills as they relate to PMT have not been systematically identified by Patterson and his colleagues to date, preliminary analyses of therapy process data show that therapist behaviors such as Support and Facilitate are accompanied by decreases in client noncooperativeness. In addition, skilled therapists have been shown to engage in a higher rate of "joining" behavior than novice therapists (as reported in Patterson 1985). "Joining" has to do with therapist behaviors that establish a relationship with the client and engage him or her in the therapy process. These and other preliminary analyses have prompted Patterson to propose three critical therapist skills for reducing client noncooperativeness: 1) skills for "joining" with or engaging the client in the therapy process, 2) skills for reframing in a supportive way the problems or obstacles that parents bring up in therapy, and 3) persistence of the therapist in teaching and confronting parents. The work of Patterson and his colleagues has increasingly been concerned with identifying, evaluating, and providing training in skills such as these to enhance the likelihood that PMT strategies will be accepted and carried forward by parents.

Specialized treatment approaches.   In early PMT research, all referred children received the same treatment, regardless of differences in their characteristics or presenting problems. However, a study in 1979 by Moore et al. found that of children treated at Patterson's center, those who were referred for stealing had a much poorer long-term outcome than children referred for other problems.

Studies such as this prompted Reid et al. (1980) to develop additions to standard PMT when the target child displays covert, predelinquent, antisocial behavior such as stealing. Changes in treatment are based on the notion that stealing is a behavior that is normally concealed from parents and is less likely to be monitored by them. Therefore, after learning standard parenting skills, parents whose children steal are taught to apply specific, negative consequences whenever they suspect that stealing has occurred. The actual behavior does not have to be observed. Therefore, it becomes the child's responsibility not only to refrain from stealing but also to remain above suspicion. Finally, to improve monitoring and parental supervision of the child, a check-in system is negotiated. Daily phone calls are made to the home by the therapist to support the parents and to remind them to apply consequences for each and every suspected stealing event, no matter how minor or insignificant.

Reid et al. (1980) evaluated the effectiveness of this enhanced approach to PMT for youngsters who steal. Parent reports of stealing and of other referral problems decreased significantly. Total Aversive Behavior, measured during home observations, decreased nonsignificantly, although it was not high at baseline for this group of children, whose aggressive behaviors were primarily low frequency and covert.

However, to conclude that the enhanced treatment program results in significant improvements over standard PMT, research needs to employ a control group of stealers receiving standard treatment and to utilize assessments outside the family system (e.g., court and police records). Until this happens, the results of Reid et al. (1980) are very encouraging but not confirmatory.

In a more recent study, which further extends and enhances the basic treatment program of Patterson, Reid, and their associates, Bank et al. (1991) treated delinquent adolescents and compared their treatment with treatment provided by other community agencies that normally offer services for such cases. To be accepted into the study, boys had to be repeat offenders with at least two offenses recorded on police files. One of these had to be a nonstatus offense. This process ensured that the study involved a seriously aggressive subject population.

For this seriously delinquent group, the treatment was modified to target not only prosocial and antisocial behaviors but also other behaviors believed to put the child at risk for further delinquency (e.g., class attendance, homework, curfew violations, congregating with delinquent friends). Parents learned to track and monitor these behaviors to facilitate supervision. In addition, families were involved as a unit in developing behavioral contracts. Instead of time-out procedures, parents were taught to use more age-appropriate punishment procedures such as work details, point loss, and restitution. Parental monitoring of the child's whereabouts and activities was emphasized, because lack of monitoring has been strongly related to delinquency.

The results of this important study showed that the expanded PMT and community control groups were comparable at baseline on all categories of official offenses. By the end of the first year, however, nonstatus offense rates had been significantly lowered for the PMT group. The difference between the PMT and the community control groups was significant at the first-year follow-up. At the second-, third-, and fourth-year follow-ups, offenses in the PMT group remained low, but offenses in the community control group had also decreased. Thus, the difference between the two groups was not significant at the follow-ups. The striking finding of the study was the difference in time required for the respective approaches to have an effect on offense rates: PMT therapy was clearly superior in this regard.

Another notable finding of the study had to do with the savings to the community of the treatment approach. There was a highly significant difference in institution time between the two groups in both the first and the second year after treatment.

Adolescents in the PMT group spent 1,287 fewer days in institutional confinement than did community-treated adolescents, with a savings to the community of $100,000.00 over the 3-year period. This means that even though the PMT group had about 14% more time available to commit offenses during the treatment and follow-up years, its members nevertheless committed 24% fewer offenses. These results offer support that PMT may be one of the most viable treatments available for outpatient care of delinquent youths. It seems to be more effective than treatment available from typical community resources on an outpatient basis. This is not to say that the PMT approach is a panacea for delinquency, however: only 18% of the subjects in the PMT group completely dropped out of the delinquency process (whereas only one of the community control subjects did so). Once adolescents reach the point of delinquency, PMT may slow the path to chronicity rather than reverse it. Nevertheless, the study did demonstrate this approach to be more effective than other available treatments in the first year of intervention.

Summary

This chapter has presented a review of empirically based theoretical work linking dysfunctional parenting to child aggression, and a therapy model—PMT—that has arisen out of that work. At present, there remains little doubt that dysfunctional parenting is directly related to aggressive behavior on the part of children. In addition, recent reviews indicate that PMT is the most promising treatment for childhood oppositional disorder and CD tested to date (Kazdin 1987).

In addition to the direct relationship between dysfunctional parenting and child aggression, it is clear that other parent and child dysfunctions, as well as ecosystemic variables, impact on the child's behavior. While acknowledging the potential impact of genetic, temperamental, biological, and psychological influences, the social learning model focuses on the controlling influences of microscopic and macroscopic behavioral processes in parent-child interactions.

PMT is a dyadic model (parent ↔ child) that intervenes directly at the level of dysfunctional parenting to alter aggressive child behavior. A more broad-based model addresses other context variables that themselves may impact on dysfunctional parenting. The treatment approach arising out of such a model has been called behavioral family therapy by some authors; this approach represents an expansion from PMT into other family targets. The reader is referred to Chapter 10 for a discussion of this expanded model.

References

American Psychiatric Association: Diagnostic and Statistical Manual of Mental Disorders, 3rd Edition. Washington, DC, American Psychiatric Association, 1980

Arnold JE, Levine AG, Patterson GR: Changes in sibling behavior following family intervention. J Consult Clin Psychol 43:683–688, 1975

Bank L, Marlowe J, Reid JB, et al: A comparative evaluation of parent-training interventions for families of chronic delinquents. J Abnorm Child Psychol 19:15–33, 1991

Barret CL, Hampe IE, Miller LC: Research on child psychotherapy, in Handbook of Psychotherapy and Behavior Change: An Empirical Analysis. Edited by Garfield SL, Bergin AE. New York, Wiley, 1978, pp 411–435

Baum CG, Forehand R: Long-term follow-up assessment of parent training by use of multiple-outcome measures. Behavior Therapy 13:16–26, 1981

Bernal ME, Klinnert MD, Schultz LA: Outcome evaluation of behavioral parent training and client-centered parent counseling for children with conduct problems. J Appl Behav Anal 13:677–691, 1980

Breiner JL, Forehand R: An assessment of the effects of parent training on clinic-referred children's school behavior. Behavioral Assessment 3:31–42, 1981

Chamberlain P, Patterson GR, Reid JB, et al: Observation of client resistance. Behavior Therapy 15:144–155, 1984

Dumas JE: Indiscriminate mothering: empirical findings and theoretical speculations. Advances in Behavior Research and Therapy 6:13–27, 1984

Dumas JE, Wahler RG: Indiscriminate mothering as a contextual factor in aggressive-oppositional child behavior: "damned if you do and damned if you don't." J Abnorm Child Psychol 13:1–17, 1985

Emery RE: Interparental conflict and the children of discord and divorce. Psychol Bull 92:310–330, 1982

Eyberg SM, Johnson SM: Multiple assessment of behavior modification with families: effects of contingency contracting and order of treated problems. J Consult Clin Psychol 42:594–606, 1974

Fauber RL, Long N: Children in context: the role of the family in child psychotherapy. J Consult Clin Psychol 59:813–820, 1991

Fauber RL, Forehand R, Thomas AM, et al: A meditational model of the impact of marital conflict on adolescent adjustment in intact and divorced families: the role of disrupted parenting. Child Dev 61:1112–1123, 1990

Ferber H, Keeley SM, Shemberg KM: Training parents in behavior modification: outcome of and problems encountered in a program after Patterson's work. Behavior Therapy 5:415–419, 1974

Fleischman MJ: A replication of Patterson's "intervention for boys with conduct problems." J Consult Clin Psychol 49:342–351, 1981

Fleischman MJ, Szykula SA: A community setting replication of a social learning treatment for aggressive children. Behavior Therapy 12:115–122, 1981

Forehand R, King HE: Preschool children's noncompliance: effects of short-term therapy. Journal of Community Psychology 2:42–44, 1974

Forehand R, Long N: Outpatient treatment of the acting out child: procedures, long-term follow-up data, and clinical problems. Advances in Behavior Research and Therapy 10:129–177, 1988

Forehand R, McMahon RJ: Helping the Noncompliant Child: A Clinician's Guide to Parent Training. New York, Guilford, 1981

Forehand R, Cheney T, Yoder P: Parent behavior training: effects on the noncompliance of a deaf child. J Behav Ther Exp Psychiatry 5:281–283, 1974

Forehand R, King HE, Peed S, et al: Mother-child interactions: comparison of a non-compliant clinic group and a non-clinic group. Behav Res Ther 13:79–85, 1975

Forehand R, Sturgis ET, McMahon RJ, et al: Parent behavioral training to modify child noncompliance: treatment generalization across time and from home to school. Behav Modif 3:3–25, 1979

Forehand R, Lautenschlager GJ, Faust J, et al: Parent perceptions and parent-child interactions in clinic-referred children: a preliminary investigation of the effects of maternal depressive moods. Behav Res Ther 24:73–75, 1986

Griest DL, Wells KC: Behavioral family therapy with conduct disorders in children. Behavior Therapy 14:37–53, 1983

Hetherington EM, Cox M, Cox R: Effects of divorce on parents and children, in Nontraditional Families. Edited by Lamb M. Hillsdale, NJ, Lawrence Erlbaum, 1982, pp 233–288

Humphreys L, Forehand R, McMahon R, et al: Parent behavioral training to modify child noncompliance: effects on untreated siblings. J Behav Ther Exp Psychiatry 9:235–238, 1978

Kazdin AE: Treatment of antisocial behavior in children: current status and future directions. Psychol Bull 102:187–203, 1987

Levitt EE: The results of psychotherapy with children: an evaluation. Journal of Consulting Psychology 32:286–289, 1957

Levitt EE: Psychotherapy with children: a further evaluation. Behav Res Ther 60:326–329, 1963

Loeber R: Development and risk factors of juvenile antisocial behavior and delinquency. Clinical Psychology Review 10:1–41, 1990

Loeber R, Dishion TJ: Early predictors of male delinquency: a review. Psychol Bull 94:68–99, 1983

Loeber R, Schmaling KB: Empirical evidence for overt and covert patterns of antisocial conduct problems: a meta-analysis. J Abnorm Child Psychol 13:337–352, 1985

Maccoby EE, Martin JA: Socialization in the context of the family: parent-child interaction, in Handbook of Child Psychology, Vol 4: Socialization, Personality, and Social Development. Edited by Hetherington EM. New York, Wiley, 1983, pp 1–101

McMahon RJ, Wells KC: Conduct disorders, in Treatment of Child Disorders. Edited by Mash EJ, Barkley RA. New York, Guilford, 1989, pp 73–132

McMahon RJ, Forehand R, Griest DL: Effects of knowledge of social learning principles on enhancing treatment outcome and generalization in a parent training program. J Consult Clin Psychol 49:526–532, 1981

Miller GE, Prinz RJ: Enhancement of social learning family interventions for childhood conduct disorder. Psychol Bull 108:291–307, 1990

Moore D, Chamberlain P, Mukai L: Children at risk for delinquency: a follow-up comparison of aggressive children and children who steal. J Abnorm Child Psychol 7:345–355, 1979

Nichols WC, Everett CA: Systemic Family Therapy: An Integrative Approach. New York, Guilford, 1986

Parke RD, Slaby RG: The development of aggression, in Handbook of Child Psychology, Vol 4: Socialization, Personality, and Social Development. Edited by Hetherington EM. New York, Wiley, 1983, pp 569–642

Patterson GR: Interventions for boys with conduct problems: multiple settings, treatments and criteria. J Consult Clin Psychol 42:471–481, 1974

Patterson GR: Coercive Family Processes. Eugene, OR, Castalia, 1982

Patterson GR: Beyond technology: the next stage in developing and empirical base for parent training, in Handbook of Family Psychology and Therapy, Vol 2. Edited by L'Abate L. Homewood, IL, Dorsey Press, 1985, pp 1344–1379

Patterson GR: Performance models for antisocial boys. Am Psychol 41:432í444, 1986

Patterson GR, Forgatch MS: Therapist behavior as a determinant for client noncompliance: a paradox for the behavior modifier. J Consult Clin Psychol 53:846–851, 1985

Patterson GR, Reid JB: Intervention for families of aggressive boys: a replication study. Behav Res Ther 11:383–394, 1973

Patterson GR, Stouthamer-Loeber M: The correlation of family management practices and delinquency. Child Dev 55:1299–1307, 1984

Patterson GR, Cobb JA, Ray RS: A social engineering technology for retraining the families of aggressive boys, in Issues and Trends in Behavior Therapy. Edited by Adams HE, Unikel IP. Springfield, IL, Charles C Thomas, 1973, pp 283–295

Patterson GR, Reid JB, Jones RR, et al: A Social Learning Approach to Family Intervention, Vol 1: Families With Aggressive Children. Eugene, OR, Castalia, 1975

Patterson GR, Chamberlain P, Reid JB: A comparative evaluation of parent training procedures. Behavior Therapy 13:638–650, 1982

Patterson GR, DeBaryshe BD, Ramsey E: A developmental perspective on antisocial behavior. Am Psychol 44:329–335, 1989

Peed S, Roberts M, Forehand R: Evaluation of the effectiveness of a standardized parent training program in altering the interactions of mothers and their noncompliant children. Behav Modif 1:323–350, 1977

Reid JB, Hinojosa Rivera G, Lorber R: A social learning approach to the outpatient treatment of children who steal. Eugene, OR, Oregon Social Learning Center, April 1980

Russo DC, Cataldo MF, Cushing PJ: Compliance training and behavioral covariation in the treatment of multiple behavior problems. J Appl Behav Anal 14:209–222, 1981

Wahler RG: The insular mother: her problems in parent-child treatment. J Appl Behav Anal 13:207–219, 1980

Wahler RG, Dumas JE: Maintenance factors in coercive mother-child interactions: the compliance and predictability hypotheses. J Appl Behav Anal 19:13–22, 1986

Wahler RG, Dumas JE: Family factors in childhood psychopathology: a coercion-neglect model, in Family Interaction and Psychopathology: Theories, Methods, and Findings. Edited by Jacob T. New York, Plenum, 1987, pp 581–627

Wahler RG, Dumas JE: Attentional problems in dysfunctional mother-child interactions: an interbehavioral model. Psychol Bull 105:116–130, 1989

Walter HI, Gilmore SK: Placebo versus social learning effects in parent training procedures designed to alter the behavior of aggressive boys. Behavior Therapy 4:361–377, 1973

Wells KC: *Coercive Family Processes*, Vol 3: A Social Learning Approach (Patterson GR, ed) (book review). Behavior Therapy 15:121–127, 1984

Wells KC: Behavioral family therapy, in Dictionary of Behavior Therapy Techniques. Edited by Bellack AS, Hersen M. New York, Pergamon, 1985, pp 25–30

Wells KC: Family therapy, in Handbook of Treatment Approaches in Childhood Psychopathology. Edited by Matson JL. New York, Plenum, 1988, pp 45–61

Wells KC, Egan J: Social learning and systems family therapy for childhood oppositional disorder: comparative treatment outcome. Compr Psychiatry 29:138–146, 1988

Wells KC, Forehand R: Child behavior problems in the home, in Handbook of Clinical Behavior Therapy. Edited by Turner SM, Calhoun KS, Adams HE. New York, Wiley, 1981, pp 527–567

Wells KC, Forehand R: Conduct and oppositional disorders, in Handbook of Clinical Behavior Therapy With Children. Edited by Bornstein PH, Kazdin AE. Homewood, IL, Dorsey Press, 1985, pp 218–265

Wells KC, Forehand R, Griest DL: Generalizability of treatment effects from treated to untreated behaviors resulting from a parent training program. J Consult Clin Psychol 9:217–219, 1980a

Wells KC, Griest DL, Forehand R: The use of a self-control package to enhance temporal generality of a parent training program. Behav Res Ther 18:347–358, 1980b

Wiltz NA, Patterson GR: An evaluation of parent training procedures designed to alter inappropriate aggressive behavior of boys. Behavior Therapy 5:215–221, 1974

Chapter 12

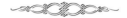

Group Therapy

Saul Scheidlinger, Ph.D.
Seth Aronson, Psy.D.

T he significant role of group life in the personality development of both children and adolescents is unquestioned. In fact, the propensity of youths for such group involvements, including the unique motivational factors inherent in the normative peer group, constitutes the basis for child and adolescent group therapy wherein these factors are strategically harnessed to undo dysfunction and to promote change and growth.

In this chapter we address the use of group therapy methods in the treatment of children and adolescents with conduct disorder (CD). Most of this work has been applied to youth with mild to moderate CD (DSM-III-R; American Psychiatric Association 1987) who have demonstrated at least a minimal capacity for group attachments and who are responsive to a nondirective treatment approach (P. F. Kernberg and Chazan 1991).

Historical Background

Antisocial children and adolescents were once labeled as having primary behavior disorders or impulsive personalities, or as ego-deficient or predelinquent. The consensus was that such youths were not readily amenable to traditional one-on-one treatments. Instead, group interventions were frequently advocated. In fact, Aichhorn's (1935) book on his work with "wayward" youths in a group context first appeared in 1925 and carried a foreword by Sigmund Freud—hardly a proponent of group therapy methods! The thrust of Aichhorn's "reeducational" approach was to restore an "unsatisfied need for tenderness and love" (p. 148) coupled with a rebuilding of "a socially directed ego ideal" (p. 236) in his charges.

Aichhorn's approach was emulated by his psychoanalytic disciples in the United States. Thus, Eissler (1949) proposed a psychological definition of delinquency as "behavior, thoughts and feelings that tend to infringe upon values" (p. 9), coupled with outside-directed aggression. His treatment aimed essentially at transforming a self-centered, acting-out individual into a neurotic one. This goal entailed forming "a tight, foolproof attachment between the psychoanalyst and the delinquent in the shortest possible time" (p. 17), followed by adopting a therapeutic stance leading to the adult's becoming an ego ideal. Direct gratifications—giving money or displaying an unfailingly helpful attitude, even in the face of provocative behavior—were all designed to counter the youth's fixed expectations of negative reactions from adults. In time, the delinquent repressed his aggressive, antisocial behavior in order "not to lose the gratification derived from the love object" (p. 22). Lippman's (1949) work in a child guidance clinic embodied a similar approach. He found that "one of the greatest obstacles to effective psychotherapy with seriously delinquent youngsters is the narcissistic defense which they have set up. This narcissism is very likely due to early profound rejection, and the secondary rejections which result from the behavior occasioned by their early trauma" (p. 160). Oberndorf (1949) extended these concepts to group work with delinquent youths, stressing the role of the peer group in fostering healthy identifications. In his words, "in any group . . . one finds not only imitation and substitution but true identification as well. One of the very important effects of identification is its powerful influence on the formation of the ego quality of the personality of the child and, equally important, of the quality of his slowly developing conscience (superego)" (p. 166).

Slavson's (1943) activity group therapy, begun in the 1930s and followed by Redl's (1944, 1966) group work with ego-disturbed children, provided the basic psychodynamic conceptual and methodological models for most of today's outpatient and residential group treatment of antisocial youths. These group therapies were offered within the broader spectrum of services designed for all categories of disturbed children and adolescents. Scheidlinger (1947) indicated how activity group therapy could be used with children with primary behavior disorders—"children who react by means of undesirable behavior patterns characterized by hostility and aggression to early emotional deprivation in a family setting" (p. 43). The classical, permissive group treatment model, Scheidlinger argued, was appropriate for severely impulsive and egocentric children.

——— ——— ——— ——— ——— ——— ——— ——— ——— ——— ——— ———

General Principles of Group Therapy

Although many types of group interventions can exert a corrective influence on people, in this chapter we will view group therapy as "a specific field of clinical practice" wherein a specially trained mental health practitioner "utilizes the emotional interaction in small, carefully planned groups to effect amelioration of personality dysfunction in individuals specifically selected for this purpose" (Scheidlinger 1982, p. 7). Most of the therapeutic factors identified by Yalom (1975) as characteristic of group therapy in general—universality, instillation of hope, corrective recapitulation of the primary family group, and development of socializing techniques, interpersonal learning, and imitative behavior—are salient in working with youngsters with CD. The accepting, supportive, and consistent climate of the treatment group, akin to Winnicott's (1965) "holding environment," stands in stark contrast to these youth's typically disorganized, punitive, and depriving family settings. The group's manual activities, games, and snacks serve as symbolic and direct gratifications coupled with opportunities for the building of self-esteem, competence, and social skills. Because group interactions abound in both interpersonal conflicts and scapegoating, the therapist uses these events to confront and to explain the motivations and the ensuing consequences at work, stressing always the learning of prosocial attitudes and behaviors.

As noted by Schamess (1986), group therapists need to adapt their particular group's structure to the phase-specific, developmental needs of the group members. In well-functioning groups, nonverbal, experimental approaches give way, in time, to more insight-oriented discussions.

Groups for Latency-Aged Children

The predilection of latency-aged children for peer group experiences and for making things with their hands, coupled with their strong urges to be independent, to socialize and, above all, to learn, was noted by Erikson (1959). It is therefore no accident that the first model of group therapy, termed *activity group therapy* (Slavson and Schiffer 1975), was designed for this age group. Such groups usually consist of about eight boys or girls of similar age and complementary behavior patterns who provide a "group balance." The balance applies in ethnic and racial backgrounds as well as intellectual and sophistication levels. These groups are run along permissive lines and cannot accommodate children who are devoid of internal controls or who lack even a minimal capacity to relate to others and to experience shame and guilt. The groups in our clinic are frequently short-term (Scheidlinger 1986), heterogeneous, and not limited to children with CD. An optimal group climate usually dictates that no more than half of a group's members should be youth with CD. P. F. Kernberg and Chazan (1991), in contrast, developed specific criteria for their treatment groups, which are designed exclusively for children with CD. Among these are children 1) whose behavioral problems focus primarily around the peer group, 2) who are not responsive to individual therapy, 3) who relate negatively to adult authority figures, 4) who are in need of feedback about their group behavior, and 5) who lack social skills.

Schamess (1986) placed the DSM-III (American Psychiatric Association 1980) category of child CD within O. F. Kernberg's (1970) broader typology of "intermediate level of character pathology." Kernberg believed that with still-undifferentiated ego and superego functions, "intense wishes for love, power, and admiration coexist with contradictory and relatively primitive demands for perfection and goodness . . . ego defenses are organized primarily around repression, although reaction formation, regression, acting out, dissociation, splitting, denial, and projection may all be present to varying degrees" (Schamess 1986, p. 38). Schamess also thought that about one-half of such children referred for treatment would respond well to either exclusive activity or play groups, or to group treatment combined with one-to-one therapy. Furthermore, most such children, when given a choice, prefer the group context to individual work.

In our clinic, all candidates for group therapy are screened before the group's beginning. The parents are interviewed about the child's functioning and are invited to cooperate in the group procedures. The child's interview explores his or her expectations, ideas, and fantasies about the group. As elaborated by Siepker and Kandaras (1985), specific treatment goals may be formulated at this point, such as talking instead of fighting, learning how to trust and to make friends, and accepting feedback about one's behavior.

A simply furnished room with arts and crafts as well as play materials is set aside for the group. Materials are chosen to promote interaction and fantasy while also allowing for lone pursuits. Snacks contribute to the nurturant and "feeding" atmosphere of the group. We have found that for children with CD, as for all prepubertal youths, the division of the group session into three distinct phases is helpful in counteracting overstimulation and undue regression. "Talk time" is thus followed by snacks, and the session concludes with a planned activity or game.

Groups for Adolescents

Given the pivotal role of the peer group in adolescence, the group modality is frequently not only the treatment of choice but also the only treatment acceptable to many older youths with CD. Notwithstanding the initial disclaimers that group therapy "sucks" and that the leaders are part of a "conspiracy" with the referral sources, there is usually also curiosity about the group and especially about the members of the opposite sex.

In this connection, early adolescents (ages 12–14 years) do best with peers and with a therapist of the same sex. A group setting that allows for free motility and that combines activities, games, and snacks with periods of discussion has been found to be the most appropriate for this population. Even in a group setting, as we have noted elsewhere (Scheidlinger and Aronson 1991), "younger adolescents are likely to be self-conscious. There is much squirming, kidding around, and whispering to pals. Warm feelings addressed to the adult can be supplanted by anger within a short timespan" (p. 107).

Our older adolescent groups (ages 15–18 years) contain both girls and boys. The presence of the girls (and of a female co-therapist) serves to dampen the frequently raw hostility exhibited by boys with CD. The medium of communication is talking—"to talk about problems and share them." As mentioned earlier, our treatment groups for adolescents are heterogeneous and balanced, which means that they contain youths from varied diagnostic categories who are deemed to be responsive to a nondirective group process.

As in all adolescent therapy, the group therapist has to find a way to avoid being "sucked in" to the role of the real parent, of other hated adults, or of "one of the gang." The task is also to help the group members verbalize their resurfacing negative feelings toward the adults, as well as toward the group's authority, as soon as these feelings occur, so as to preserve the therapeutic alliance. In this connection, interventions by peers tend to carry more weight than those offered by the group therapist.

Group Treatment of Delinquents

In a chapter devoted to clinical group psychotherapy of delinquents, Raubolt (1983) noted a common problem in this sphere: distinguishing between the legal and the clinical (i.e., delinquent versus CD) aspects of treating antisocial youths. In fact, many of his citations from the literature referred to generic group therapies for adolescents, some of whom happened to be hard-to-reach "acter-outers."

A number of authors have described group treatment models for adolescents who have been adjudged delinquent by the legal system. In this work, as might be expected, the legal system became a significant "player" in the therapeutic transactions. The literature tends to differentiate between so-called neurotic delinquents (anxious and internally conflicted) and CD delinquents (externalized, guiltless, and antisocial). As we had noted earlier, Aichhorn (1935) and Eissler (1949) tried to promote neurotic anxiety in their adolescent delinquents so as to render them accessible to psychodynamic psychotherapy. Slavson (1947) asserted early on that nondirective group therapy was not suitable for delinquents with "extreme behavior disorders or psychopathic states" (p. 423). Peck and Bellsmith (1954), on the contrary, used a permissive group approach in a juvenile court clinic and found that such groups could accommodate one or two psychopathic or even schizophrenic youngsters.

More recent reports suggest the feasibility of a more directive approach with frequent reliance on therapist activity, structure, and firm limits in treatment groups for nonneurotic delinquents. This approach was prompted by an increasing realization that only firm controls can ensure a basic climate of safety—a *sine qua non* for any therapy group! As Shellow et al. (1958) pointed out, "Group therapy must be tailor-made to the problems of these patients because of their desperate struggle against authority and the intensification of that struggle in an institutional society" (p. 271).

A rare example of group work with 13-year-old court-involved delinquent boys in a private practice setting was reported by Madonna and Caswell (1991). Using "flexible techniques" (i.e., aggressive and cooperative play), they were able to evoke in these youngsters some anxiety as well as a greater readiness to verbalize feelings and to engage in self-observation.

Regrettably, notwithstanding all of the above clinical efforts, follow-up studies of delinquents have failed to prove the long-term effectiveness of group treatment, with the possible exception of behavior modification groups (Kazdin 1985).

Group Therapists

Given that individual youths with CD "are no fun to work with," facing an entire group of such children, replete with ever-present emotional lability, subversive alliances ("we against you"), and contagious acting out, is bound to evoke anxiety even in the sturdiest and most optimistic of therapists. On a realistic level, the adult often is dealing with a treatment-resistant and provocative group of children with few effective techniques at his or her command. Accordingly, the required stance of self-assured competence and calm firmness calls for practitioners capable of containing raw emotions and of depersonalizing "below the belly" provocations. In addition, such therapists require prior training in how to work with child and adolescent groups. Furthermore, even experienced practitioners should have ongoing supervision to help them deal with their understandable countertransference reactions, which may range on a continuum from inner feelings of rage against being demeaned by "kids" in front of a group to fears of being insufficient in oneself to fill the tragic void in these children's lives. Similar countertransference themes are also likely to extend to the patients' caretakers (Rey and Plapp 1990).

A co-therapy team of male and female workers is desirable. In addition to providing mutual support and enhanced consensual validation, such a structure addresses the frequent practical need of one therapist to remain with the group when another is required to deal with a group member individually outside the group (Davis and Lohr 1971).

However, as noted by Anthony (1957), despite its stressfulness, such group work does carry its gratifications. "The tolerance of the therapist is put to a stern test, especially early on, but if [the therapist] can survive the repeated crises that punctuate the progress of the group, [he or she] will find the experience among the more rewarding in the field of group work" (p. 217).

Stages of Group Development

Various schemata have been proposed for the progressive phases in therapy groups. Garland et al. (1973) postulated a detailed five-stage model beginning with 1) preaffiliation, and including such issues as 2) power and control, 3) intimacy-cohesion and, ultimately, 4) termination. Most clinicians, however, rely on a rougher breakdown of three main phases: a group formative phase, a working phase, and a termination phase.

Group formative phase.   Predictably, there is much anxiety and testing of limits at the group's beginning. The therapists, having already met the youths during the individual screening sessions, reintroduce themselves. Each member introduces himself or herself in turn, indicating the reasons for having come to the clinic. The "rules" of the group are discussed, with special emphasis on the prohibitions on hurting one another and destroying property. The therapists maintain an active and focused role throughout.

> In the first session of a pubertal boys' group, Mike, a boy with a CD, suggested that the introductions include each member's ethnic background. One therapist asked: "Oh, is that so you should know not to call people hurting names?" Mike, a Hispanic boy, nodded. This led to a discussion of name calling in general and a decision not to permit it in the group.

This early group phase is usually tension-laden, abounding in acting out and testing of limits. One therapist of a younger adolescent boys' group described the situation as follows: "Pulled in many directions by the acter-outers, I had to limit behavior, explain, support and occasionally exclude individuals temporarily from the room 'to calm down and get a hold of yourself.' "

A firm and calm adult stand in the face of what often feels like chaos leads eventually to a workable group climate. Needless to say, empathic reflections to the youngsters about the understandable discomfort felt in a new group situation are very helpful.

Confidentiality, too, requires early discussion and a necessary caveat that it will be broken by the therapists if confronted with dangerous behavior (e.g., substance abuse, suicidal ideas).

Youths with CD need constant help with basic social skills. Accordingly, the adult roles of healer and teacher frequently become indistinguishable. The following example comes from a therapy group run in a day treatment school for older adolescents:

> All group members began to talk at once, rushing to tell Monique, a newcomer, what the school rules were, about the other groups in the school, and about last year's group. The therapist noted the members' eagerness to "fill Monique in" on the facts. However, how could Monique possibly understand them unless they spoke one at a time?

Reassurance, encouragement, and support are essential here, given that the most innocuous comment by an adult can be construed by these youths as criticism. P. F. Kernberg and Chazan's (1991) psychotherapy manual contains a "hierarchy" of helpful verbatim suggestions for such therapist interventions.

Working phase.   The second phase usually begins when a degree of group cohesiveness has evolved. "We" references now outnumber "I" comments, and the therapists are acknowledged (though not always respected) as authority figures. Themes of dependency and of rebellion emerge intermittently in the transference, together with group roles such as that of "clown," "instigator," and "assistant therapist."

> Harry usually positioned himself next to the male therapist. When the latter at times had trouble maintaining even a semblance of quiet, he would say, "Guys, cut it out. Keep it down, will you." Once silence was restored, he would "hand the reigns" of the group back to the leader.

In this middle phase, together with manifestations of defensiveness and of resistance, the group may have poignant periods of self-disclosure about physical or sexual abuse experienced at home. There can also be meaningful and even insightful discussion by the "toughest" kids about people within and outside the group, including discussions about the human condition in general. Touches of delightful humor abound, which include the therapists, who will hopefully laugh with—but never at—the kids.

We view resistances as any individual- or group-level behavior used defensively rather than in the service of the stated group task of sharing personal and interpersonal issues, feelings, and concerns. Examples of such resistances are remaining silent, moving around the room, engaging in horseplay, scapegoating, or talking about irrelevant subjects. Rosenthal (1971) and Redl (1966) discussed such resistances in detail. Once basic rapport is established, group-level resistances are addressed as well as individual defenses. As a result, members blame others less and, especially, learn to accept their own and others' shortcomings. In groups for younger adolescents, symbolic communications tend to emerge through play with Nerf balls, pillows, or jousting pads. Rage against hurtful adults may thus gain sublimated expression and anger can be talked about rather than acted out. Events in the here-and-now life of the group become the subject of general scrutiny, with a focus on the cause and effect in interpersonal behavior.

> Frank, who had been very protective of Sean when the latter first entered the group, now began to pick fights with him. The therapist wondered aloud what brought about this change. When Frank denied any change in his attitude, the other boys urged him to tell the truth. Frank finally related an upsetting incident that had occurred between Sean and him outside the group.

Termination phase.   In the final phase, feelings of separation, loss, and mourning are evident. The group members who have improved the most can now separate their positive and realistic relationships with the therapists from those with authority figures outside the groups. The group's past, including stressful events, is recalled with feelings of nostalgia and gratification. The youths are now a cohesive unit with a positive history to be internalized. Individuals are encouraged to talk about plans for the future and about ways to maintain their progress. Those in need of further treatment are helped to recognize both the gains they have already achieved and what remains to be worked on further. With younger groups, a special party or trip, with photographs, is useful as a ritual that helps to signal the group's end.

Research

Dies and Riester (1986), as well as Azima and Dies (1989), have outlined the current meager status of child and adolescent group therapy research. Rigorous studies are rare, with the majority of reports rendering only impressionistic and qualitative outcome reports. Process studies geared toward objectively scrutinizing the what and the how in the therapeutic group situation are regrettably absent.

A welcome exception was offered by Feldman et al. (1983), who introduced an effective group treatment model for antisocial youths that was supported by a sophisticated research design. Known as the St. Louis Experiment, this program involved the use of a prosocial environment (settlement house) and the placement of selected youngsters with designated behavioral problems in groups composed of prosocial children. This study demonstrated the "therapeutic" effect of "normal" peers on antisocial children in groups led by trained group therapists.

In the broader assessment of the variety of group treatment methods applied with youths with CD, the frequent overlap of the clinical term *conduct disorder* with the legal term *delinquency* in the literature represents, as previously noted, a serious handicap. Axelrod (1965) examined, in this connection, the relationship between concepts of psychoanalysis and sociology. Rinsley (1978) provided an overview of juvenile delinquency from the perspective of a clinician, whereas Gordon and Arbuthnot (1987) delineated the group approaches employed in working with delinquent youths. There is some research support to suggest that, with older delinquents, learning and behavior modification groups are more effective than groups that operate on sociopsychological principles (Akers et al. 1979).

A Look at the Future

Given the fact that the typical individual "case-by-case" clinical interventions have been proven to be woefully inadequate in stemming the tide of CD in childhood (Reiss 1991), the need for small-group modalities and for preventive large-scale community interventions is paramount. In this connection, Boyle and Offord (1990) called for an identification of effective interventions that promise success and are cost effective. Such interventions are, at present, virtually nonexistent.

In the clinical context (outpatient and inpatient), we would hope that the current pragmatic practice of utilizing combined individual, group, family, and pharmacological interventions with children with CD, when available, will be subjected to more systematic scrutiny. In our view, no single treatment approach (including group therapy) has been proven to be definitively more effective than any other. Building on the all-too-few earlier successful experiments with group therapy in children with CD, P. F. Kernberg and Chazan (1991) have most recently incorporated a play group therapy component into their systematic tripartite model of treatment for such children and their parents. The results from this work will be eagerly awaited. Although such interventions are obviously more applicable to work with children, it is our hope that similar programs will be developed for adolescents with relevant evaluation measures included.

An important additional direction might well lead to the preventive sphere. Given the increasing psychosocial stressors in children's lives, psychoeducational group measures—for example, "rap" or counseling groups—might be regularly employed in schools to help young people deal with such normative "crises" as divorce, bereavement, physical abuse, and substance abuse. Needless to say, a research component would need to be a part of such work.

Because small groups represent major motivational forces in the normative life of both children and adolescents, there is good reason to believe that group processes can eventually be successfully employed in the service of therapy in general and of therapy with patients with CD in particular.

References

Aichhorn A: Wayward Youth. New York, Viking, 1935

Akers RL, Krohn MD, Lanza-Daduce L, et al: Social learning and deviant behavior: a specific test of a general theory. American Sociological Review 44:636–655, 1979

American Psychiatric Association: Diagnostic and Statistical Manual of Mental Disorders, 3rd Edition. Washington, DC, American Psychiatric Association, 1980

American Psychiatric Association: Diagnostic and Statistical Manual of Mental Disorders, 3rd Edition, Revised. Washington, DC, American Psychiatric Association, 1987

Anthony EJ: Group analytic psychotherapy with children and adolescents, in Group Psychotherapy: The Psychoanalytic Approach. Edited by Foulkes SH, Anthony EJ. New York, Penguin, 1957, pp 186–233

Axelrod S: Juvenile delinquency: a study of the relationship between psychoanalysis and sociology. Smith College Studies in Social Work 35:89–108, 1965

Azima FJC, Dies RR: Clinical research in adolescent group psychotherapy: status, guidelines and directions, in Adolescent Group Psychotherapy. Edited by Azima FJC, Richmond L. Madison, CT, International Universities Press, 1989, pp 193–223

Boyle MH, Offord DK: Primary prevention of conduct disorder: issues and prospects. J Am Acad Child Adolesc Psychiatry 29:227–233, 1990

Davis F, Lohr N: Special problems with the use of co-therapists in group psychotherapy. Int J Group Psychother 21:943–958, 1971

Dies RR, Riester AE: Research in child group therapy: present status and future directions, in Child Group Psychotherapy—Future Tense. Edited by Riester AE, Kraft I. Madison, CT, International Universities Press, 1986, pp 193–220

Eissler K: Some problems of delinquency, in Searchlights on Delinquency. Edited by Eissler K. New York, International Universities Press, 1949, pp 3–25

Erikson E: Identity and the Life Cycle: Selected Papers. New York, International Universities Press, 1959

Feldman RA, Caplinger TE, Wodarski JS: The St. Louis Conundrum: The Effective Treatment of Antisocial Youths. Englewood Cliffs, NJ, Prentice-Hall, 1983

Garland J, Jones H, Kolodny R: A model for stages in development in social work groups, in Explorations in Group Work: Essays in Theory and Practice. Edited by Bernstein S. Boston, MA, Milford House, 1973, pp 17–71

Gordon DA, Arbuthnot J: Individual, group and family interventions, in Handbook of Juvenile Delinquency. Edited by Quay HC. New York, Wiley, 1987, pp 290–319

Kazdin AE: Treatment of Antisocial Behavior in Children and Adolescents. Homewood, IL, Dorsey Press, 1985

Kernberg OF: A psychoanalytic classification of character pathology. J Am Psychoanal Assoc 18:800–821, 1970

Kernberg PF, Chazan SE: Children With Conduct Disorders: A Psychotherapy Manual. New York, Basic Books, 1991

Lippman HS: Difficulties encountered in the psychiatric treatment of chronic juvenile delinquents, in Searchlights on Delinquency. Edited by Eissler K. New York, International Universities Press, 1949, pp 156–165

Madonna JM, Caswell P: The utilization of flexible techniques in group therapy with delinquent adolescent boys. Journal of Child and Adolescent Group Therapy 1:147–158, 1991

Oberndorf CP: Psychotherapy in a residential children's group, in Searchlights on Delinquency. Edited by Eissler K. New York, International Universities Press, 1949, pp 165–174

Peck HB, Bellsmith V: Treatment of the Delinquent Adolescent. New York, Family Service Association of America, 1954

Raubolt RR: The clinical practice of group psychotherapy with delinquents, in Adolescent Group Psychotherapy. Edited by Azima FJC, Richmond LH. Madison, CT, International Universities Press, 1983, pp 143–162

Redl F: Diagnostic group work. Am J Orthopsychiatry 14:53–67, 1944

Redl F: When We Deal With Children. Glencoe, IL, Free Press, 1966

Reiss D: Conduct disorders in childhood. Psychiatry 54:113–115, 1991

Rey JM, Plapp J: Quality of perceived parenting in oppositional and conduct disordered adolescents. J Am Acad Child Adolesc Psychiatry 29:382–385, 1990

Rinsley DB: Juvenile delinquency—a review of the past and a look at the future. Bull Menninger Clin 42:252–260, 1978

Rosenthal L: Some dynamics of resistance and therapeutic management in adolescent group therapy. Psychoanal Rev 58:353–366, 1971

Schamess G: Differential diagnosis and group structure in the outpatient treatment of latency-age children, in Child Group Psychotherapy—Future Tense. Edited by Riester A, Kraft I. Madison, CT, International Universities Press, 1986, pp 29–68

Scheidlinger S: Activity group therapy with primary behavior disorders in children, in The Practice of Group Therapy. Edited by Slavson SR. New York, International Universities Press, 1947, pp 43–58

Scheidlinger S: Focus on Group Psychotherapy: Clinical Essays. New York, International Universities Press, 1982

Scheidlinger S: Short-term group psychotherapy for children: an overview. Int J Group Psychother 34:573–585, 1986

Scheidlinger S, Aronson S: Group psychotherapy of adolescents, in Adolescent Psychotherapy. Edited by Slomowitz M. Washington, DC, American Psychiatric Press, 1991, pp 101–119

Shellow R, Ward J, Rubenfeld S: Group therapy and the institutionalized delinquent. Int J Group Psychother 8:265–275, 1958

Siepker B, Kandaras C: Group Therapy With Children and Adolescents. New York, Human Sciences Press, 1985

Slavson SR: An Introduction to Group Therapy. New York, International Universities Press, 1943

Slavson SR: An elementaristic approach to the understanding and treatment of delinquency. The Nervous Child 6:413–424, 1947

Slavson SR, Schiffer M: Group Psychotherapies for Children—A Textbook. New York, International Universities Press, 1975

Winnicott DW: The Maturational Processes and the Facilitating Environment. New York, International Universities Press, 1965

Yalom I: The Theory and Practice of Group Psychotherapy. New York, Basic Books, 1975

Chapter 13

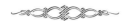

Behavior Therapy

Ronald J. Prinz, Ph.D.

The field of behavior therapy has contributed much research on the treatment of childhood antisocial behavior and conduct disorder (CD). Several reasons can be offered to explain the proliferation of behavior therapy research for childhood conduct problems:

1. Antisocial behaviors, which are readily observable and quantifiable, lend themselves to an assessment and therapy approach that emphasizes observational data.
2. The high incidence of CD in the population facilitates the identification of treatment samples.
3. Behavior therapy emphasizes the role of the social environment in the maintenance and modification of behavior problems (e.g., childhood social isolation, adult anxiety), and childhood conduct problems are best understood within a social context.
4. As the new area of behavior therapy developed in the 1960s and 1970s, it was applied to problem areas that had not previously met with widespread treatment success, such as alcoholism, schizophrenia, autism, and delinquency.

Much of the published behavior therapy research on childhood antisocial problems has focused on preschool and elementary school–aged children and, to a lesser extent, on adolescents. Consequently, behavior therapy approaches to antisocial behavior have been more thoroughly tested with children who would qualify within the current classification system (i.e., DSM-IV [American Psychiatric Association 1994]) for a diagnosis of oppositional defiant disorder (ODD), which would have placed them at pronounced risk for CD even though they were not old enough at the time of treatment to display all of the qualifying features for CD. The behavior therapy literature on childhood conduct problems can be separated into three relatively independent domains: classroom interventions, family interventions, and social/cognitive skills interventions. These three domains have several concepts in common, including the specification of target behaviors, an emphasis on positive reinforcement processes, and the assumptions that aggressive and antisocial behaviors are controlled by the same environmental variables as socially acceptable behaviors and that child behaviors are best understood within an environmental context.

Classroom Interventions

The behavior therapy movement pioneered a major direction of research on classroom behavioral management that has blossomed into a large and significant body of literature (O'Leary and O'Leary 1977). Much of this work has general applicability to regular and special education classroom settings and to various child populations, including normative, CD, attention-deficit hyperactivity disorder (ADHD), developmentally disabled, and learning disabled children. Classroom programming is a necessary ingredient to comprehensive interventions for children with CD but is generally not construed as addressing underlying causes for the development of CD. Classroom interventions for aggressive and disruptive children are usually employed to prevent misconduct from escalating into more serious situations (e.g., violence, suspension or expulsion, school failure) and to maintain a classroom environment conducive to learning for all of the children in the class. The more ambitious classroom interventions also undertake skills acquisition as a major objective.

Several principles underlie classroom behavioral approaches, both in specific programming for children with CD and in general classroom application:

1. **Positive environment.** Child cooperation and academic performance are best promoted by teachers who rely heavily on positive reinforcement, avoid harsh punishment and criticism, and use corrective feedback in place of general criticism.
2. **Contingent reinforcement.** A positive environment is not sufficient: reinforcement needs to be applied contingently to specific target behaviors immediately after they occur. Reinforcement serves at least two functions: to strengthen behaviors by reinforcing consequences and to inform children of which behaviors are desired.
3. **Successive approximation (shaping).** Acquisition of new behaviors typically needs to be accomplished in steps. A concept underlying most

successful academic and behavior management programs is that of successive approximation: new skills are carved out of behaviors already in a child's repertoire. Programming needs to begin with what a child is able to do and then to shape the child's behavior by gradually changing the target goal to require greater (or longer) performance of the reinforced behavior.

4. **Reinforcement of incompatible behaviors.** When children engage in behavioral excesses (as is typical of youths with CD), a program that focuses exclusively on the negative behavior is likely to fail. A more effective goal is to target positive behaviors that can take the place of—and that are incompatible with—the negative behaviors. For example, staying in one's seat and working on class assignments is incompatible with roaming around the classroom; speaking nicely to other children is incompatible with making derogatory remarks; keeping one's hands to oneself is incompatible with hitting others.

5. **Avoiding reinforcement of inappropriate behaviors.** Classroom behaviors that are disruptive or otherwise inappropriate are subject to inadvertent reinforcement through social attention and other influential consequences in the environment. Successful classroom programs evaluate and then eliminate or minimize competing reinforcement patterns.

6. **Modeling and prompting of appropriate behavior.** Contingent reinforcement is typically not sufficient to promote and maintain positive classroom behavior. Teachers and classmates are important sources of modeling. A teacher who frequently yells at and criticizes children in the classroom is likely to find some children imitating this behavior in other contexts. Additionally, children who are just beginning to acquire positive classroom behavior will need prompting to know what they must do to optimize reinforcement.

7. **Social/attentional reinforcement.** Positive social contacts between teacher and child and among children in the class provide the "glue" that makes behavioral programs successful. A reinforcement program that is administered without enthusiasm and frequent use of sincere, warm praise is doomed to failure.

Classroom programming to promote positive conduct has taken many forms. Perhaps the most common approach is a token reinforcement program. In a token program, rather than frequently disrupting academic lessons to provide a reinforcing activity or other positive consequence every time some child earns it, the teacher dispenses symbolic reinforcers (in the form of points, stars, chips, and so forth) that can be accumulated and exchanged periodically for backup reinforcers at designated times. Many variations of token programs are possible. A token program can have one or several behavioral goals, which can be standardized for the entire class or tailored to each child. The behavioral goals can remain constant throughout the academic year or can be modified or replaced at regular intervals. Tokens can be dispensed freely throughout the day or at the end of designated time blocks (e.g., class periods). A token program can consist solely of the dispensing of tokens or can also include the removal of tokens—commonly called *response cost*. Tokens can be pooled for the entire class and exchanged for classwide reinforcers, or children can earn their own tokens and pursue individually administered reinforcers. For extended discussions of classroom token reinforcement programs, the reader is referred to reviews by Kazdin (1977), Kazdin and Bootzin (1972), and O'Leary (1978).

Time-out procedures have commonly been employed, particularly in special education classrooms, as part of an overall classroom intervention strategy to ameliorate conduct problems at school. The rationale for time-outs is based on the assumption that when children are in a classroom or other environment that is truly reinforcing to them, brief removal from that setting (i.e., time-out from reinforcement) for misconduct will lower the probability of a repeat offense. In practice, time-outs can be easily misapplied if the classroom is not sufficiently reinforcing to the child, if the time-out period is unduly long (e.g., longer than 10 minutes), if the time-out situation actually contains sources of reinforcement (e.g., the child can interact with others or has access to entertaining objects) or permits the child to escape an activity such as a difficult academic assignment, or if the child is not adequately reinforced for a prosocial alternative to the behavior that earned the time-out.

Another classroom intervention strategy is the home-based reinforcement system. Home-based school reinforcement programs have been implemented in several different forms and have met with general success in improving classroom conduct and academic effort (Atkeson and Forehand 1979; Ayllon et al. 1975; Blechman et al. 1981a, 1981b; Budd et al. 1981; DuPaul et al. 1991; Kent and O'Leary 1976).

Classroom intervention methods are necessary but not sufficient to address the problems associated with CD and high-risk youth. However, intervention packages that overlook the classroom are not only missing an opportunity to positively impact much of a child's week but also contributing to the acceleration of CD brought on by unaddressed failure at school.

Family Interventions

Behavior therapy has made unique contributions to the development of family-based interventions for children and adolescents with CD. These contributions have resulted in the accumulation of an impressive body of research (Atkeson and Forehand 1978; Dangel and Polster 1984; Dumas 1989; Fleischman et al. 1983; Kazdin 1987; Miller and Prinz 1990; Patterson

1982; Sanders and Glynn 1981; Sanders and James 1983). Although several approaches to family intervention for conduct problems can be found in the behavioral literature, all of them share certain primary features and goals:

— The interventions are structured and usually well specified.
— Behavioral goals are pinpointed.
— Child behavior is assessed and understood within its environmental context.
— An overriding goal is to change the social atmosphere at home and to improve the parent-child relationship.
— Positive reinforcement processes are recognized as preferable to coercive and punitive modes of interacting.

Much, but not all, of the family-based behavior therapy work with children with CD falls under the rubric of what Kazdin (1987) has labeled parent management training (PMT). In a comprehensive review of all approaches to treatment of childhood antisocial behavior, Kazdin (1987) concluded that structured, family-based interventions in general—and PMT in particular—showed the most promise to date.

Within the general category of PMT are a number of variations in approach. Some parent training approaches include the parents but not necessarily the child/children in all sessions (Barkley 1987; Bernal et al. 1980; Fleischman et al. 1983; Forehand and McMahon 1981; Kent and O'Leary 1976; Webster-Stratton 1985). Other approaches include the children as an integral part of every session (Blechman 1985; Patterson et al. 1982). Treatment protocols vary in length from as few as 8 to as many as 30 (or more) sessions. Some approaches (e.g., Forehand and McMahon 1981) emphasize acquisition of general skills and abstract principles, whereas others (e.g., Blechman 1985) organize the regimen around concrete problems. All of the PMT approaches attempt to increase positive parental attention for child prosocial behaviors and to help parents cope more effectively with child noncompliance and aggression. There seems to be a general consensus that PMT produces short-term changes in most children and families and leads to long-term change in some (Kazdin 1987). However, there is also acute awareness that treatment gains are not maintained for a significant proportion of families (Dumas 1989; Miller and Prinz 1990; Patterson and Fleischman 1979). Several factors have been implicated in this failure, including social stressors (Dumas and Wahler 1983; Patterson 1983; Wahler and Dumas 1989), parental resistance (Chamberlain et al. 1984), and possible intervention deficiencies (Dumas 1989; Miller and Prinz 1990).

Recognizing that parent training in its most basic form is not sufficiently strong to produce lasting improvement in multiple-problem families with children who have CD, investigators have augmented and enhanced existing treatment protocols. The additions to PMT have included conflict-resolution skills (Martin 1977), parent-taught child self-control skills (Wells et al. 1980), simultaneous marital intervention (Dadds et al. 1987; Kelly et al. 1979), and interventions addressing parental needs for social support (Wahler and Dumas 1984, 1987).

Other behaviorally oriented family interventions for children with CD have been noted, although the number of published evaluations is considerably fewer. For example, functional family therapy (FFT) was developed specifically to address delinquency and associated conduct problems (Alexander and Parsons 1982; Barton and Alexander 1981; Parsons and Alexander 1973). FFT differs from PMT in two important ways. First, in FFT, the therapist meets with the entire family and works to improve family communication and support. Second, the therapist interprets family interactions using a broader systemic schema rather than a dyadic model. Nonetheless, FFT targets social reinforcement patterns and helps family members hone their communication skills, which are goals not at odds with parent training. Although promising, FFT has met with only limited evaluation or adoption.

Another example of a behaviorally oriented alternative to parent training is problem-solving communication training (Robin and Foster 1989). Although created for a broader population than just families with a child with CD, problem-solving communication training is a directive and skill-oriented intervention designed to help families learn more effective ways of resolving disputes. Like FFT, this intervention targets family communication and allows the therapist to adapt the model to fit the unique issues that each family presents. The approach has undergone some evaluation (Foster and Robin 1989; Foster et al. 1983; Robin et al. 1977) but needs to be tested with a homogeneous population of children with CD and their families. The model seems to be most appropriate for families with children in the 10- to 15-year-old age range.

In summary, behavior therapy approaches to family intervention for children with CD are generally promising and very well researched. A multicomponent intervention that fails to take advantage of the available behavioral treatment protocols is overlooking a valuable asset.

Social/Cognitive Skills Interventions

A third line of research has focused on social and cognitive-behavioral skills interventions that are administered individually or in groups. Reviews by Michelson (1987), Kazdin (1987), and Dush et al. (1989) identified several treatment outcome studies that applied either social skills training or cognitive-behavioral problem solving (or both) to samples of socially maladjusted children, including those exhibiting high rates of aggressive and antisocial behavior. The basic tenet of social skills training is that children with CD have identifiable behavioral/social deficits that can be altered by teaching them new and socially acceptable interpersonal behaviors through coaching, instruction, repeated practice, modeling, and reinforcement. These interventions focus on teaching friendship-making, conversation, and cooperation as well as the microskills that contribute to social adaptation, such as eye contact, listening, and smiling.

Social skills training has proven effective with socially isolated children (Wanlass and Prinz 1982) and has been extended to socially rejected children who exhibit varying degrees of disruptive and aggressive behavior (Bierman 1986; Bierman et al. 1987; Coie and Krehbiel 1984; Krehbiel and Milich 1986; Pelham et al. 1987). Results of social skills interventions with rejected children do not completely generalize to the antisocial CD population. Bierman (1986) found that although some rejected children display aggressive behavior, social rejection is not synonymous with aggression and conduct problems. Krehbiel and Milich (1986) have noted that social skills training has been shown to increase prosocial behavior and peer acceptance in rejected children who did not have CD but has produced less change in children who are both severely aggressive and peer-rejected. In a study by Coie and Krehbiel (1984), for example, a 12-session social skills training program failed to yield significant improvement in classroom behavior and social acceptance in a group of preadolescent children referred for aggressive/disruptive social interactions and peer rejection. In another example, Pelham et al. (1987) found that social skills training for peer-rejected ADHD children failed to enhance the effect of either parent training or medication on measures of peer acceptance, reported aggression, or classroom behavior. Much of the social skills programming was originally developed with the intent of increasing positive social interaction in withdrawn and shy children and was subsequently extended, first to socially rejected children and then to aggressive children with CD. Although there is no doubt that aggressive children have poorly developed social skills, the particular tactics previously tested have not met with much success in modifying aggressive behavior and skills deficits in youth with CD.

An alternate approach to skills interventions has emerged based on the view that deficits in cognitive processes and verbal mediation skills produce social maladjustment in children with CD. Support for this assumption is found in a growing body of research on cognitive processes in aggressive children. Aggressive children have been shown to differ substantially from nonaggressive children in perceptions of hostile intent by others (Dodge 1980; Dodge and Frame 1982), selective use and retention of cues in conflict situations (Dodge et al. 1984; Lochman 1987; Lochman and Lampron 1986; Milich and Dodge 1984), overlabeling of affective arousal as anger (Garrison and Stolberg 1983), self-control deficits associated with an impulsive cognitive style (Camp 1977; Kendall and Finch 1979), and failure to develop adequate problem-solving skills (Deluty 1981; Shure and Spivack 1979,

1982). Generally, the cognitive-behavioral interventions have emphasized either self-instruction strategies (Camp et al. 1977; Goodwin and Mahoney 1975; Kendall and Braswell 1982; Kendall and Zupan 1981; Kettlewell and Kausch 1983; Meichenbaum and Goodman 1971) or interpersonal problem-solving training (Lochman 1985; Lochman and Curry 1986; Lochman et al. 1981, 1984, 1985; Shure and Spivack 1982; Spivack et al. 1976), or a combination of both (Camp and Bash 1981; Kazdin et al. 1987; Michelson et al. 1983). Across the three approaches, short-term benefits were reported with respect to observed classroom behavior, teacher and parent reports of aggression and social adjustment, and academic performance. Most of the investigations targeted samples that were not composed exclusively of children exhibiting marked aggression and conduct problems, and most did not assess long-term effects. Notable exceptions to these limitations can be found in the work of Kazdin, Lochman, and Michelson and their respective colleagues.

In a sample of preadolescent children with severe CD, Michelson et al. (1983) compared Interpersonal Cognitive Problem Solving (ICPS with a multidimensional skills-training package emphasizing specific adaptive behaviors and a Rogerian treatment that controlled for nonspecific effects. Children received 12 weekly 1-hour sessions in each of the three conditions. Michelson et al. found that ICPS clearly outperformed the Rogerian treatment at 6-month and 1-year follow-ups on teacher, peer, self-report, and academic performance measures, and produced gains equivalent to those obtained with the multidimensional skill-training package. Inconsistent improvement on direct observation measures caused the investigators to recommend a more intensive and comprehensive intervention to enhance the efficacy of their cognitive-behavioral approach.

Over several years, Lochman and his colleagues have refined a comprehensive treatment program aimed at children's cognitive processing during interpersonal conflict situations (Lochman 1985; Lochman and Curry 1986; Lochman et al. 1981, 1984, 1985). In this program, children are taught to interrupt their deficient responses to perceived threats by inhibiting initial aggressive reactions, cognitively relabeling stimuli perceived as threatening, recognizing situations that call for improved problem solving, and generating and evaluating alternative coping strategies. The samples selected by Lochman and colleagues were characterized by marked aggression and conduct problems. The inclusion of a goal-setting procedure into the context of the original intervention (Lochman et al. 1984) and the extension of treatment from 12 to 18 sessions (Lochman 1985) produced greater short-term and long-term gains in terms of reduced aggression, improved self-esteem, and improved classroom behavior in comparison with either a shortened form of the program or a control condition. It is also apparent from the work of Lochman and others (Lochman et al. 1991) that social problem solving in aggressive children and children with CD is a complex topic with significant implications for improving our understanding of etiology and intervention.

Kazdin and his colleagues tested cognitive-behavioral interventions with preadolescent inpatients with severe antisocial behavior problems (mostly CD) in two outcome studies. Kazdin et al. (1987) found that children who received problem-solving skills training showed significantly greater immediate and 1-year follow-up improvement in prosocial behavior and reduction of aggression at home and in school when compared with children receiving either nondirective relationship therapy or an activity–contact control condition. In the second study, Kazdin et al. (1989) compared two types of interpersonal problem-solving interventions administered over 25 sessions to children with CD 7–13 years of age and found significantly greater improvement for both variations compared with a nondirective relationship therapy. However, Kazdin et al. (1989) lamented the fact that despite significant improvements, the majority of children receiving the experimental interventions remained within the clinical range of deviant behavior.

Future Directions

Behavior therapy researchers have tackled childhood conduct problems by using three distinct intervention modes: classroom programming, family-based interventions, and social/cognitive skills training. Interventions in all three domains have shown some success, although none can be offered by itself as a sufficient answer for the most severely disordered children. Future intervention research with CD as well as at-risk youth will need to consider the following parameters for ideal intervention programs:

— **Intervene early**—Postponing intervention for CD until adolescence is clearly undesirable. It is difficult to intervene successfully with adolescents with severe CD who have extended histories of conduct problems. Children with early onset of conduct problems present a higher risk for serious and chronic CD (Loeber 1990) and can benefit from intervention as early as age 5 or 6. However, because some CD or CD-prone youth do not come to the attention of service providers until they are adolescents, alternative treatment models are needed for these individuals, even if success rates are not optimal.

— **Intervene in multiple settings**—Most of the intervention research with childhood conduct problems has been with a single intervention mode, typically in only one setting. To optimize impact, interventions should take place in multiple settings—ideally including the home, the school, the peer group, and the neighborhood/community.

— **Address multiple targets**—Children at risk for CD exhibit a range of problems and are affected by a range of contexts. Full-impact interventions need to target child aggression, child impulsivity, academic difficulties, peer relations and social skills, family dysfunction and parenting practices, and other family and child needs.

— **Sustain interventions over time**—Sixteen-week and even 6-month programs are too brief for youths with more severe CD or who are CD-prone. Interventions over multiple years with phases matched to developmental level are needed to achieve and maintain positive outcomes.

These general goals are slowly being adopted by the field. The next 5 years should see more rigorous evaluations of multifaceted interventions administered in trials of longer duration to address the complex problem of CD.

References

Alexander JF, Parsons BV: Functional Family Therapy. Monterey, CA, Brooks/Cole, 1982

American Psychiatric Association: Diagnostic and Statistical Manual of Mental Disorders, 3rd Edition, Revised. Washington, DC, American Psychiatric Association, 1987

Atkeson BM, Forehand R: Parents' behavioral training for problem children: an examination of studies using multiple outcome measures. J Abnorm Child Psychol 8:449–460, 1978

Atkeson BM, Forehand R: Home-based reinforcement programs designed to modify classroom behavior: a review and methodological evaluation. Psychol Bull 86:1298–1308, 1979

Ayllon T, Garber S, Pisor K: The elimination of discipline problems through a combined school-home motivational system. Behavior Therapy 6:616–626, 1975

Barkley RA: Defiant Children: A Clinician's Manual for Parent Training. New York, Guilford, 1987

Barton C, Alexander JF: Functional family therapy, in Handbook of Family Therapy. Edited by Gurman AS, Kniskern DP. New York, Brunner/Mazel, 1981, pp 403–443

Bernal ME, Klinnert MD, Schultz LA: Outcome evaluation of behavioral parent training and client-centered parent counseling for children with conduct problems. J Appl Behav Anal 13:677–691, 1980

Bierman KL: The relationship between social aggression and peer rejection in middle childhood, in Advances in Behavioral Assessment of Children and Families, Vol 2. Edited by Prinz RJ. Greenwich, CT, JAI Press, 1986, pp 151–178

Bierman KL, Miller CL, Stabb SD: Improving the social behavior and peer acceptance of rejected boys: effects of social skill training with instructions and prohibitions. J Consult Clin Psychol 55:194–200, 1987

Blechman EA: Solving Child Behavior Problems at Home and at School. Champaign, IL, Research Press, 1985

Blechman EA, Kotanchik NL, Taylor CJ: Families and schools together: early behavioral intervention with high-risk students. Behavior Therapy 12:308–319, 1981a

Blechman EA, Taylor CJ, Schrader SM: Family problem solving vs. home notes as early intervention with high-risk children. J Consult Clin Psychol 49:919–926, 1981b

Budd KS, Liebowitz JM, Riner LS, et al: Home-based treatment of severe disruptive behaviors: a reinforcement package for preschool and kindergarten children. Behav Modif 5:273–298, 1981

Camp BW: Verbal mediation in young aggressive boys. J Abnorm Psychol 86:145–153, 1977

Camp BW, Bash BW: Think Aloud: Increasing Social and Cognitive Skills, a Problem-Solving Program for Children. Champaign, IL, Research Press, 1981

Camp BW, Blom GE, Herbert F, et al: "Think Aloud": a program for developing self-control in young aggressive boys. J Abnorm Child Psychol 5:157–169, 1977

Chamberlain P, Patterson G, Reid J, et al: Observation of client resistance. Behavior Therapy 15:144–155, 1984

Coie JD, Krehbiel G: Effects of academic tutoring on the social status of low-achieving, socially rejected children. Child Dev 55:1400–1416, 1984

Dadds MR, Schwartz S, Sanders MR: Marital discord and treatment outcome in behavioral treatment of child conduct disorders. J Consult Clin Psychol 55:396–403, 1987

Dangel RF, Polster RA (eds): Parent Training. New York, Guilford, 1984

Deluty RH: Adaptiveness of aggressive, assertive, and submissive behavior for children. J Clin Child Psychol 10:155–158, 1981

Dodge KA: Social cognition and children's aggressive behavior. Child Dev 51:162–170, 1980

Dodge KA, Frame CL: Social cognitive biases and deficits in aggressive boys. Child Dev 53:620–635, 1982

Dodge KA, Murphy RR, Buchsbaum K: The assessment of intention-cue detection skills in children: implications for developmental psychopathology. Child Dev 55:163–173, 1984

Dumas JE: Treating antisocial behavior in children: child and family approaches. Clinical Psychology Review 9:197–222, 1989

Dumas JE, Wahler RG: Predictors of treatment outcome in parent training: mother insularity and socioeconomic disadvantage. Behavioral Assessment 5:301–313, 1983

DuPaul GJ, Guevremont DC, Barkley RA: Attention-deficit hyperactivity disorder, in The Practice of Child Therapy, 2nd Edition. Edited by Kratochwill TR, Morris RJ. New York, Pergamon, 1991, pp 87–112

Dush DM, Hirt ML, Schroeder HE: Self-statement modification in the treatment of child behavior disorders: a meta-analysis. Psychol Bull 106:97–106, 1989

Fleischman MJ, Horne AM, Arthur JL: Troubled Families: A Treatment Program. Champaign, IL, Research Press, 1983

Forehand R, McMahon RJ: Helping the Noncompliant Child: A Clinician's Guide to Parent Training. New York, Guilford, 1981

Foster SL, Robin AL: Parent-adolescent conflict, in Treatment of Childhood Disorders. Edited by Mash EJ, Barkley RA. New York, Guilford, 1989, pp 493–528

Foster SL, Prinz RJ, O'Leary KD: Impact of problem-solving communication training and generalization procedures on family conflict. Child and Family Behavior Therapy 5:1–23, 1983

Garrison SR, Stolberg AL: Modification of anger in children by affective imagery training. J Abnorm Child Psychol 11:115–130, 1983

Goodwin SE, Mahoney MJ: Modification of aggression through modeling: an experimental probe. J Behav Ther Exp Psychiatry 6:200–202, 1975

Kazdin AE: The Token Economy: A Review and Evaluation. New York, Plenum, 1977

Kazdin AE: Treatment of antisocial behavior in children: current status and future directions. Psychol Bull 102:187–203, 1987

Kazdin AE, Bootzin RR: The token economy: an evaluative review. J Appl Behav Anal 5:343–372, 1972

Kazdin AE, Esveld-Dawson K, French NH, et al: Problem-solving skills training and relationship therapy in the treatment of antisocial child behavior. J Consult Clin Psychol 55:76–85, 1987

Kazdin AE, Bass D, Siegel T, et al: Cognitive-behavioral therapy and relationship therapy in the treatment of children referred for antisocial behavior. J Consult Clin Psychol 57:522–536, 1989

Kelly ML, Embry LH, Baer DM: Skills for child management and family support: training parents for maintenance. Behav Modif 3:373–329, 1979

Kendall PC, Braswell L: Cognitive-behavioral self-control therapy for children: a components analysis. J Consult Clin Psychol 50:672–689, 1982

Kendall PC, Finch AJ: Developing nonimpulsive behavior in children: cognitive-behavioral strategies for self-control, in Cognitive-Behavioral Interventions: Theory, Research and Procedures. Edited by Kendall PC, Hollon SD. New York, Academic Press, 150–182, 1979

Kendall PC, Zupan BA: Individual vs group application of cognitive-behavioral self-control procedures with children. Behavior Therapy 12:344–359, 1981

Kent RN, O'Leary KD: A controlled evaluation of behavior modification with conduct problem children. J Consult Clin Psychol 44:586–596, 1976

Kettlewell PW, Kausch DF: The generalization of the effects of a cognitive-behavioral treatment program for aggressive children. J Abnorm Child Psychol 11:101–114, 1983

Krehbiel G, Milich R: Issues in the assessment and treatment of socially rejected children, in Advances in Behavioral Assessment of Children and Families, Vol 2. Edited by Prinz RJ. Greenwich, CT, JAI Press, 1986, pp 249–270

Lochman JE: Effects of different treatment lengths in cognitive behavioral interventions with aggressive boys. Child Psychiatry Hum Dev 16:45–56, 1985

Lochman JE: Self and peer perceptions and attributional biases of aggressive and nonaggressive boys in dyadic interactions. J Consult Clin Psychol 55:404–410, 1987

Lochman JE, Curry JF: Effects of social problem-solving training and self-instruction training with aggressive boys. Journal of Clinical Child Psychology 15:159–164, 1986

Lochman JE, Lampron LB: Situational social problem-solving skills and self esteem of aggressive and nonaggressive boys. J Abnorm Child Psychol 14:605–617, 1986

Lochman JE, Nelson WM, Sims JP: A cognitive behavioral program for use with aggressive children. Journal of Clinical Child Psychology 10:146–148, 1981

Lochman JE, Burch PR, Curry JF, et al: Treatment and generalization effects of cognitive-behavioral and goal-setting interventions with aggressive boys. J Consult Clin Psychol 52:915–916, 1984

Lochman JE, Lampron LB, Burch PR, et al: Client characteristics associated with behavior change for treated and untreated aggressive boys. J Abnorm Child Psychol 13:527–538, 1985

Lochman JE, Meyer BL, Rabiner DL, et al: Parameters influencing social problem-solving of aggressive children, in Advances in Behavioral Assessment of Children and Families, Vol 5. Edited by Prinz RJ. London, Jessica Kingsley, 1991, pp 31–63

Loeber R: Development and risk factors of juvenile antisocial behavior and delinquency. Clinical Psychology Review 10:1–41, 1990

Martin B: Brief family intervention: effectiveness and the importance of including the father. J Consult Clin Psychol 45:1002–1010, 1977

Meichenbaum DH, Goodman J: Training impulsive children to talk to themselves: a means of developing self-control. J Abnorm Psychol 77:115–126, 1971

Michelson L: Cognitive-behavioral strategies in prevention and treatment of antisocial disorders in children/adolescents, in Prevention of Delinquent Behavior. Edited by Burchard JD, Burchard SN. Beverly Hills, CA, Sage, 1987, pp 190–219

Michelson L, Mannarino T, Marchione K, et al: Comparative outcome study of behavioral social skills training, cognitive problem-solving, and Rogerian treatments for child psychiatric outpatients: process, outcome, and generalization effects. Behav Res Ther 21:545–556, 1983

Milich R, Dodge KA: Social information processing in child psychiatric populations. J Abnorm Child Psychol 12:471–490, 1984

Miller GE, Prinz RJ: Enhancement of social learning family interventions for childhood conduct disorder. Psychol Bull 108:291–307, 1990

O'Leary KD: Token reinforcement programs in the classroom, in Handbook of Applied Behavior Analysis: Social and Instructional Processes. Edited by Catania AC, Brigham TA. New York, Irvington, 1978, pp 247–273

O'Leary KD, O'Leary SG: Classroom Management: The Successful Use of Behavior Modification, 2nd Edition. New York, Pergamon, 1977

Parsons BV, Alexander JF: Short-term family intervention: a therapy outcome study. J Consult Clin Psychol 41:195–201, 1973

Patterson GR: Coercive Family Processes. Eugene, OR, Castalia, 1982

Patterson GR: Stress: a change agent for family process, in Stress, Coping and Development in Children. Edited by Garmezy N, Rutter MP. New York, McGraw-Hill, 1983, pp 235–264

Patterson GR, Fleischman MJ: Maintenance of treatment effects? some considerations concerning family systems and follow-up data. Behavior Therapy 11:168–185, 1979

Patterson GR, Chamberlain P, Reid JB: A comparative evaluation of parent training procedures. Behavior Therapy 13:638–650, 1982

Pelham W, Schnedler R, Miller J, et al.: The combination of behavior therapy and methylphenidate in the treatment of attention deficit disorder: a therapy outcome study, in Attention Deficit Disorder. Edited by Bloomingdale L. New York, Spectrum, 1987, pp 56–74

Robin AL, Foster SL: Negotiating Parent-Adolescent Conflict: A Behavioral-Family Systems Approach. New York, Guilford, 1989

Robin AL, Kent R, O'Leary KD, et al: An approach to teaching parents and adolescents problem-solving communication skills: a preliminary report. Behavior Therapy 8:639–643, 1977

Sanders MR, Glynn T: Training parents in behavioral self-management: an analysis of generalization and maintenance. J Appl Behav Anal 14:223–237, 1981

Sanders MR, James JE: The modification of parent behavior: a review of generalization and maintenance. Behav Modif 7:3–27, 1983

Shure MB, Spivack G: Interpersonal cognitive problem solving and primary prevention: programming for preschool and kindergarten children. Journal of Clinical Child Psychology 2:89–94, 1979

Shure MB, Spivack G: Interpersonal problem-solving in young children: a cognitive approach to prevention. Am J Community Psychol 10:341–356, 1982

Spivack G, Platt JJ, Shure MB: The Problem-Solving Approach to Adjustment. San Francisco, CA, Jossey-Bass, 1976

Wahler RG, Dumas JE: Changing the observational coding styles of insular and noninsular matters: a step toward maintenance of parent training affects, in Parent Training. Edited by Dangel RF, Polster RA. New York, Guilford, 1984, pp 379–416

Wahler RG, Dumas JE: Stimulus class determinants of mother-child coercive interchanges in multidistressed families: assessment and intervention, in The Prevention of Delinquent Behavior. Edited by Burchard JD, Burchard SN. Beverly Hills, CA, Sage, 1987, pp 190–219

Wahler RG, Dumas JE: Attentional problems in dysfunctional mother-child interactions: an interbehavioral model. Psychol Bull 105:116–130, 1989

Wanlass RL, Prinz RJ: Methodological issues in conceptualizing and treating childhood social isolation. Psychol Bull 92:39–55, 1982

Webster-Stratton C: Predictors of treatment outcome in parent training for conduct disordered children. Behavior Therapy 16:223–243, 1985

Wells KC, Griest DL, Forehand R: The use of a self-control package to enhance temporal generality of parent training. Behav Res Ther 18:347–358, 1980

Appendix: Catalogue of Specific
Behavior Therapy Techniques and Terms

A number of the same concepts and techniques are commonly used in many behavior therapy treatment regimens. Some of the more frequently encountered terms are described below:

Contingency contracting   A contingency contract (sometimes called a "behavioral contract") is an agreement between two or more individuals that specifies a behavior change and the positive and negative consequences that will result if that agreement is or is not honored.

Differential reinforcement of other behavior (DRO)   A key concept in behavior therapy is DRO, the differential reinforcement of behavior incompatible with a problem behavior. By reinforcing a desirable behavior that cannot co-occur with the problem behavior, the problem behavior can be weakened and more appropriate behavior strengthened without the use of aversive procedures.

Extinction   The process of extinction refers to the gradual weakening of a behavior by the withdrawal of reinforcing consequences. This concept has clear application to family and school interventions with children with conduct disorder (particularly in the early elementary school years); behaviors such as temper tantrums and verbal disruption that are maintained by social reinforcement can be reduced through the systematic application of extinction.

Fading   Fading refers to the gradual withdrawal of aids used in training. Prompts, other antecedent stimuli provided by the change agent, and artificial reinforcers are gradually eliminated and replaced by naturally occurring stimuli and reinforcers.

Modeling   Modeling involves the demonstration of a target behavior as a means of instruction. The second part of the modeling process is reinforcement of accurate imitation.

Prompting   In teaching new behaviors, it is often the case that a child does not exhibit the desired behavior without help. Prompting is a procedure antecedent to the target behavior that makes it easier for a child to exhibit the behavior and earn the reinforcer. For example, if a child is learning to ask another child to share an activity, the change agent could prompt the child with the first part of the question ("May I . . . ?"). The goal behind the use of prompting is to promote errorless learning and a high rate of reinforcement in skills acquisition.

Punishment   Just as reinforcement is the process that strengthens behavior, punishment is the process in nature that weakens behavior. When behavior therapists work with families that include youth with conduct disorder, an important goal is to help parents replace either harsh punishment (e.g., corporal punishment, intimidation, coercion) or absence of punishing consequences for serious misconduct with socially acceptable and consistent punishment (e.g., 2-hour chore, earlier bedtime, restriction of television access). However, punishment as the sole means of intervention is improper and must be recommended only in the context of a strong reinforcement program.

Reinforcement contingency   To effectively reinforce a particular behavior, it is preferable that the reinforcer be earned only when the target behavior is emitted. A reinforcement contingency is in effect when the occurrence of the target behavior accurately predicts the reinforcing consequence and the nonoccurrence of the target behavior does not result in delivery of the selected reinforcer.

Response cost   Response cost is the retraction of a positive reinforcer contingent upon the occurrence of a (presumably unwanted) behavior. Response cost can be combined with either a simple reinforcement contingency or an entire token program.

Self-reinforcement and self-control   An alternative to reliance on external reinforcement is the development of self-reinforcement. The change agent can teach a child to accurately self-evaluate and appropriately self-reinforce (i.e., with tangible and cognitive consequences).

Shaping   The premise underlying the concept of shaping is that the change agent begins with behaviors that are already in a child's repertoire rather than imposing standardized behavioral requirements that might be out of reach for some children. Shaping involves the acquisition of a skill or other behavior by rewarding successive approximations of a target behavior, beginning with a similar behavior the child can already do.

Time-out from reinforcement   Removing a child from a rewarding situation for specific misconduct can potentially weaken the problem behavior. Time-out from reinforcement is the temporary (e.g., 10-minute) removal of a child from a setting in which reinforcers are readily available to a setting in which reinforcers are not available. However, if the primary setting does not provide sufficient reinforcement for desired behavior, then a time-out procedure is likely to fail or perhaps even to intensify the problematic behavior.

Token program Reinforcement for one behavior is often not sufficient to cope with the multiple needs of children. A token program is an organizing system for delivering multiple token or symbolic reinforcers for a few or even several behaviors and then permitting children to exchange these tokens for activity or tangible backup reinforcers. Token programs can be implemented at home, in the classroom, in training groups, or in other settings.

Chapter 14

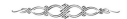

Pharmacotherapy

Jacquelyn Miller Zavodnick, M.D.

Conduct disorder (CD) is a ubiquitous problem with probable multiple origins. It is currently included as one of the disruptive behavior disorders in the DSM-III-R (American Psychiatric Association 1987) classification. The disruptive behavior disorders also include attention-deficit hyperactivity disorder (ADHD) and oppositional defiant disorder (ODD), both of which have been postulated as possible precursors to at least some forms of CD. ODD and CD that begin in childhood usually have a poorer prognosis (see Chapter 2) than behavioral disorder that first appears in adolescence, unless the behavioral disorder is part of a major mental illness. Biological vulnerabilities have been implicated in CD (Lewis et al. 1989), especially if the CD is accompanied by aggression. In addition, sociocultural and family violence factors have shown a marked association with CDs in general—aggressive and nonaggressive types as well as childhood and adolescent varieties. It is difficult to state the role of medication in CD because the definition of the disorder varies widely in the literature, and research studies in behavioral problems rarely focus on CD per se.

Drug studies dealing with conduct problems can be divided into several categories. There are "pure" studies dealing with DSM-III (American Psychiatric Association 1980) or DSM-III-R–defined CD. Other studies look at aggression as a factor independent of diagnosis. Still other studies examine the disruptive behavior disorders as a group. Finally, there are studies that look at comorbidity and treatment for children with CD who have some other additional diagnosis.

Comorbidity of CD with depression and with ADHD have received the most attention. When aggression is examined as an issue, however, the literature shows far wider implications. Especially of interest to clinicians are the many anecdotal, open, and controlled studies of aggression in the men-

269

tally retarded population. Also of heuristic value are the studies of self-injurious behavior in CD, autism, and mental retardation. Suicide studies are important because of the association of suicide with CD, depression, and aggression. Studies that look at irritability, aggression, and impulse control as behavioral dimensions in both patients and control subjects may eventually clarify issues related to CD. Although the relationship of CD and aggression to juvenile delinquency is ill defined, these populations clearly share many characteristics. Researchers in behavior find associations between anxiety (or lack of it) and possible biological differences children with CD. Epilepsy—in particular, partial complex phenomena—has been associated with conduct problems (Kim 1991). Although some behaviorally disordered children with epilepsy improve both behaviorally and in seizure control with medication, there is no clear association between "temporal lobe" phenomena and CD subtype (Apter et al. 1991). Finally, deafness has been linked with conduct problems.

Association of CD With ADHD

Of the disruptive behavior disorders, ADHD is the condition most clearly associated with CD. British clinicians generally diagnose the large majority of cases of what Americans call ADHD as CD. However, such diagnostic fine points may become irrelevant in light of some evidence that the disruptive behavior disorders can be viewed either as a whole or as a continuum of disorders. Many ADHD children also have ODD and CD symptoms. Children who display aggression and oppositional behavior in preschool may exhibit hyperactivity and conduct problems at school age. The relationship between these disorders is complex. Clearly, children who have attentional problems elicit frequent criticism from adults. Some develop feelings of being "bad," and as a result "act bad" because they feel hopeless and angry. Children on methylphenidate tend to receive less criticism from caregivers (Barkley 1988; Schacher et al. 1987), and this may prevent some of them from "feeling bad" and then "acting bad." However, self-esteem is an individual matter: even with successful medication, many hyperactive children remain angry, feel "bad," and "act bad."

A few studies of CD in children have demonstrated improvements with methylphenidate (Kaplan 1990; Klorman et al. 1990; Simeon 1991); however, this finding is confounded by the fact that most of those children also had ADHD. Interestingly, at least one study of methylphenidate in CD-ADHD adolescents (Kaplan 1990) showed a greater improvement in aggression than in attention. Although some reports actually discourage the use of methylphenidate in CD, the successful use of methylphenidate with ADHD-CD children is well documented (Stewart et al. 1990). No study has shown that CD decreases the likelihood of positive treatment responses for ADHD, although clinically the children referred by primary care physicians for treatment of hyperactivity are often referred because of failure to respond to methylphenidate and/or because of concurrent conduct problems—a phenomenon that may lead to a perception of CD-ADHD children as less responsive to methylphenidate.

ADHD treatment has expanded beyond stimulants not only because of treatment failures but also because of pressures from parents who do not wish their children to use stimulants. Serendipitous findings in other disorders have also led to novel uses. Clonidine (Hunt et al. 1985, 1986, 1990) was tried in ADHD because it was found to reduce concurrent hyperactivity when used in the treatment of Tourette's syndrome children. That an alpha-adrenergic agonist could help a disorder of attention may be related to noradrenergic mechanisms in ADHD, although stimulants specifically target dopamine effects. Clonidine, a profoundly sedating agent, might reduce hyperactivity or impulsivity on simpler grounds—that is, by sedating. However, Kemph et al. (1991) found that plasma gamma-aminobutyric acid (GABA) levels were significantly increased with clonidine and postulated a role for GABA in aggressive, cruel, and destructive child behavior. Fifteen of 17 children exhibiting such behavior improved on modest doses. Clonidine has been used with a disparate group of adult disorders, including addiction withdrawal and manic depression, with some success.

Tricyclic antidepressants (TCAs) have long been used for ADHD (Biederman et al. 1989a, 1989b, 1985) as well as depression in children with CD. Puig-Antich (1982) noted that conduct symptoms disappeared in prepubertal depressive children administered TCAs, who also became undepressed if their conduct symptoms had appeared secondarily to the depression. The relationship of depression and ADHD to CD has long been noted, whereas that between ADHD and depression is less elucidated. Some might argue that antidepressants make so-called resistant ADHD children more attentive because their attention problem is related to depressive concentration problems. Others argue that because of the shorter time course to improvement and the lower doses needed with antidepressants, the fact that a child's ADHD fails to respond to stimulants does not necessarily prove that the ADHD was "masked depression" when it responds to antidepressants. Although blood-level studies have been correlated with antidepressant response in depressed children, it would be of interest to know how blood levels in hyperactive children on antidepressants correlate with attention effects. The antidepressants bupropion (Casat 1989; Casat et al. 1987) and fluoxetine (Barrickman et al. 1991) have been successfully used with ADHD in recent trials; they may have a better side effect profile than the TCAs for ADHD.

In the past, neuroleptics were also among the drugs used for hyperactivity. Although not usually recommended for that use today, neuroleptics are still extensively used with CD and aggression.

Association of CD With Anxiety

In Chapter 2 of this volume, Lahey and colleagues define an early-onset group of children with CD who may differ biologically from control subjects without CD. The prognosis for this group is poor for both adult adjustment and adult antisocial behavior. Lahey et al. divide these children into two groups: CD-ASN children are anxious, socialized, and nonaggressive, whereas CD-NUA children are nonanxious, undersocialized, and aggressive. These groups differ from one another as well as from control subjects. Lahey and colleagues describe Borkovec's (1970) work, which showed CD-ASN children's skin conductance responses to tones to be higher than those of control subjects, which in turn were higher than those of CD-NUA children. This finding is consistent with the commonsense notion that unsocialized or antisocial people are able to lie without detection on a polygraph. Lahey et al. also quote studies of serotonin (5-HT) in whole blood that showed high levels of 5-HT in CD-NUA children, whereas the 5-HT levels of CD-ASN children did not differ from those of control subjects.

Many different biological and neurotransmitter systems have been implicated in behaviors exhibited by persons with CD (Plizka et al 1988; Rogeness et al. 1982). There are intriguing, often confusing, and sometimes contradictory findings. Taking Lahey et al.'s lead, one could identify "anxious" youth with CD as a possible subgroup. Some support exists for such a distinction. One hypothesis is that anxious children in a noxious environment use acting-out behavior as a defense against internal trait feelings or states. A child experiencing anxiety may throw chairs at school in response to a perceived threat. Children experiencing separation anxiety can become severely oppositional and aggressive if their verbalized or unverbalized wishes to stay home are not fulfilled. Thus, separation anxiety could present as school conduct problems if children feel they cannot ask to stay home, or as oppositional problems with parents if they ask directly and are thwarted. When the anxiety is addressed, the oppositional and conduct symptoms sometimes are alleviated. Thus, children with anxiety disorders can present with conduct symptoms. Likewise, children with CD can be anxious. Often, they are extremely sensitive to every nuance of their environment and take offense at everything, even as they are offending others. Children with CD frequently appear to be in a high state of arousal that has been compared to a panic state. "Anger attacks" have also been described in depressed adult patients. Others have compared "anger attacks" to panic attacks in adults (Fava et al. 1990). Kashani et al. (1991) found that children were significantly more anxious if they had high levels of verbal or physical aggression. Anxiety may be less frequently diagnosed in children with CD because of parental and professional tendencies to focus on behavior with "bad" kids. Yet many a young child appears in the clinician's office who acts bad all day and worries all night. It is important to look for anxiety symptoms and anxiety disorders in misbehaving children and adolescents with CD. Perhaps we need a new diagnosis called "masked anxiety" to make us more ready to look for anxiety in bad kids, just as "masked depression" was the first attempt at prompting professionals to consider that children might be depressed. We will probably find that anxious children can be diagnosed similarly.

Association of CD With Depression and Aggression

Children with CD often present with concurrent or preceding depression. When conduct symptoms appear after depressive symptoms, they often disappear when the depression resolves with TCAs (Puig-Antich 1982). Many children with CD later develop depression as well. In the older concept of masked depression, conduct problems were viewed as a manifestation of depression; however, it is now felt that core depressive symptoms—typical or atypical—are present in even the youngest depressed children if they are carefully examined. Irritability is becoming a factor to be reckoned with in the study of childhood depression and CD as well as of adult depression, suicidality, self-injurious behavior, and aggression. This symptom is more prominent in childhood depression than in adult depression. Irritability may be a link to the seemingly contradictory finding that depressive and aggressive cohorts share neurochemistry. Suicidal behavior is common to both depression and CD. Researchers in aggression see commonalities between inwardly directed aggression (self-abuse, suicide) and outwardly directed aggression (violence). Both suicidal and aggressive subjects show decreased cerebrospinal fluid (CSF) levels of 5-hydroxyindoleacetic acid (5-HIAA) (Kreusi et al. 1990). Aggressive, depressive, Down's syndrome, and phenylketonuria patients show decreased plasma 5-HT (Marazziti and Conti 1991), whereas obsessive-compulsive disorder (OCD) patients show increased levels and autistic patients show variable levels.

Autistic patients have been given fenfluramine without overall success, although some children did have decreases in stereotypy and withdrawal. Fenfluramine was used because a subset of autistic children have high levels of plasma 5-HT. Interestingly, the patients who did best were high-functioning individuals with or without hyperserotonemia. Hyperserotonemia is usually correlated with low functioning in autism. Because fenfluramine depletes serotonin, long-term administration of this agent is problematic on toxic grounds. Fenfluramine does not appear to decrease aggression in autistic patients, so it is paradoxical that this drug has been tried in patients with low plasma, blood, and platelet 5-HT levels, such as suicidal patients. Suicidal individuals show a decrease in suicidality (Meyendorff et al. 1986) when given fenfluramine regardless of whether their primary diagnosis improves. The suicidality of depressed patients usually tends to decrease before the depression improves when serotonergic antidepressants such as fluoxetine are administered, whereas the depression is the first symptom to improve when noradrenergic compounds are administered to such patients. Paradoxically, subjects given fluoxetine may experience an upsurge of suicidality (Riddle et al. 1990), a phenomenon that may be linked to fluoxetine's agitating/anxiety-increasing qualities if initial doses are too high. This effect may also be linked to akathisic symptoms. Akathisia in neuroleptic-treated patients has been associated with increased suicidality, and this link may possibly explain the paradoxically increased suicidality in rare patients on fluoxetine. The effects of serotonin reuptake inhibitors on the neuronal axis are not yet fully understood, and research findings are incomplete and contradictory. It is clear that early responses are different from longer-term responses with all antidepressants, a finding that could relate to these agents' sequential effects on the neuronal axis at different times as well as to the state of receptor sensitivity in different individuals at different times. This differential response could also relate to the locus of action, which can be presynaptic or postsynaptic at different doses.

Buspirone and other azapirones have been examined for their specificity for 5-HT$_{1A}$. At low doses (15–25 mg), buspirone decreases akathisia. For this reason as well as because of its effect in reducing irritability, buspirone has been suggested as a useful adjunct to fluoxetine (Neppe 1991). Reduction of irritability is an early effect of buspirone at low doses, which may make it a useful drug for syndromes in which irritability is a component (e.g., childhood depression, adult agitated depression, CD). Buspirone is felt to work presynaptically at these doses, and thus works antagonistically at the receptor. At higher doses (25–60 mg), buspirone may work postsynaptically as an "agonist," which might explain its usefulness in obsessive-compulsive phenomena. At very large doses (60–90 mg), buspirone has been postulated by Neppe (1991) to have a 5-HT$_2$ effect as a 5-HT$_{1A}$ receptor agonist, making it antimanic (because lithium essentially acts as a 5-HT$_{1A}$ agonist). At megadoses (120–240 mg), buspirone may be useful in treating tardive dyskinesia. Work on antiaggressive factors in the serotonin system has been somewhat stymied by the fact that rats have 5-HT$_{1B}$, which is precisely correlated with aggression. Rat aggression is nicely stopped by "serenics" such as the benzodoxines (Neppe 1991), which act specifically at this receptor. However, humans do not appear to share this 5-HT$_{1B}$ site (Neppe 1991). This difference may explain many of the discrepancies between human studies and animal research (Van Praag 1986), which shows clear antiaggressive properties of serotonin reuptake inhibitors that have not yet been shown or that have even been contradicted in humans (Winchel and Stanley 1991). Thus, although serotonin reuptake inhibitors such as fluoxetine or partial agonists such as buspirone may eventually play a role in decreasing aggression, irritability, or hyperactivity, their role is currently investigational.

The lithium cation is known to affect serotonergic functioning, because it is "effectively" a 5-HT_{1A} agonist (Neppe 1991). It is also known to raise CSF levels of 5-HIAA. Kreusi et al. (1990) found decreased CSF 5-HIAA levels in aggressive versus OCD children. They did not find impulsivity, however, to be related to 5-HIAA levels. Wetzler et al. (1991) found decreases in CSF levels of 5-HIAA in both self-directed (suicidal) and outwardly directed (violent) aggression, regardless of the subject's diagnosis. These authors ruled out 5-HT receptor hypersensitivity as being related to aggression but did not rule out hyposensitivity as postulated by Coccaro et al. (1991).

Of course, theoretical reasoning at its current state does not translate directly to treatment. Clinical judgment, patient response, and serendipity still play major roles in treatment outcome. The role of fluoxetine and buspirone and their as-yet-unreleased cousins in the treatment of CD remains to be clarified.

Lithium, on the other hand, has a long track record in aggression and a probable promising future with CD (Campbell 1991, in press; Campbell and Spencer 1988; Campbell et al. 1972, 1984, 1990a; Stewart et al. 1990). Neuroleptics, however, remain the primary agents used by clinicians (Campbell 1985; Campbell et al. 1972, 1984; Teicher and Glod 1990). Neuroleptics have considerable and serious drawbacks for managing aggression (Campbell et al. 1983a, 1983b), whether in youngsters with CD, aggressive mentally retarded children, or children with episodic dyscontrol. These populations all suffer from long-term and chronic behavioral disorders. The long-term risk of tardive dyskinesia—as well as the short-term risks of dystonias, akathisias, and parkinsonian side effects, and especially of neuroleptic malignant syndrome (Joshi et al. 1991; Turk and Laske 1991), which is neither dose nor time related—are so severe as to seriously call into question the use of neuroleptic drugs unless psychosis is clearly documented. The advantage of neuroleptics, on the other hand, is that the risks are very well known and can be monitored if not avoided. However, the use of neuroleptics for sedation alone is highly questionable.

Benzodiazepines have become extremely popular in the treatment of adult schizophrenic patients as an adjunct for sedation to neuroleptics. They have also been used in intermittent explosive disorder in adults. It has long been stated anecdotally that children can acquire "behavioral disinhibition" from benzodiazepines. The addictive potential of these agents makes their use unheard-of in the pediatric community, and they would thus appear to be an unlikely choice for children with CD. However, benzodiazepines have been used in children by hospitals and residential centers to supplement sedation or to be administered on an as-needed basis, as in adults. An alternative agent for sedation and acute aggression control may be the antihistamines, which share a brain H_2 receptor effect on sedation with the neuroleptics and therefore may offer a useful substitute.

Other drugs that may be of interest in CD include propranolol, carbamazepine, naltrexone, trazodone, and bupropion. As noted previously, fenfluramine, fluoxetine (and other 5-HT reuptake inhibitors), and the azapirones (Neppe 1991; Quiason et al. 1991) have theoretical appeal. Monoamine oxidase inhibitors (MAOIs) have been used in depression in adolescents and in "personality disorders" in adults, but most adolescents do not follow the diet even if the drug is successful (Ryan 1990). Until safer MAOIs are available, they cannot prudently be considered for use in depressed children and adolescents with CD. Bupropion, on the other hand, has been reported by several authors to be useful in ADHD (Casat 1989; Casat et al. 1987; Simeon et al. 1986; Wender and Reimherr 1990), and it may also be a useful antidepressant for CD.

Naltrexone (Bernstein et al. 1987; Campbell et al. 1990b; Herman and Chatoor 1991) has been seen as a theoretically helpful treatment for self-injurious behavior (SIB) in autism because of its effect on the opiate system. Some theories of SIB (Campbell et al. 1990a; Winchel and Stanley 1991) postulate that an opiate antagonist may be useful in reducing SIB, because individuals who exhibit SIB may have high cerebral levels (either intrinsically or self-induced) of opiate-type neuropeptides (Pies 1991). SIB is also found in youths with CD (Chowanec et al. 1991), although such behavior appears more purposeful when initials are carved on the arm or suicidal when wrists are slashed. Unfortunately, naltrexone has not proved particularly effective for the SIB of autism, although it does appear to improve overall performance, especially by reducing hyperactivity (Campbell et al. 1990a, 1990b). The possibility of trying this drug in impulsive/destructive children who appear "immune" to discipline is theoretically tantalizing. There are children who fulfill criteria for both a pervasive developmental disorder and CD; these children are often unresponsive to standard treatments of any kind.

Fenfluramine was initially seen as possibly effective in SIB in autism (Campbell et al. 1986; Donnelly et al. 1986; Ritvo et al. 1986); however, its results have been disappointing, both for SIB and for autism's other symptoms (Campbell et al. 1988; Donnelly et al. 1989; Varley and Holm 1990; Viesselman et al. 1994). Toxicity may also limit fenfluramine's usefulness (Schuster et al. 1986). Buspirone continues to be clinically tested (Gualtieri 1991; Quiason et al. 1991) for possible usefulness in irritability, aggression, depression, and pervasive developmental disorder.

Treatment

Many drugs have been tried in various patient subgroups (Brizer 1988), but the studies in children are limited and sometimes contradictory. The clinician should take a commonsense approach to treatment choices based on the behaviors and needs of the child. Environmental adjustments, behavioral techniques, family interventions, individual psychotherapy, and other possible interventions need to be factored into the risk-benefit ratio when making medication decisions. The risks of medication, both short- and long-term, must be weighed against the limitations of our knowledge of therapeusis.

Except for sedation with antihistamines as an early adjunct to more target symptom–specific medication, medication should always be begun as monotherapy so that effects, lack of effects, and side effects can be clear. Appropriate precautions should be taken and prescreening and follow-up studies performed. Specific contraindications such as allergies should be sought. Medications should be dosed in an appropriate manner for the particular class of drug. Increases should be implemented to upper limits or until side effects are prohibitive. The appropriate time for effect should then be allowed (e.g., 6 weeks for antidepressant effect, 4 weeks for antipsychotic effect, 4 hours for methylphenidate). If the drug is ineffective, it should be discontinued as necessary and a new trial instituted. Modern therapeusis should mean that no one gets too little or too much of a drug that doesn't work. If a drug works, it should be used; if it doesn't, something else should be tried in a logical way. If side effects are prohibitive, a different medication should be tried.

Table 14–1 illustrates possible drug regimens within categories or types of children with CD. The following sections summarize the classes of drugs used in CD.

Neuroleptics

Haloperidol and thioridazine are the most commonly used neuroleptics in children. Chlorpromazine has been less frequently used because of sedation and lowering of the seizure threshold. Trifluperazine, molindone, and thiothixene have been approved for all ages. Molindone and thioridazine are said to be less likely to cause neuroleptic malignant syndrome. Neuroleptic malignant syndrome is quite possible in childhood and is especially associated with affective disorder. Thioridazine causes less general acute side effects such as parkinsonism (extrapyramidal symptoms) but can cause tardive dyskinesia and ocular damage. Ocular effects limit thioridazine's dosage to 800 mg/day. All neuroleptics can cause agranulocytosis and seizures. Infrequently, galactorrhea and breast enlargement may occur, which is especially problematic for boys. The anticholinergic effects of neuroleptic drugs can be exaggerated by antiparkinsonian drugs, producing confusional states. Hepatotoxicity is possible. Orthostatic hypotension is a significant problem with chlorpromazine and thioridazine. All neuroleptics can produce parkinsonian signs, akathisia, tardive dyskinesia, withdrawal dyskinesia, dystonias, and oc-

Table 14–1. Possible drug regimens for types of conduct disorder

Possible indication	Drug	Dosage	Blood level	Cautions
CD-ADHD	Methylphenidate	0.3–0.5 mg/kg/dose	—	—
	D-Amphetamine	0.15–0.25 mg/kg/dose	—	—
	Pemoline citrate	56.25–112.50 mg/day	—	Blood dyscrasia; liver dysfunction
	Clonidine	0.025–0.05 mg/day to start; gradually increase every 3 days to 0.2–0.6 mg daily in divided dosage	—	Sedation; hypotension
	Antidepressants	(See CD-Depression)	(See CD-Depression)	Antidepressants not first choice (see CD-Depression)
CD-Anxiety	Diphenhydramine	25–500 mg/day	—	Idiosyncratic agitation
	Clonazepam (representative of benzodiazepines)	0.5–8.0 mg/day	—	Benzodiazepines can cause inhibition
	Buspirone	Anxiety 10–25 mg/day; OCD or depression 30–60 mg/day	—	Nonsyncopal dizziness; delay of action
CD-Depression	Fluoxetine	5–40 mg/day	—	Not studied for *depression* in children; delay of action; sensitivity to side effects
	Imipramine	Enuresis 2.5 mg/kg/day; hyperactivity 25–200 mg/day; depression 3.0–5.0 mg/kg/day or higher	Therapeutic lab levels combined 150–250 ng/ml; therapeusis combined > 155 ng/ml, > 200 ng/ml; toxicity combined > 225 ng/ml, > 500 ng/ml, > 1,000 ng/ml	Tricyclics can have 38- to 72-fold differences in blood level on same dose; all tricyclics are cardiotoxic and baseline and follow-up ECGs are necessary

		Therapeutic level	Side effects/monitoring
	Desipramine	100–200 mg/day (depression)	150–300 ng/ml; toxic > 1,000 ng/ml	—
	Nortriptyline	50–100 mg/day (depression)	50–150 ng/ml (therapeutic window)	—
	Bupropion	Up to 400 mg/day	—	Seizures; no studies with childhood depression
CD-Aggression (including self-injurious behavior)	Lithium carbonate	600–1,800 mg or 2,100 mg/day	0.8–1.5 mEq/L	Antithyroid, kidney
	Neuroleptics	Equivalent to 0.1–10.0 mg/day haloperidol	—	EPS, TD, NMS, akathisia; must do pre- and posttreatment movement assessment (AIMS)
	Propranolol	20–1,000 mg (give 20–40 mg twice daily; increase every 3 days if blood pressure stable; anxiety—low doses; aggression—high doses)	—	Hypotensive effects
	Carbamazepine	400–800 mg/day (1,000 mg below 15 years of age; 1,200 mg above age 15)	0.5–0.9 µg/ml (Campbell); Seizures—0.9–12 µg/ml alone; 0.5–0.9 µg/ml with other drugs	Rare—aplastic anemia, agranulocytosis, Lyell's syndrome, Stevens-Johnson syndrome; common—leukopenia; baseline complete blood count and differential; follow-up if symptoms (See CD-Depression)
	Antidepressants	Unknown (see CD-Depression)	Unknown (see CD-Depression)	(See CD-Depression)
	Buspirone	Irritability 10–25 mg/day; mania 60–80 mg/day	—	—

Note. ADHD = attention-deficit hyperactivity disorder. AIMS = abnormal involuntary movement scale. CD = conduct disorder. ECG = electrocardiogram. EPS = extrapyramidal symptoms. NMS = neuroleptic malignant syndrome. OCD = obsessive-compulsive disorder. TD = tardive dyskinesia.

ulogyric crises (Gualtieri et al. 1984; Richardson et al. 1991). All can also produce enuresis and sexual dysfunction. These last symptoms need to be specifically asked about because adolescents are usually too embarrassed to bring them up. Haloperidol has been reported to cause separation anxiety in children with tics (this author has also observed that symptom in one explosive mentally retarded youth on molindone). Parkinsonian symptoms respond to anticholinergic drugs; however, because these agents produce their own side effects, the lowest effective dosage should be used. Anticholinergics are not usually necessary after 6 months. Akathisia is a significant problem that may respond to a lowered dosage or the use of a beta-blocking agent such as propranolol. It is important to note that thioridazine can interact with beta-blockers to increase the levels of both drugs. Acute dystonias respond readily to diphenhydramine, especially by intramuscular route. Tardive dyskinesia is best prevented by using the smallest dose for the least time necessary. Mentally retarded individuals may be more at risk for tardive dyskinesia. An abnormal involuntary movement scale (AIMS) or similar rating of abnormal movements taken while the child sits, stands, walks, and talks is important before starting neuroleptics. This test should be repeated at regular intervals.

In adult schizophrenic patients, daily dosages greater than 10 mg of haloperidol have no more antipsychotic effects than a 10-mg daily dosage (Rifkin et al. 1991), although more sedation may be needed. This has been especially borne out by studies in children, which have shown small doses of haloperidol to be very effective in both autism (Campbell et al. 1983a) and CD (Campbell et al. 1984). Large doses are simply not warranted. If sedation rather than an antipsychotic effect is desired, then other sedating agents, especially the antihistamines, should be tried.

Droperidol, an ultrashort-acting anesthetic phenothiazine, was recently reported as an effective "tantrum aborter" in intramuscular dosing for hospitalized, violently acting-out children (Walkup et al. 1991). However, because it has been used only in surgical settings, droperidol's long-term consequences as a behavioral controller need assessment before inpatient use in children can be recommended.

Although the efficacy of neuroleptics in schizophrenia is unquestionable (Campbell 1985; Teicher and Glod 1990), the use of these agents for aggression in CD and even autism must be weighed against their long-term consequences. Although there is no question that neuroleptics can effectively decrease aggressiveness, other treatments with less long-term toxicity continue to be sought. Short-term and long-term side effects, however, are not unique to neuroleptics. In fact, side effects and unknown long-term risks continue to thwart attempts at finding replacements for neuroleptics. The value of neuroleptics cannot be underrated, but they require constant vigilance and willingness to judge their effects objectively. Aggression in institutions is clearly related to concrete variables such as patient mix and staffing patterns (Chowanec et al. 1991; Winchel and Stanley 1991). When considering a neuroleptic for behavioral control, all such variables should be assessed as possible targets for intervention. Dosages should be limited to the equivalent of 10 mg haloperidol unless blood levels document hyporesponsiveness (Rifkin et al. 1991). Patients already on high doses must have these titrated down extremely slowly to avoid rebound psychosis or aggression.

Lithium

Lithium has been used recently for children and adolescents with CD. Campbell (1984, 1985, 1987) found its effect equal to that of haloperidol but with less sedation. A 6-month follow-up, however, revealed that almost half of the subjects had withdrawn from the study because of side effects. Younger children seem to have more side effects and less improvement even when such factors as lithium level are controlled (Campbell, in press; Silva et al. 1991). Effects were seen in some children at levels below 0.50 mEq/L, however. Common side effects include weight gain (77% of one population), nausea, stomachache, vomiting, headache, tremor, enuresis, acne, and occasional weight loss. Lithium has been seen as specifically antiaggressive (Scassi 1982) and as especially useful in CD that has an affective component (Youngerman and Canino 1978). Strober (1991) has advocated lithium's usefulness in bipolar adolescents to prevent relapse. He noted that early treatment before the third episode is necessary to avoid treatment resistance. Strober also reported that 15 of the 50 bipolar adolescents in his study had experienced childhood problems with hyperactivity, emotional lability, and boisterousness—symptoms commonly seen in children with CD. Bipolar disorder should be considered if there is a cyclical behavioral problem in retarded or nonretarded misbehaving individuals; it should also be suspected if there is a sudden, unexplained onset of behavioral problems.

Lithium can interact with neuroleptics to reduce the levels of both drugs. It has also been used to augment antidepressants. Lithium levels are not affected by aspirin but can be by ibuprofen; they are definitely increased by indomethacin and other nonsteroidal antiinflammatory drugs (NSAIDs) (Ragheb 1990).

Lithium steady-state plasma levels can be difficult to maintain in children because of this population's variable salt ingestion patterns. Lithium salts are reduced by high salt intake, leading to what has been called the "taco tantrums" (Coffey et al. 1991). Exercise can affect lithium levels dramatically. In addition, children and adolescents are clearly prone to be overexposed to sun and sweating, and fluid and salt replacement may become necessary. Lithium toxicity must be carefully monitored, therefore, especially in the summer or during sports seasons. Fever can also increase lithium levels through dehydration.

Although saliva lithium level is reliable when individually calibrated to the patient's blood level, few if any laboratories do this routinely. Most children with CD, fortunately, do not find blood drawing noxious. Levels need to be determined at each dosage change until stable. Periodic checks, especially when side effects emerge, are necessary. Drug levels should be measured 8–12 hours after the last therapeutic dose. Therapeutic levels usually run between 0.8 and 1.5 mEq/L (but laboratories vary).

Gastrointestinal complaints sometimes respond to timing the dose to meals. Tremor requires dose reduction. Children and adolescents tend to skip doses if they experience ill effects, and such skipping leads to unreliable serum levels. If simple measures do not resolve side effects, other drugs should be considered, especially when noncompliance is an issue. Children have rapid renal clearance of lithium, which might require closer monitoring of blood levels and higher mg/kg dosage. Lithium often causes polydypsia and polyuria due to central nervous system (CNS) effects. It is thyrotoxic, and thyroid hormones should be monitored. Rarely, lithium can cause pseudotumor cerebri, requiring termination. Kidney disorder must be ruled out and renal function monitored over time.

More investigation is required regarding the use of lithium in children under 12 years of age. The long-term effects of lithium on the growing organism are unknown, and, therefore, treatment should be reserved for severe, refractory CD or bipolar disorder. Lithium is available in pill or liquid formulations.

Stimulants

Stimulants, primarily methylphenidate, have long been the backbone of treatment for hyperactivity (Jacobvitz et al. 1990), a problem often present in children with CD. Although some authors have not recommended the use of stimulants for CD, others have (Gadow et al. 1990). Dosages of methylphenidate range from 0.3 mg/kg/dose for attention to 0.5 mg/kg/dose for hyperactivity. Hunt et al. (1990) have recommended augmentation with other drugs such as clonidine or antidepressants if adequate relief is not obtained from stimulant monotherapy. They state that clonidine reduces the total dosage of stimulant required by 40%.

Methylphenidate's safety is enhanced by its short half-life, but this quality also leads to problems in smoothness of effect in some children. Midday dosing can be a considerable problem in some schools. Sustained-release forms offer some lengthening of treatment response. Although, clinically, the sustained-release form does not usually last the full 6–8 hours suggested, it may last long enough to get the child through the school day. Sustained-release methylphenidate can be useful in children who would otherwise require three-times-a-day dosing of regular methylphenidate, because compliance is increased by twice-a-day dosing.

Some children may have sleep difficulties secondary to late-day dosing of stimulants; others can finally pay enough attention to fall asleep normally for the first time. Although methylphenidate definitely affects weight and—at least temporarily—height, this is usually not a problem except in very thin children. Some parents find that they can overcome the anorexogenic effect by feeding the child before a dose is due. If the child loses his or her appetite, the sustained-release form would interfere with lunch; thus, regular-strength methylphenidate should be used with such children. Some children get stomachaches that do not improve over time. Other children develop headaches. Tearfulness, overtalkativeness, and dysphoria can also be seen. Children who have a suspected CNS disorder may respond to the drug with a "zombielike" overattention. Occasionally, children develop hallucinosis. Allergic reactions are possible. Parents should be warned of all of these possible consequences. Fortunately, stimulants are usually taken without any of these untoward effects. The most serious contraindication at present is presence of or family history of a tic disorder. The relationship of stimulants to the onset of tics is uncertain.

Methylphenidate can be easily monitored for effectiveness by teacher or caregiver reports (such as the Conners scales [Conners 1969]). Heart rate and blood pressure should be normal before beginning the drug and should be monitored periodically.

Although methylphenidate can be used in children and adolescents with ADHD, its use in preschool children is unclear. Interestingly, adolescents with CD and ADHD were reported to have more improvement of their impulsivity than of their inattention in one study (Kaplan 1990). In all age groups, methylphenidate appears to affect level of activity. There have been occasional reports of abuse of prescribed methylphenidate by adolescents. Prescribing of this drug can be limited by parental drug abuse or by parental uneasiness regarding the child's use of a controlled substance.

Dextroamphetamine has been less frequently used of late because of the difficulty for families in obtaining it (i.e., many pharmacies choose not to stock this medication). It is the drug of choice for preschoolers. Dextroamphetamine's side effects are similar to those of methylphenidate, and it can produce psychosis with chronic usage. Dosage ranges from 0.15 mg/kg/dose to 0.25 mg/kg/dose.

Pemoline citrate, a long-acting stimulant, can be used for a longer lasting effect, but is less effective then methylphenidate. It can have the same problem side effects as all stimulants; in addition, it has been infrequently associated with aplastic anemia and less rarely found to cause reversible liver enzyme abnormalities and hepatitis that require termination. Dosages range from 56.25 mg/day to 112.5 mg/day, with weekly additions of 18.75 mg to therapeutic levels.

Antidepressants

Tricyclic Antidepressants

The most commonly used antidepressants in children are the TCAs (Viesselman et al. 1994). The tricyclic imipramine was originally studied and approved for enuresis. Multiple studies of imipramine (Barrickman et al. 1991; Puig-Antich 1982; Ryan et al. 1987; Strober et al. 1990), desipramine (Barrickman et al. 1991; Biederman et al. 1989a, 1989b; Boulos et al. 1991; Gualtieri 1991), and nortriptyline (Geller et al. 1985, 1990) have led to controversial conclusions regarding the usefulness of TCAs in other disorders—particularly depression, but also ADHD. The controversies revolve around efficacy and safety (Riddle et al. 1991; Ryan et al. 1987).

Effectiveness may be contingent on dosage sufficient to produce blood levels in the therapeutic range. On the other hand, Popper (1992) notes that occasional children respond only to doses that produce blood levels *above* the therapeutic range. Dosing can thus be tricky with children and adolescents, because some children require high dosages to achieve therapeutic blood levels, whereas others become cardiotoxic on very low doses (Bartels et al. 1991; Giesler et al. 1991). In general, one cannot rely on dosage as a guide to treatment of depression. Also, effectiveness must be judged after sufficient time. As long as 6 weeks are required to judge therapeusis on sufficient dosage to produce a therapeutic blood level. Children and families desperate for relief may not be willing or able to wait this long for results. Effectiveness for ADHD (Gualtieri et al. 1991) and for panic anxiety may require lower dosages of TCAs; therapeutic levels have not been established to correlate with response in these conditions.

Safety, on the other hand, requires cardiac studies to be obtained on all children, regardless of condition or dosage. Blood levels may or may not correspond to cardiovascular effects. Imipramine plus desipramine levels vary as much as 36-fold on the same dosage, and monotherapy desipramine levels vary on an even wider scale. Children have more cardiovascular side effects than adults, and recent concerns about sudden death (Riddle et al. 1991; Wiles et al. 1991) make the study of safety correlations more urgent. TCAs tend to increase heart rate (Giesler et al. 1991). Because children have higher heart rates already, Ryan (1990) advises using a heart rate of 100 as the highest for children above 11 years of age and a cutoff of a 110 heart rate for children below 11 years of age. These ceilings are lower than previous recommendations in the literature. Twelve-lead electrocardiograms (ECGs) must be obtained before beginning therapeusis with TCAs. In addition to heart rate changes, tricyclics will prolong PR intervals, increase QRS duration (leading to bundle blockade), shorten QT intervals, and increase QTc levels

(Tingelstad 1991; Wiles et al. 1991). Tingelstad (1991) and others (Riddle et al. 1991; Wiles et al. 1991) recommend the QTc as the most important variable because its levels predict tachyrhythmia associated with sudden death. In addition, there are ST segment and T wave changes. ECG parameter changes with treatment should not exceed the following (Bartels et al. 1991; Tingelstad 1991):

— PR < 0.18 (ages 4–16 years)
— PR < 0.20 (over age 16 years)
— QRS < 0.12 or < 130% of change from baseline
— QTc < 0.45
— Blood pressure < 130/90

Blood pressure should not be raised to abnormally high levels. Blood pressure increases should be correlated with baseline blood pressure. The child's history may be of importance in ruling out increased susceptibility to arrhythmias. Riddle et al. (1991) have suggested that a family history of sudden death, cardiac disease, or paroxysmal atrial tachycardia may be related to sudden deaths in children. Dosage is not related. Blood level may or may not be related, although, theoretically, toxic changes could take place below, at, or above the therapeutic blood level. Tingelstad (1991) adds other risks, such as the association of some types of deafness with arrhythmias; this is important to remember because CD has been linked with deafness.

In addition to obtaining baseline and follow-up ECG, heart rate, and blood pressure at major dosage adjustments, baseline blood work should include a thyroid profile to rule out thyroid disease as a possible treatable problem. In addition, a routine complete blood count with differential, urinalysis, and blood sugar should be done to rule out anemia and other possible causes of tiredness or other symptoms. As with all children, routine pediatric care should be maintained, and a thorough history of medical problems is essential before beginning any program.

Currently, studies are available on the use of three TCAs: imipramine and desipramine in depression; imipramine, desipramine, and nortriptyline in ADHD; and imipramine in separation anxiety disorder. Results have been more positive in noncontrolled than in controlled studies, but there are many variables to account for the lack of consistent confirmation of effect. Therapeutic blood levels in use in most laboratories are as follows when obtained 8–12 hours after the last dose (the child should not eat or drink before the test):

— Imipramine combined: 150–250 ng/ml
— Desipramine: 150–300 ng/ml
— Nortriptyline: 50–150 ng/ml (therapeutic window)

Ambrosini and Puig-Antich (1985) suggested that levels of imipramine combined (i.e., imipramine and desipramine) of greater than 200 ng/ml may be necessary for the full antidepressant effect. Unfortunately, toxic effects are often seen beginning at 225 ng/ml, according to Preskorn et al. (1983). Other authors note therapeusis for depression at about 155 ng/ml. The child's tolerance for the drug may be unrelated to dosage or blood level. It has been suggested that divided doses may reduce toxicity (Ryan et al. 1987).

Limiting factors for the TCAs go beyond cardiotoxicity. Children may not tolerate other side effects such as orthostatic hypotension, sedation, or dry mouth. Suicidal ideation can emerge with any antidepressant, usually in children with previous episodes of such ideation (Mann and Kapur 1991). Because withdrawal effects (e.g., vomiting, nausea) can be quite pronounced in children, withdrawal should be as slow as possible. TCAs are very problematic in overdose and thus should be kept well out of access by suicidal children or their young siblings. Tancer et al. (1991) demonstrated the high rate of atypicality in adolescent depression and its low responsiveness to TCAs. Ryan et al. (1988; Ryan 1990) have suggested lithium augmentation as useful to increase tricyclic effectiveness. Use of MAOIs is not recommended.

Nontricyclics (Novel Antidepressants)

Bupropion, a novel nontricyclic, nonserotonergic antidepressant, has already been tried—specifically, in children with CD who have attention-deficit disorder (Simeon et al. 1986) and in ADHD children (Casat 1989; Casat et al. 1987) and adults (Wender and Reimherr 1990)—with positive results. Seizures were observed in adult studies with eating disorder subjects. Bupropion is not recommended for individuals with preexisting seizures. It is not known whether the proneness of younger children to febrile seizures would make them more susceptible to seizures on this drug. Dosages cannot exceed 400 mg/day in adults; parameters are not known for children.

A single report, by Zubieta and Alessi (1991), found that trazodone decreased hyperactivity, impulsivity, and aggressiveness in refractory disruptive, behaviorally disordered children. Trazodone's effect on sexual functioning in adult men may make it a problematic choice for males with CD.

Fluoxetine has been used in childhood hyperactivity but not in CD per se. Anecdotal reports of fluoxetine's side effects actually exceed the number of treatment studies. Treatment studies (Barrickman et al. 1991; Riddle et al. 1990) in children have been limited to OCD, Tourette's syndrome, and hyperactivity. Adverse reactions reported in children have included mania and self-destructive ideation (King et al. 1991; Mann and Kapur 1991). Other reported negative effects include regression, silliness, and hypomania.

Side effects reported with fluoxetine in adults include amotivational syndrome (Hoehn-Saric et al. 1990), agitation, and akathisia; side effects can also include nausea, diarrhea, constipation, restlessness, headache, and sexual dysfunction. Most side effects can be reduced by starting with the smallest doses (5 mg/day or less) and working up to higher doses only as side effects are tolerated. The major disadvantage of fluoxetine is its extremely long delay of action and its very long half-life. Dosage can range from 5 mg/day to 80 mg/day. Fluoxetine decreases liver enzyme breakdown; therefore, blood levels of other drugs (e.g., benzodiazepines) may be increased. In addition, because it is tightly bound to plasma protein, fluoxetine may displace or be displaced by other tightly bound drugs such as warfarin.

Antianxiety Agents

Benzodiazepines

There are very few studies on the use of benzodiazepines in children. With CD populations, these agents have come into increasing use as a sedating alternative to neuroleptics, especially for crisis use. However, the possibility of behavioral disinhibition renders such usage problematic. Children and adolescents who have tantrums will often resist the sedation vigorously, which can then lead to a "high" rather than sedation. Whereas in hospital settings, restraint and higher dosages may produce the desired sedation, achieving optimal sedation in home and residential settings may not be possible. Disinhibition can be a problem as an aftereffect even when the child does not resist the medication. Clonazepam does not appear to offer any particular advantage in this regard.

A study by Milner and colleagues (1991) seriously calls this usage into question. In a double-blind crossover design study of clonazepam in 11 children with anxiety disorders, symptoms of disinhibition, liability, irritability, and oppositional behavior became significant problems for many of the children with "pure" anxiety disorders. It would seem logical that such effects might be even more of a problem for children with CD, who already have these symptoms.

Benzodiazepines may be more helpful for acute anxiety in short-term treatment. Their use in chronic disorders needs to be weighed against the risks of disinhibition, memory effects, tolerance, and dependency. Withdrawal from chronic use must be gradual to prevent seizures.

Antihistamines

Diphenhydramine has been used for years in child psychiatry without any systematic reports of efficacy. Magda Campbell (1985) has recommended this drug for acute and chronic sedation, especially in psychosis. Except for idiosyncratic behavioral arousal, diphenhydramine appears to be uniquely safe. It is useful for extrapyramidal symptoms (EPS) and dystonic reactions. Dosages range from 12.5 mg to 500 mg; pill, liquid, and intramuscular forms are available.

Hydroxyzine is also available as an antianxiety agent. It potentiates CNS depression by other drugs and alcohol. High doses have been reported to cause seizures. Dosage is 50–100 mg in divided doses for anxiety and higher dosages up to 500 mg/day for sedation. Hydroxyzine is available in tablet, syrup, and intramuscular forms.

Buspirone

Buspirone, although marketed as an antianxiety drug, shows some promise in depression, OCD, CD, and possibly aggression. For anxiety, doses start at 5 mg three times a day and commonly go up to 10 mg three times a day. Because of buspirone's short half-life, multiple dosing is desirable. For anxiety and (depressive or nondepressive) irritability, and possibly for "short fuse" aggressivity or impulsivity and hyperactivity, small doses between 15 mg/day and 25 mg/day may be useful. For depression and OCD, larger doses (30–60 mg/day) may be needed. These ideas clearly require further testing.

Common side effects are nonsyncopal dizziness, nonspecific chest pain, ringing in the ears, and dysphoria. Some patients report restlessness, a symptom that may or may not relate to buspirone's moderate dopamine-binding-site affinity. Paradoxically, small doses (5–15 mg/day) of buspirone have been used to combat the restlessness produced by fluoxetine.

Antiepileptic Drugs

Carbamazepine, valproate (and valproic acid), and clonazepam are currently being extensively explored for nonseizure uses. Phenytoin enjoyed a flurry of popularity in research in the 1950s and 1960s but was subsequently abandoned as a useful behavioral drug. Valproate has not been studied in CD, but carbamazepine has been, both in retrospective reports (Evans et al. 1987) and in one prospective trial (Campbell 1991).

Carbamazepine is effective for CD and is also used successfully for intermittent explosive disorder; it is a logical theoretical choice for severe conduct problems. Reportedly, it is most successful in children with abnormal electroencephalograms (EEGs), but actual results in anecdotal reports are mixed. Carbamazepine has been reported to induce mania. In children who have documented partial complex seizures, carbamazepine may secondarily improve behavior. In an open-label study in children with CD, Campbell (1991) reported positive results in 6 of 10 subjects at a median dose of

641 µg/day with blood levels of 5–9 µg/ml.

Although carbamazepine's hematopoietic effects have been overrated, it can rarely cause aplastic anemia and agranulocytosis. It commonly causes leukopenia. A baseline complete blood count and differential should be obtained. Patients and parents should be warned to call if there is a sore throat, unusual bleeding, fever, easy bruising, or malaise, and a complete blood count should be reordered at that time. The drug must be stopped and treatment instituted if a disorder exists. Even weekly follow-up complete blood counts will not detect a true agranulocytosis as easily as will careful observation of symptoms, and children should not be traumatized by unnecessary needle sticks.

Stevens-Johnson syndrome and Lyell's syndrome of toxic epidermal necrolysis can occur rarely and require immediate drug cessation. Infrequently, carbamazepine can cause as well as treat seizures. It can also induce mania, hypomania, and hypersexuality (Myers and Carrera 1989; Pleak et al. 1988). Urinalysis and blood urea nitrogen measurement should be done to rule out renal dysfunction both before beginning administration and periodically afterward to monitor renal function. Like other tricyclics, carbamazepine can affect cardiac function and it can cause arrhythmia and atrioventricular block. It can cause liver dysfunction and hepatitis as well; therefore, baseline liver function tests with follow-up should be done. Commonly, carbamazepine can cause gastrointestinal distress in children. Theoretically, eye changes are possible, although reports have included only possible lens opacities.

There are no current guidelines for carbamazepine's use in nonepileptic conditions such as CD. The dosages and blood levels used by Campbell (1991) were lower than those commonly used for seizure monotherapy. Carbamazepine induces liver enzyme oxidation, leading to lowering or raising of various other drug levels and autoinduction of carbamazepine. The drug's initial half-life is 25–65 hours, whereas later it decreases to 12–17 hours. The blood level in seizure monotherapy is 9–12 ng/ml; in multidrug therapy it is 4–9 ng/ml. The half-lives of phenytoin, warfarin, doxycycline, and theophylline are significantly shortened by carbamazepine. Haloperidol levels can be reduced. On the other hand, levels of erythromycin, cimetidine, propoxyphene, isoniazid, nifedipine, and verapamil are elevated by carbamazepine and can lead to toxicity. Carbamazepine can increase the side effects and levels of lithium. Carbamazepine levels are lowered by other anticonvulsants but remain therapeutic. Tricyclic levels are affected (Brown et al. 1990).

Usual doses of carbamazepine for CD have not been established, nor have blood levels. Starting dosage can be 100–200 mg twice daily; this can be increased to approximately 800 mg (maximum 1,000–1,100 mg) per day in divided doses. Anecdotally, neurologists prefer the brand name to the generic form. Carbamazepine is available as a chewable tablet and a pill.

Clonidine

Clonidine appeared to hold special promise as a result of early reports by Hunt et al. (1985, 1986) of its special efficacy for impulsivity, which is clearly a problem for youngsters with CD. However, no studies with clonidine have been done in CD per se, although Hunt and colleagues specifically reported on clonidine's effectiveness in children with hyperactivity plus CD who were characterized by hyperarousal. However, these authors also state that clonidine is not useful for CD (Hunt et al. 1990) without hyperactivity, in spite of its use in adults as an antiaggressive agent.

This alpha-adrenergic drug is marketed as an antihypertensive agent but is used in Tourette's syndrome and hyperactivity. It may be useful for impulsiveness. Clonidine is clearly hypotensive and can reduce pulse rate significantly. It can cause oversedation, orthostatic hypotension, depression, tearfulness, vivid dreams, and other behavioral problems; it can also cause nausea and vomiting, anorexia, or weight gain. Rarely, clonidine can cause cardiac conduction problems, arrhythmias, and cardiac ischemia. Allergic reactions to both the tablet and the skin patch can occur.

Workup must include blood pressure and heart rate and a general physical examination with an ECG as necessary. Dosage should be started at 0.025–0.05 mg at bedtime, with increments of no more than 0.5 mg added every 3 days up to a maximum of 0.4–0.6 mg/day in divided doses. The most common side effect is sleepiness, which can inhibit clonidine's usefulness. Interestingly, sometimes bedtime dosing can eliminate this problem while still maintaining behavioral effects. If this regimen does not produce the desired behavioral effects, withdrawal from clonidine should be done as slowly as dosing (i.e., reducing no more than 0.05 mg every 3 days) to avoid rebound hypertension. The skin patch (Hunt 1987) can be used after a daily dose is established with pills. Pulse should not go below 55–60.

Clonidine tablets are available in generic form, whereas the skin patch is a brand name product.

Propranolol

In smaller doses, propranolol can be used for "stage fright," such as that occurring in examination anxiety or generalized performance anxiety. It has also been used to treat akathisia. In larger doses, propranolol has been used in behavioral aggressiveness and dyscontrol such as that found in CD and intermittent explosive disorder (Williams et al. 1982). It acts peripherally to reduce the autonomic behavioral equivalents of anxiety. In large doses, propranolol may act on other systems such as 5-HT, which may explain its antiaggressive effects. Yudofsky et al. (1981) warn that it may take 5–8 weeks to obtain full effect. Kuperman and Stewart (1987) found this drug useful in undersocialized aggressive CD children in an uncontrolled study.

Propranolol should not be used in asthmatic children, and it can mask thyrotoxicosis. Chlorpromazine increases the level of both drugs if used concomitantly. Propranolol can induce congestive heart failure in susceptible patients. Caution should be used with diabetic patients. Propranolol can commonly cause hypotension, epigastric discomfort, and lightheadedness, and can also cause depression. Allergic skin, hematopoietic, and laryngeal reactions, as well as other rare reactions, can occur.

Propranolol should be given at 20–40 mg twice daily and be increased at 20-mg intervals, depending on blood pressure stability in children. Dosage can be twice daily or three times daily. Doses of up to 1,000 mg have been used for aggressiveness. Dosages over 300 mg do not usually alter blood pressure any more than 300 mg. The drug should be discontinued slowly to avoid rebound hypertension and other cardiovascular problems. If blood pressure or pulse lowers with a dosage change, the clinician should wait for stability before initiating further increases. Dosages for anxiety are as low as 40 ng/day. Baseline blood pressure and heart rate should be monitored at each dosage change.

Summary

Although a variety of drugs have been explored for use with CD, medication remains primarily adjunctive to behavioral and parent management techniques. If CD co-occurs with a diagnosable disorder such as depression or ADHD, treatment of that disorder may render management of the CD far more effective. It is very important to look diligently for depression, anxiety, and other conditions because of the tendency to miss such symptoms due to these children's overt behavioral problems.

Aggression in CD must also be examined carefully. Although lithium and antiepileptic drugs hold promise as specific antiaggressive agents, their long-term consequences in children are as yet unknown. Neuroleptics may not be the only drugs to cause long-term consequences in children.

Finally, children with CD can have developmental disorders, including pervasive developmental disorders. These must be searched out and planned for in treatment.

References

Ambrosini P, Puig-Antich K: Major depression in children and adolescents, in The Clinical Guide to Child Psychiatry. Edited by Shaffer D, Ehrhardt A, Greenhill L. New York, Free Press, 1985, pp 182–192

American Psychiatric Association: Diagnostic and Statistical Manual of Mental Disorders, 3rd Edition. Washington, DC, American Psychiatric Association, 1980

American Psychiatric Association: Diagnostic and Statistical Manual of Mental Disorders, 3rd Edition, Revised. Washington, DC, American Psychiatric Association, 1987

Apter A, Arun A, Yaminer Y: Behavioral profile and social competence in temporal lobe epilepsy of adolescents. J Am Acad Child Adolesc Psychiatry 30:887–892, 1991

Barkley RA: The effects of methylphenidate on the interactions of preschool ADHD children with their mothers. J Am Acad Child Adolesc Psychiatry 27:336–341, 1988

Barrickman L, Noyes R, Kuperman S, et al: Treatment of ADHD with fluoxetine: a preliminary trial. J Am Acad Child Adolesc Psychiatry 30:762–767, 1991

Bartels MG, Varley CK, Mitchell J, et al: Pediatric cardiovascular effects of imipramine and desipramine. J Am Acad Child Adolesc Psychiatry 30:100–103, 1991

Bernstein G, Hughes J, Mitchell J, et al: Effects of narcotic antagonists on self-injurious behavior: a single case study. J Am Acad Child Adolesc Psychiatry 27:886–889, 1987

Biederman J, Gastfriend D, Jellinek MS, et al: cardiovascular effects of desipramine in children and adolescents with attention deficit disorder. J Pediatr 106:1017–1020, 1985

Biederman J, Baldessarini RJ, Wright V, et al: A double-blind placebo controlled study of desipramine in the treatment of ADD, I: efficacy. J Am Acad Child Adolesc Psychiatry 28:777–784, 1989a

Biederman J, Baldessarini RJ, Wright V, et al: A double-blind placebo controlled study of desipramine in the treatment of ADD, II: serum drug levels and cardiovascular findings. J Am Acad Child Adolesc Psychiatry 28:903–911, 1989b

Boulos C, Katcher S, Marton P, et al: Response to desipramine treatment in adolescent major depression. Psychopharmacol Bull 27:59–65, 1991

Brizer DA: Psychopharmacology and the management of violent patients. Psychiatr Clin North Am 11:531–568, 1988

Brown C, Wells BG, Cold JA, et al: Possible influence of carbamazepine on plasma imipramine concentrations in children with attention deficit hyperactivity disorder. J Clin Psychopharmacol 10:359–362, 1990

Campbell M: The role of neuroleptics in children and adolescents. Psychiatric Annals 15:101–107, 1985

Campbell M: Psychopharmacology of conduct disorder. Institute on Conduct Disorder, American Academy of Child and Adolescent Psychiatry Annual Meeting, San Francisco, CA, October 1991

Campbell M: Predictors of side effects associated with lithium administration in children. Psychopharmacol Bull 27 (in press)

Campbell M, Spencer EK: Psychopharmacology in child and adolescent psychiatry: a review of the past five years. J Am Acad Child Adolesc Psychiatry 27:267–279, 1988

Campbell M, Fish B, Jorein J, et al: Lithium and chlorpromazine: a controlled crossover study in hyperactive severely disturbed young children. Journal of Autism and Childhood Schizophrenia 2:234–263, 1972

Campbell M, Perry R, Bennett W, et al: Long-term therapeutic efficacy and drug-related abnormal movement: a prospective study of haloperidol in autistic children. Psychopharmacol Bull 19:80–83, 1983a

Campbell M, Grega DM, Green WH, et al: Neuroleptic-induced dyskinesias in children. Clin Neuropharmacol 6:207–227, 1983b

Campbell M, Small AM, Green WH, et al: Behavioral efficacy of haloperidol and lithium carbonate: a comparison in hospitalized aggressive children with conduct disorder. Arch Gen Psychiatry 41:650–656, 1984

Campbell M, Deutsch SI, Perry R, et al: Short-term efficacy and safety of fenfluramine in hospitalized preschool-age autistic children: an open study. Psychopharmacol Bull 22:141–147, 1986

Campbell M, Adams P, Small AM, et al: Efficiency and safety of fenfluramine in autistic children. J Am Acad Child Adolesc Psychiatry 27:434–439, 1988

Campbell M, Malone RP, Kanfantaris V: Autism and aggression: treatment strategies in child and adolescent psychiatry, in Treatment Strategies in Child and Adolescent Psychiatry. Edited by Simeon JG, Ferguson HB. New York, Plenum, 1990a, pp 77–98

Campbell M, Anderson L, Small AM: Naltrexone in autistic children: a double-blind and placebo-controlled study. Psychopharmacol Bull 26:130–133, 1990b

Casat CD: Bupropion in children with attention deficit disorder. Psychopharmacol Bull 25:198–201, 1989

Casat CD, Pleasants DZ, VanWyk FJ: A double blind trial of bupropion in children with attention deficit disorder. Psychopharmacol Bull 215:127–134, 1987

Chowanec GD, Josephson AM, Coleman C, et al: Self-harming behavior in incarcerated male delinquent adolescents. J Am Acad Child Adolesc Psychiatry 30:202–207, 1991

Coccaro EF, Harvey PD, Kupsaw-Lawrence E: Development of neuropharmacologically based behavioral assessments of impulsive aggressive behavior. Journal of Neuropsychiatry 3:544–551, 1991

Coffey B, Dulcan M, Ryan N, et al: Psychopharmacology. American Academy of Child and Adolescent Psychiatry Annual Meeting Symposium, San Francisco, CA, October 1991

Conners CK: A teacher rating scale for use in drug studies with children. Am J Psychiatry 126:152–156, 1969

Donnelly M, Rapoport J, Ismond DR: Fenfluramine treatment of childhood attention deficit disorder with hyperactivity: a preliminary report. Psychopharmacol Bull 22:152–154, 1986

Donnelly M, Rapoport JL, Potter WZ, et al: Fenfluramine and dextroamphetamine treatment of childhood hyperactivity: clinical and biochemical findings. Arch Gen Psychiatry 46:205–212, 1989

Evans RW, Clay TH, Gualtieri CT: Carbamazepine in pediatric psychiatry. J Am Acad Child Adolesc Psychiatry 26:2–8, 1987

Fava M, Anderson K, Rosenbaum JF: "Anger attacks": possible variants of panic and major depressive disorders. Am J Psychiatry 147:867–870, 1990

Gadow KD, Nolan EE, Sverd J, et al: Methylphenidate in aggressive-hyperactive boys, I: effects on peer aggression in public school settings. J Am Acad Child Adolesc Psychiatry 29:710–718, 1990

Geller B, Cooper TB, Farooke Q, et al: Serial ECG measurements at controlled plasma levels of nortriptyline in depressed children. Am J Psychiatry 142:1095–1097, 1985

Geller B, Cooper TB, Graham DL: Double-blind placebo controlled study of nortriptyline in depressed adolescents using a "fixed plasma level" design. Psychopharmacol Bull 26:85–90, 1990

Giesler J, Reeve E, Borchardt CM: Low dose tricyclic tachycardia (letter). J Am Acad Child Adolesc Psychiatry 30:151, 1991

Gualtieri CT: Buspirone for the behavior problems of patients with organic brain disorders (letter). J Clin Psychopharmacol 11:280–281, 1991

Gualtieri CT, Quade D, Hicks RE, et al: Tardive dyskinesia and other clinical consequences of neuroleptic treatment in children and adolescents. Am J Psychiatry 141:20–21, 1984

Gualtieri CT, Kennan RA, Chandler M: Clinical and neuropsychological effects of desipramine in children with attention deficit hyperactivity disorder. J Clin Psychopharmacol 11:155–159, 1991

Herman BH, Chatoor I: Naltrexone shown to decrease frequency of self-injurious behavior. The Psychiatric Times, August 22, 1991, pp 32–39

Hoehn-Saric R, Lipsey JR, McLeod DR: Apathy and indifference in patients on fluvoxamine and fluoxetine. J Clin Psychopharmacol 10:343–345, 1990

Hunt RD: Treatment effects of oral and transdermal clonidine in relation to methylphenidate: an open pilot study in ADDH. Psychopharmacol Bull 23:111–114, 1987

Hunt RD, Minderaa RB, Cohen DJ: Clonidine benefits children with attention deficit disorder: report of a double-blind placebo crossover trial. J Am Acad Child Adolesc Psychiatry 24:617–629, 1985

Hunt RD, Minderaa RB, Cohen DJ: The therapeutic effect of clonidine in attention deficit disorder and hyperactivity: a comparison with placebo. Psychopharmacol Bull 22:229–236, 1986

Hunt RD, Capper L, O'Connell P: Clonidine in child and adolescent psychiatry. Journal of Child and Adolescent Psychopharmacology 1:87–101, 1990

Jacobvitz D, Sroufe A, Steward M, et al: Treatment of attentional and hyperactivity problems in children with sympathomimetic drugs: a comprehensive review. J Am Acad Child Adolesc Psychiatry 29:677–688, 1990

Joshi PT, Capozzoli JA, Coyle JT: Neuroleptic malignant syndrome: life-threatening complication of neuroleptic treatment in adolescents with affective disorder. Pediatrics 87:235–239, 1991

Kaplan SL: Effect of methylphenidate on adolescents with aggressive conduct disorder and ADDH: a preliminary report. J Am Acad Child Adolesc Psychiatry 29:719–723, 1990

Kashani JH, Deuser W, Reid JC: Aggression and anxiety: a new look at an old notion. J Am Acad Child Adolesc Psychiatry 30:218–223, 1991

Kemph JP, DeVane CL, Levin GL: Plasma gamma-amino butyric acid (GABA) levels in aggressive children treated with clonidine (NR132). American Academy of Child and Adolescent Psychiatry Annual Meeting Research Abstracts, 1991, p 74

Kim WJ: Psychiatric aspects of epileptic children and adolescents. J Am Acad Child Adolesc Psychiatry 30:874–886, 1991

King RA, Riddle MA, Chappell PB, et al: Emergence of self-destructive phenomena in children and adolescents during fluoxetine treatment. J Am Acad Child Adolesc Psychiatry 30:179–186, 1991

Klorman R, Brumaghim J, Fitzpatrick P, et al: Clinical effects of a controlled trial of methylphenidate on adolescents with attention defect disorder. J Am Acad Child Adolesc Psychiatry 29:702–709, 1990

Kreusi MJP, Rapoport JL, Hamburger S, et al: Cerebrospinal fluid monoamine metabolites, aggression, and impulsivity in disruptive behavior disorders of children and adolescents. Arch Gen Psychiatry 47:419–426, 1990

Kuperman S, Stewart MA: Use of propranolol to decrease aggressive outbursts in younger patients. Psychosomatics 28:315–319, 1987

Lewis DO, Lovely R, Yeager C, et al: Toward a theory of the genesis of violence: a follow-up study of delinquents. J Am Acad Child Adolesc Psychiatry 28:431–436, 1989

Mann JJ, Kapur S: The emergence of suicidal ideation and behavior during antidepressant pharmacotherapy. Arch Gen Psychiatry 48:1027–1033, 1991

Marazziti D, Conti L: Aggression, hyperactivity and platelet imipramine binding. Acta Psychiatr Scand 84:209–211, 1991

Meyendorff E, Jain A, Traskman-Bendz L, et al: The effect of fenfluramine on suicidal behavior. Psychopharmacol Bull 22:155–159, 1986

Milner J, Rozzotto L, Klein RL: Clonazepam and childhood anxiety disorders: a pilot study (NR72). American Academy of Child and Adolescent Psychiatry Annual Meeting Research Abstracts, 1991, p 62

Myers WC, Carrera F: Carbamazepine induced mania with hypersexuality in a 9-year-old boy (letter). Am J Psychiatry 146:400, 1989

Neppe V: The clinical psychopharmacologic probe: serotonin 1A. Philadelphia, PA, Grand Rounds, Jefferson Medical College, December 11, 1991

Pies R: The biology of self-injurious behavior. The Psychiatric Times, December 19, 1991, pp 19–20

Pleak RR, Birmaher B, Gavrilescu A, et al: Mania and neuropsychiatric excitation following carbamazepine. J Am Acad Child Adolesc Psychiatry 27:500–503, 1988

Plizka SR, Rogeness GA, Renner P, et al: Plasma neurochemistry in juvenile offenders. Journal of the American Academy of Child Psychiatry 27:588–594, 1988

Popper CW: Disregarding antidepressant blood levels. AACAP Newsletter (Winter):19–20, 1992

Preskorn S, Weller E, Weller R, et al: Plasma levels of imipramine and adverse effects in children. Am J Psychiatry 140:1332–1335, 1983

Puig-Antich J: Major depression and conduct disorder in prepuberty. Journal of the American Academy of Child Psychiatry 21:118–128, 1982

Quiason J, Ward D, Kitchen T: Buspirone for aggression (letter). J Am Acad Child Adolesc Psychiatry 30:102, 1991

Ragheb M: The clinical significance of lithium–nonsteroidal anti-inflammatory drug interactions. J Clin Psychopharmacol 10:350–354, 1990

Richardson MA, Cray TJ, Haugland G: Children found to have a wide range of neuroleptic side effects. APA Meeting, New Orleans, LA, July 1991. Clinical Psychiatry News 19:7, 1991

Riddle MA, Harden MT, King R, et al: Fluoxetine treatment of children and adolescents with Tourette's and obsessive-compulsive disorders: preliminary clinical experience. J Am Acad Child Adolesc Psychiatry 29:45–48, 1990

Riddle MA, Nelson C, Kleinman CJ, et al: Sudden death in children receiving norpramin: a review of three reported cases and commentary. J Am Acad Child Adolesc Psychiatry 30:104–108, 1991

Rifkin A, Dodde S, Karaygi B, et al: Dosage of haloperidol for schizophrenia. Arch Gen Psychiatry 48:166–170, 1991

Ritvo ER, Freeman BJ, Yuwiler A, et al: Fenfluramine treatment of autism: UCLA collaborative study of 81 patients at nine medical centers. Psychopharmacol Bull 22:133–140, 1986

Rogeness GA, Hernandez JM, Macedo CA: Biochemical differences in children with conduct disorder socialized and undersocialized. Am J Psychiatry 139:307–311, 1982

Ryan ND: Pharmacotherapy of adolescent major depression: beyond TCAs. Psychopharmacol Bull 26:75–79, 1990

Ryan ND, Puig-Antich J, Cooper T, et al: Relative safety of single vs. divided dose imipramine in adolescent major depression. J Am Acad Child Adolesc Psychiatry 26:400–406, 1987

Ryan ND, Meyer V, Dachille S, et al: Case study: lithium antidepressant augmentation in TCA-refractory depression in adolescents. J Am Acad Child Adolesc Psychiatry 27:755–758, 1988

Scassi I: Lithium treatment of impulsive behavior in children. J Clin Psychiatry 43:482–484, 1982

Schacher R, Taylor E, Wieselberg M, et al: Changes in family functions and relationships in children who respond to methylphenidate. J Am Acad Child Adolesc Psychiatry 26:728–732, 1987

Schuster CR, Lewis M, Seuden LS: Fenfluramine: neurotoxicity. Psychopharmacol Bull 22:148–151, 1986

Silva R, Gonzalez NM, Kanfantaris V, et al: Long-term use of lithium in aggressive conduct disorder children (NR131). American Academy of Child and Adolescent Psychiatry Annual Meeting Research Abstracts, 1991, p 74

Simeon JG: Ritalin may curb conduct disorders in children. Paper presented at the Fifth World Congress of Biological Psychiatry, Florence, Italy, August 1991. Clinical Psychiatry News 19:8, 1991

Simeon JG, Ferguson HB, VanWyck FJ: Bupropion effects in children with attention deficit and conduct disorders. Can J Psychiatry 31:581–585, 1986

Stewart JT, Myers WC, Burket RC, et al: A review of the pharmacotherapy of aggression in children and adolescents. J Am Acad Child Adolesc Psychiatry 29:269–277, 1990

Strober M: Course of bipolar illness in teens, adults. APA Meeting, New Orleans, LA, May 1991. Clinical Psychiatry News 19:27, 1991

Strober M, Freeman R, Rigale J: The pharmacotherapy of depressive illness in adolescence, I: an open label trial of imipramine. Psychopharmacol Bull 26:80–84, 1990

Tancer NK, Klein RG, Koplewicz HS, et al: Rate of atypical depression and tricyclic drug response in adolescents (NR115). American Academy of Child and Adolescent Psychiatry Annual Meeting Research Abstracts, 1991, p 71

Teicher MA, Glod CA: Neuroleptic drugs: indications and guidelines for their rational use in children and adolescents. Journal of Child and Adolescent Psychopharmacology 1:33–55, 1990

Tingelstad JB: The cardiotoxicity of the tricyclics. J Am Acad Child Adolesc Psychiatry 30:845–846, 1991

Turk J, Laske B: Neuroleptic malignant syndrome. Arch Dis Child 66:91–92, 1991

Van Praag HM: Affective disorder and aggression disorder: evidence for a common biological mechanism. Suicide Life Threat Behav 16:103–132, 1986

Varley CK, Holm VAA: A two-year follow-up of autistic children treated with fenfluramine. J Am Acad Child Adolesc Psychiatry 29:137–140, 1990

Viesselman JO, Weller EB, Weller RA, et al: The psychopharmacologic treatment of depressed children and adolescents, in The Transmission of Depression in Families and Children. Edited by Sholevar GP, Schwoeri L. Northvale, NJ, Jason Aronson, 1994, pp 285–317

Walkup JT, Pizzo M, DeTornes R, et al: Droperidol in the acute management of agitated children and adolescents (NR93). American Academy of Child and Adolescent Psychiatry Annual Meeting Research Abstracts, 1991, pp 66–67

Wender PH, Reimherr FW: Bupropion treatment of attention-deficit hyperactivity disorder in adults. Am J Psychiatry 147:1018–1020, 1990

Wetzler S, Kahn RS, Asnis GM, et al: Serotonin receptor sensitivity and aggression. Psychiatry Res 37:271–279, 1991

Wiles CP, Harden MT, King RA, et al: Antidepressant-induced prolongation of QTc interval of ECG in two children (NR109). American Academy of Child and Adolescent Psychiatry Annual Meeting Research Abstracts, 1991, pp 70–71

Williams DT, Mehl R, Yudofsky S, et al: The effect of propranolol on uncontrolled rage outbursts in children and adolescents with organic brain dysfunction. Journal of the American Academy of Child Psychiatry 21:129–135, 1982

Winchel RM, Stanley M: Self-injurious behavior: a review of the behavior and biology of self-mutilation. Am J Psychiatry 148:306–317, 1991

Youngerman J, Canino IA: Lithium carbonate use in children and adolescents: a survey of the literature. Arch Gen Psychiatry 35:216–224, 1978

Yudofsky SC, Williams D, Gorman J: Propranolol in the treatment of rage and violent behavior in patients with chronic brain syndrome. Am J Psychiatry 138:218–220, 1981

Zubieta JK, Alessi N: Trazodone in the treatment of refractory disruptive behavioral disorders (NR130). American Academy of Child and Adolescent Psychiatry Annual Meeting Research Abstracts, 1991, p 74

Chapter 15

Hospitalization and Inpatient Treatment

John E. Meeks, M.D.

The hospitalization of youngsters with conduct disorder (CD) has been a source of some controversy in the field. Some reports have suggested that these patients are not appropriate candidates for inpatient treatment. Other, more scientific studies have shown that the diagnosis of CD includes many youngsters with treatable psychiatric illness (Alessi et al. 1984; Buydens-Branchey et al. 1989; Coccaro et al. 1989; Kazdin 1990). Still other studies have shown that failure to treat youngsters with CD is correlated with extremely adverse long-term outcomes for these patients (Loeber 1991; Robins 1966).

Most of the complex psychopathological syndromes that manifest a symptom picture justifying the diagnosis of CD are chronic illnesses that often include major elements of family dysfunction and ineffective parenting (Patterson 1982). Effective treatment needs to be long-term and must include assistance to the parents. Brief hospitalization plays a specific and limited role in the comprehensive treatment of youngsters with CD and their families. Indeed, if these youngsters' difficulties can be recognized early, many of the severe personality distortions of full-blown CD can often be prevented. Turecki (1989) has built on the research work of Thomas et al. (1968) to provide a practical and usable approach to this task.

Unfortunately, clinicians often encounter these youngsters after years of failure and maladaptive defenses have led to an explosive situation in which crippled self-esteem precipitates desperate efforts to achieve a spurious sense of invulnerability. Lying, stealing, intimidation, and other unacceptable actions escalate and are met by increasingly harsh but ineffective attempts on the part of parents and other adults to control the youngster. This negative spiral often leads to situations in which the youngster or others are in real danger. Hospitalization may be the only realistic response to ensure safety.

It is important, however, to avoid misuse of the hospital. Angry parents may be tempted to hospitalize their acting-out adolescent as a punishment or as a power move to "show who's the boss," even when an objective review of the situation suggests that the youngster has sufficient self-control to work safely in outpatient treatment. Even when hospitalization is indicated, the purpose of the inpatient stay needs to be understood in the context of the overall treatment needs of the patient.

Indications for Hospitalization

The most common reason for hospitalization of a child with CD is out-of-control behavior that is extreme enough to pose a danger to the child, to others, or to valuable property. The youngster may be threatening and homicidal, particularly toward family members but sometimes toward other individuals in the community. For example, in reviewing 10 consecutive admissions to our inpatient unit for youngsters with CD, it was noted that one of the patients had actually lacerated his father with a knife, two others had threatened family members with weapons, and three had been involved in violent outbursts with peers or adults outside of their family.

The destruction of property is important, not simply because of the financial distress it creates for families, but also because such behavior often is a prodrome to violence toward people. Many emotionally disturbed youngsters with CD will "trash" their rooms, breaking furniture and smashing holes in the wall in an effort to handle a rage that is actually felt toward people.

The out-of-control behavior of the child with CD can also be a threat to his or her own well-being. Perhaps the most common example is runaway behavior, which can place youngsters in dangerous situations in which their safety is compromised. In addition, many adolescents with CD become quite suicidal and pose an immediate threat to their own safety because of suicidal acting out (Coccaro et al. 1989; Shaffer 1985). In a recent large study (Shaffer 1988), the rate of completed suicides was higher in the group with CD than in any of the other populations studied—even the depressed population.

It should be mentioned that not all out-of-control behavior in fact represents an emergency indication for hospitalization. Other interventions such as emergency family sessions or individual interviews with the patient may be sufficient to manage the crisis and to make outpatient treatment feasible and safe again. In the atmosphere of fear, anger, and uncertainty that often surrounds a crisis in the family of a youngster with CD, it is important not to move too quickly to inpatient care as a solution to everyone's anxiety. On the other hand, many out-of-control behaviors *do* pose a threat to the safety of those involved and can only be managed by emergency hospitalization.

The second most common reason for hospitalization of the youngster with CD is the failure of outpatient treatment. That failure may result from the patient's refusal to even present him- or herself for care, the family's ambivalence about treatment, or the parents' total inability to effectively direct or limit their child. This failure of treatment compliance should not immediately or automatically lead to hospital care. Other interventions, such as mobilization of probation officers or other community leaders to support the family and to place effective limits on the youngster, should always be attempted. However, if these efforts fail, inpatient treatment may remain the only alternative for initiating effective care.

Other youngsters comply with outpatient treatment but find it insufficient to contain the extremity of their disorder—that is, they come for sessions and make a sincere effort to cooperate in treatment but still find themselves overwhelmed by impulsivity, depression, rage, or other uncontrollable psychological events so that they continue to function poorly (Gerstley et al. 1989; Marohn 1981). For some of these youngsters, the addition of a brief period of inpatient care is a sufficient catalyst to permit outpatient treatment to succeed following hospital discharge.

Finally, it is important to avoid using hospital care as a punishment. Parents' threats to hospitalize their youngster if he or she engages in certain behaviors that they have forbidden, parents' pleas for hospitalization because of their anger and frustration with the child, and even a therapist's impatience or frustration are not appropriate reasons to hospitalize a child with CD.

Goals of Short-Term Hospitalization

At present, acute hospital care actually means brief hospital treatment. Depending on the hospital's locale and fiscal structure, this translates into a length of stay ranging from 2 to 6 weeks, or occasionally 60 days. This reality needs to be recognized in planning hospital programs, estimating the potential value of hospitalization for a specific youngster, and planning for aftercare. However, length of stay is only one element to be considered in determining the therapeutic impact of an inpatient treatment experience. The time should be energetically used to accomplish specific goals.

The initial purpose of hospitalization of a youngster with CD who is out of control or failing in treatment is to provide the opportunity for a comprehensive diagnostic evaluation. Such an assessment should include not only the psychiatric, psychological, and neurological evaluation of the child but also the opportunity to evaluate family functioning and to assess the youngster's behavior on a 24-hour-per-day basis. Careful monitoring of the youngster frequently provides diagnostic clues that permit treatment to be more accurately attuned to the patient's actual needs, and therefore more successful. Inpatient care also has the advantage of being able to apply these diagnostic insights rapidly in a controlled setting to see if they actually help to stabilize the patient.

The second goal of inpatient treatment of a child with CD is to provide containment and control of the acting-out behaviors. These behaviors are often defensive against a variety of other difficulties that youngsters are experiencing and that they may be avoiding through their antisocial behavior. In the study of incarcerated youngsters conducted by Lewis et al. (1979), it was discovered that many of the youngsters had remained silent about psychiatric symptoms, histories of sexual abuse, and neurological deficits of which they were aware, even though disclosing these problems would have helped in their defense. The youngsters chose to be seen as bad rather than ill, even if it cost them their freedom or even their lives.

Limit setting in the hospital is a complex process that is discussed later in this chapter. In addition to providing youngsters with an opportunity to deal with life without the disruptive behavior that characterizes their recent adjustment, the hospital setting also affords an opportunity for parents to see effective control mechanisms in place that permit dignity yet prevent self-destructiveness. The techniques developed in the course of the hospital stay are also useful in designing an appropriate aftercare containment program, including home contracts and appropriate structured school or treatment elements.

The third main goal of hospital treatment of a child with CD is the process of redefining the nature of the problem for both the child and his or her family. These patients and their families tend to define the difficulty as volitional, moral, and vindictive. Blaming, accusations, demands, and moralistic lectures are frequently the primary materials of family discourse, enlivened only by the rage, obscenities, and threats coming from the adolescent. In the process of diagnosis and limit setting, the underlying anxieties, adaptational deficiencies, depressive feelings, and misunderstandings are frequently brought to light, thereby permitting the youngster's behavior to be reframed as a misguided adaptive effort rather than a vicious attack on the parents (Aichhorn 1964; Hoffer 1949; Linnoila et al. 1989; Marohn 1974).

Of course, if the youngster and family are to redefine the problem, the hospital staff needs to have a coherent consensus about their view of the core pathology in youngsters with CD. One view that does not depart from our knowledge base and that is teachable is offered here.

It is probably true that there are multiple factors involved in the etiology of CD, including biological, social, family, and psychological contributions. Some factors are more important in one case, others in the next. However, severe CD represents a misguided and ultimately destructive effort to maintain function and self-regard. The basic problems in these youngsters include the following:

— Perceived or real deficiencies in mastery skills (Biederman et al. 1991; Birmaher et al. 1990; Brown et al. 1981; Linnoila et al. 1983; Maziade et al. 1983) and/or self-control and capacity to modulate affect. In brief, there is an absence of felt emotional competence.
— Avoidance of dependent relationships, especially with anyone who would offer guidance, instruction, or direction.
— A defensive turn to omnipotent wishes and attitudes, bolstered and maintained through denial, constriction or repudiation of realistic achievements, lying, stealing, and intimidation (Aichhorn 1935; Cloninger 1987).

The overall result is youngsters who cannot learn because they cannot admit that there are things they need to know and people they can permit to teach them. Such youngsters fall gradually further behind their same-age peers, become more anxious, increase their defensive acting out, fall still further behind, and descend into a negative spiral from which they can see no escape. Even admitting that they are troubled or dissatisfied is difficult, since admission of need is frightening and unacceptable.

These adolescents themselves often feel guilt, self-hatred, and self-doubt because they have no real grasp of the reasons behind their inability to deal with their family and their world in a competent manner. When they learn, for example, that they suffer from a learning disorder, this information permits them to redefine a number of issues, including their interactions with their parents.

> Dorothy, a 15-year-old girl, stated after her treatment that she had always considered herself to be stupid, unlovable, and inherently oversexed and wicked. In the process of her hospital evaluation and treatment, she learned that she suffered from an undiagnosed reading disability and was attempting to maintain some self-esteem by proving that she was attractive to young men. She also recognized that her expectation that her parents would be disappointed in and disapproving of her had led her to provoke them in ways that caused them to in fact display this behavior. When she ceased to view herself in a negative way, she became more open to accepting their positive regard.

Related to the process of redefining the problem is the task of reenfranchising the parents. Many of the behaviors in which youngsters with CD engage are designed to demonstrate a spurious superiority and to make others feel helpless and inferior. These defenses are frequently unleashed on the parents in a very strong fashion. Parents whose youngsters have lied to them, stolen from them, threatened them, and constantly accused them of inadequate support and care are frequently a dispirited group. Often receiving nothing but negative feedback from their child, these parents' parenting performance deteriorates, in fact, so that they retain little or no control over their child's behavior by the time the situation is severe enough to warrant hospitalization. One important goal of the hospital stay is to reenfranchise the parents by working both to improve the adequacy of their parenting skills and to help them desist from inappropriate or destructive practices, while at the same time insisting that *they* are the ones who are best able to direct the child and supporting their right to maintain a parenting role of authority in the child's life (Patterson 1982).

The final goal of the short-term hospital care of youngsters with CD is to plan and design an acceptable and practical aftercare plan and to at least take the initial steps of gaining family and patient acceptance of that plan.

Organization of Inpatient Treatment

If one sees the symptomatology of youngsters with CD as their efforts to maintain a sense of competence and safety in the face of underlying distrust of their own mastery skills and of the availability of help, the hospital treatment program needs to address two major aspects of the youngster's dilemma: 1) the youngster's maladaptive, omnipotent action-defenses must be challenged and blocked through limit setting, and 2) a plan for increasing the youngster's mastery skills and his or her capacity to trust others must be designed and implemented. Of course, the ego-building elements of the plan will be carried out over an extended period of time after the youngster's discharge.

Adolescents with CD require special attention and programs designed to meet their particular needs. Most of all, they require staff members who understand the basic nature of the child with CD. For example, staff members who are uncomfortable with setting limits or who have difficulty dealing with the tendency of the youngster with CD to challenge, manipulate, threaten, and generally test any authority system will find it very difficult to work constructively in a program of this kind. It is also important to design a program with clear behavioral expectations, consequences for failure to follow those expectations, yet generous opportunities for success and positive feedback. Because the youngster with CD has a secret need for success and approval, it is important that plentiful supplies of such nutrients for the human spirit are provided, but without excessive sentiment or fanfare.

Behavioral control is obviously a major issue in the design of programs for youngsters with CD. Almost all units are locked, both because of these youngsters' tendency to run away when faced with stressful or upsetting experiences and because of the need to contain the adolescents' motor restlessness and preoccupation with seeking new and exciting experiences. At the same time, within the structure of the unit, generous allowances must be made for the youngsters' needs for physical activity, excitement, and risk taking. It is important to design programs that allow these needs to be met without overstimulating or seducing the adolescents into further hyperaggressiveness or destructive behavior.

For example, one such program—designed to support the discharge of angry feelings and to structure the expression of such feelings in socially acceptable ways—used boxing lessons as its medium. When tested on a unit for adolescents with CD, the program had some success but tended to overstimulate some of the youngsters, who could not contain their aggressiveness within the rules and limitations of the boxing ring.

The selection of staff for programs specializing in the treatment of youngsters with CD is not an exact science. Many people who feel they would enjoy working with these youngsters do not in fact prove successful when placed on the job. Others who come with ambivalence toward or outright reluctance for the task find that they are actually quite good at meeting the special needs of this patient population. There does not seem to be any one personality type or training background that necessarily qualifies people for this work. However, it is important to provide good supervision and to suggest quickly to people who are not working well in the system that they might be wise to consider treating a different patient population. Such measures are important because youngsters with CD often are hypersensitive to rejection and disapproval as a result of having encountered these reactions so frequently in the course of their lives.

In outpatient groups, it has sometimes been recommended that a heterogeneous collection of adolescent patients may be more helpful to one another than a homogeneous group. For example, a group that includes some youngsters with CD along with other youngsters who are more compulsive or perhaps depressed is a lively admixture, because the more conventional youngsters can help the children with CD to see a different pattern of living while the youngsters with CD may support a needed increase in adventurousness on the part of the more stilted children. In the inpatient treatment of youngsters with CD, however, a homogeneous group that permits the use of a program specifically created for this population may be the only practical approach. In mixed programs, youngsters with CD are often abusive to their less-aggressive fellow patients and may—if provided insufficient structure and limitation—use the supportive and nurturing permissiveness of the adolescent unit to continue their self-destructive acting-out behaviors.

It is important to have a highly structured and very active treatment program for these youngsters. A variety of special skill-building activities and specific treatment modalities is important if the program is to truly meet the needs of youngsters with CD.

For example, special education is a crucial element in the treatment program because many of these youngsters have learning disabilities that may be undiagnosed as the result of an assumption on the part of adults that their difficulties in school are purely caused by rebelliousness and inappropriate behavior there. Activity programs designed to socialize the risk-taking element in these youngsters—for example, "Outward Bound" types of challenge programs in which safety is maintained, the element of excitement and challenge is present, and youngsters must directly face external challenges—are very effective ways to mobilize a protherapy attitude in these youngsters.

Art therapy, movement therapy, and assertiveness training may be useful experiences for these youngsters if the therapists conducting the groups are familiar with the particular sensitivities and needs of this patient population. Guided imagery, a treatment that encourages youngsters to find mythical metaphors within which to express their personal difficulties with self-image and identity formation, can be very useful with these youngsters, because they are inclined to take special interest in heroes, conflict, and adventure. Because many of these youngsters have already created their own mythical characters—their "street image"—they take readily to this kind of self-expression through the creation of myths.

In addition, special treatment interventions need to be available because they are necessary to the effective treatment of the complex problems presented by this patient group. Such special treatments include programs for chemically dependent adolescents, special treatment tracks for youngsters who have experienced physical and/or sexual abuse, and cognitive-behavioral treatments designed to assist patients in managing anger in more constructive ways.

The extent to which the "skill building" aspects of treatment can be used within the hospital will vary with the available length of stay. In very brief admissions (4–10 days), it may be impossible to even begin such interventions. However, evaluation of needs and prescription and planning for such treatment and training experiences must be done or other so-called high-impact or stabilization interventions may be wasted effort.

Admission

It is often important to support and direct the parents of these youngsters through the admission process. Frequently, the nature of the illness has eroded parental self-confidence, produced destructive countermeasures, and resulted in extreme emotional distancing from the youngster. Understanding the particular distress of these parents and providing support and direction will permit them to examine the options and—if appropriate—make the difficult decision to hospitalize their child, even in the face of the child's predictable threats and manipulations aimed at derailing the treatment process. It is important to keep the admission process as simple as possible and to eliminate as many obstacles as can practically be avoided, relegating some of the paperwork and routine matters to a period following the time when the youngster is safely on the unit.

In some cases, it is possible to gain the adolescent's cooperation, particularly if the youth has been seen in outpatient therapy, has formed some working alliances, and is able to acknowledge his or her out-of-control state and to accept the need for external structure and support to gain treatment benefit. However, some adolescents with CD need to be hospitalized quickly and without their consent. A variety of more aggressive techniques—for example, mobilizing family and neighbor support with a show of strength to require the youngster to enter the hospital or using "white lies" to lure the youngster into the hospital—are regrettable but sometimes necessary.

> Dorothy, the 15-year-old girl described above as having achieved enormous gains in self-confidence and coping skills from her hospital stay, was tricked into coming onto the unit and was initially furious with her parents. Following her successful treatment, however, she was asked if she still resented her parents' duplicity. She stated, "It was their only choice. If they had told me I was coming here, I would have run away and perhaps would not have returned."

If the admission must be done without the cooperation of the adolescent, it is important to provide early opportunities after admission for the parents and the treatment staff to explain the purpose of the hospitalization and the reasons why the adolescent was not involved in the decision, and to provide an opportunity for the adolescent to express his or her inevitable anger. It is also important to begin family work right away so that the adolescent can come to understand that the treatment program does not assume that the parents have no responsibility for needed improvements or changes in the family system, but that everyone will be held jointly responsible, and that the goal of the treatment team is to encourage growth in *all* family members.

It is also important that the newly admitted patients receive special attention from the nursing staff on the unit as well as from other patients who have accepted the program and "settled in." These conversations, which may be resisted by the new patients, are still very useful because they often bring out the adolescents' misunderstandings, anxieties, and fears regarding how they will be treated in the hospital and what the implications for their future might be.

Steven, a 14-year-old boy who was admitted because of out-of-control, violent behavior in the home, including serious physical threats toward his 10-year-old brother, was able to tell a staff member on the second night of his hospital stay that he believed his parents had placed him in the hospital with the expectation that he would remain there forever and never return to his home. He believed that this course of action had been taken in retaliation for his angry threats toward his little brother, whom he believed his parents loved better than him.

Under the circumstances that usually accompany hospital admissions with these adolescents and their parents, the ideal of a mutually acceptable treatment goal is often a fantasy. The treatment team may have to actively push a treatment plan based on compromise goals that do not entirely satisfy either the parents or the adolescent.

Evaluation

The components of the evaluation process for adolescents with CD include the traditional elements of a psychiatric evaluation (i.e., social history, medical history, psychiatric history, family history with regard to mental illnesses), a physical examination, a mental status examination, and a careful evaluation of leisure activities and social skills. In addition, a thorough educational evaluation is essential because of the high rate of learning disabilities and cognitive disorders in this patient group.

The purpose of the basic evaluation is to assess a number of elements that may contribute to the adolescent's behavior problems. These areas of investigation include neurological functioning, affective functioning, reality testing, and the quality and nature of human relationships. The evaluation of neurological intactness includes not only a basic history of damage to the central nervous system (CNS) or other evidence of CNS disability but also a careful observation of the youngster's mental status, capacity to speak clearly and communicate effectively, memory functions, and ability to think abstractly. Any questions regarding neurological processes should lead to a more thorough evaluation of CNS functioning. Such an evaluation might include a neurological examination, an electroencephalogram (EEG), or other tests as indicated; more importantly, it should also involve neuropsychological testing, which is more likely to reveal subtle dysfunctions of the brain. Some centers have used evoked potentials or procaine-activated EEGs to further refine the neurological investigation. These tests, when performed by experienced and skilled individuals, do seem to provide valuable information (Ryback and Gardner 1991).

Because some youngsters with CD in fact suffer primarily from a depressive disorder, careful assessment of emotional functioning in this area is essential as part of the complete evaluation (Alessi et al. 1984; Harrington et al. 1990; Ryan et al. 1987). Many youngsters with CD will deny depressive symptoms, preferring to act out in an effort to avoid dysphoria. Careful observation of the patient's affect as well as continued exploration for the presence of depressive symptomatology—for example, crying spells, suicidal thoughts, or somatic symptoms such as weight loss or sleep disturbance— need to continue as the patient settles into the evaluation process and becomes more trusting.

The exact relationship between affective disorder and CD is not clear. The old concept of "masked depression" is giving way to the view that there are several patterns in which the two symptom pictures co-occur (Alessi et al. 1984; Biederman et al. 1991). These include cases in which the patient seems to be acting out to avoid dysphoria, depressive states that follow from the failure of delinquent defenses to maintain narcissistic balance, and depressive states secondary to drug abuse, among others. In all cases, therapeutic response to the depressive element can only occur if the affective element is diagnosed.

The treatment team must also remember the high risk for suicidal behavior in this population. If affective elements and substance abuse make up part of the presenting syndrome, the risk is even higher. The suicidal urges in these patients may be the result of an angry and manipulative state or may reflect a hopeless despair related to their repeated failures and lack of supportive relationships. Often, both elements contribute to suicidal risk along with the previously mentioned drug use (Abel and Zeidenberg 1985; Buydens-Branchey et al. 1989; Shaffer 1988).

Units committed to treating youngsters with CD need to have a well-designed hierarchy of suicidal precaution protocols ranging from "buddy systems" and increased communication to full-scale protection of the very self-destructive youngster. Fundamental safety rules regarding "sharps" and other dangerous objects are a basic expectation on any adolescent unit. Staff members also need to be aware of the risk of self-destruction when the adolescent with CD is very angry. Rage is a powerful emotion, and if its outward expression is contained without help in its modification being provided, it can become self-directed. When a youngster with CD is infuriated by a limit or other interpersonal interaction, he or she should be observed until self-control is regained.

The careful assessment of academic achievement and learning capacity should be a routine part of the evaluation of the youngster with CD. Primary learning disabilities, often unrecognized, are quite common in this population and need aggressive remediation.

Regardless of the underlying cause of anxiety and low self-esteem in these adolescents, their life situations are greatly complicated as the result of their use of action defenses, which are designed to obscure feelings of deficiency from others and from themselves. Staff members need to assess in specific ways how a patient avoids genuine challenges and is able to deny appropriate anxiety, as well as the patient's use of action to avoid frightening feelings and to prevent a sense of disorganization. It is also important to inquire regarding the prevalence of self-injury, either self-mutilation or breaking bones by striking walls and other hard objects. Many of these youngsters will use behavior of this kind to avoid a sense of overstimulation and to provide some release from the unbearable tension that is often part of their condition.

Careful assessment of patients' patterns of interpersonal relationships is important to clarify their tendency to avoid dependency urges. These problems appear in interactions with staff, parents, and other patients. Fear of closeness and lack of trust can manifest as open suspiciousness and cynicism or can be indirectly displayed through provocative behavior. All staff members need help in understanding this typical core pathology, both to avoid taking such rejections personally and to quickly confront youngsters' anxiety about dependency as a treatment issue.

Families also require careful evaluation. It is sometimes difficult to gain an objective view of the parents. The stress of the illness and the intensity of its interpersonal expression—especially within the family—often lead to extremely dysfunctional patterns. Some parents appear to have relinquished all attempts at control and live in fearful servitude to their "Imperial Child," still trying pathetically to understand and placate a youngster who has long since lost all respect for them.

Other parents are enraged and outraged, dealing with their pain by being totally rejecting of their child. However, it is important to recognize the source of some of this unwanted behavior so that the hospital program can assist parents to behave in ways that are more constructive and useful for their child. The brief respite from direct responsibility for child care may allow such parents greater objectivity and a chance for a new start.

Finally, it is important to recognize family strengths. Self-esteem is often at a low ebb for all members of these families and they often see themselves as ineffective, destructive, and deplorable. The treatment teams' insistence on recognizing areas of competence and survival skills is a crucial element in building a therapeutic alliance with the family.

The task of supporting and reenfranchising parents is often most difficult when it is most crucial—as, for example, in the case of parents whose parenting capacities are very deficient. Even in such cases, the positive elements of parenting must be recognized and supported even as all available treatment supports are provided to strengthen parenting skills. It is important to recognize the chronicity and interactive nature of the problem. The child is often difficult to parent and has been for some time (Maziade et al. 1983; Raine et al. 1990; Turecki 1989). The parent may have less-than-average knowledge, self-control, self-esteem, and general coping skills. Both parties in the relationship have great needs and a limited capacity to give. Frustration is inevitable, and it is the treatment team's responsibility to try to prevent further erosion of the family bond.

Multidisciplinary Treatment Plan

Based on the diagnostic findings, a treatment plan is evolved that aims to address the basic biological and/or psychological problems that gave rise to the low self-esteem and poor skills underlying the CD, while at the same time continuing to maintain limit setting in a safe environment so that basic issues can be addressed. The treatment of youngsters with CD requires the services of a number of well-trained specialists, including child and adolescent psychiatrists, social workers, educators, nursing personnel, speciality therapists such as those trained to treat substance abuse or the aftermath of trauma, and expressive therapists. This multidisciplinary team is organized under the leadership of a program director, who may be the child psychiatrist or another professional member of the team. The team members' goal is to work together, using their special skills in a complementary way for the benefit of the individual youngster.

It is inevitable that a team in a treatment setting of this kind will experience considerable splitting. Youngsters with CD are remarkably skilled at manipulation, intimidation, and other techniques that can easily lead to chaos within the team. It is crucial that team members arrange time for discussion with one another and that mutual support and direction be provided under the team leader to ensure that the youngster encounters a unified treatment effort (Marohn et al. 1973; Stanton and Schwartz 1954).

The adolescents themselves will also form a group that requires active attention if it is to be constructive and basically inclined to promote therapeutic gain. Because many of these youngsters depend on an unrealistic self-image, there will usually be at least one youngster who attempts to take over as "gang leader," using intimidation, rebellion, and omnipotent posturing to gain the adoration and support of the other patients. Often there are several youngsters who adopt a stance of this kind. Staff members are very much threatened by such behavior and often see adolescents who deal with their anxiety in this way as usurping the staff's control of the unit. This leads to anxiety as well as anger, and the potential for harsh retaliation is very real (Marohn 1981). Unfortunately, if staff members respond in this way, the effect is to produce a "martyr" who is seen as even more brave and admirable than ever, if the youngster refuses to give in to punishment.

It is much wiser to reverse the usual standards for honor and bravery and to insist that the really courageous act is to talk openly and freely about one's feelings while acknowledging that there are "risks" involved. This position can be tied in with other kinds of activity programs or athletics in the treatment program that involve physical risk, in effect equating the moral courage needed to openly face and overcome one's problems (i.e., "succeed" in the treatment) with the physical courage needed to succeed in physically demanding activities. The girls with CD in the program are slightly more likely than the boys to open up with their feelings and to discuss traumatic events in their past. They often have a positive influence on the male members of the patient population by providing a model for honesty and constructive response. The staff, of course, is highly supportive of honesty, directness, and constructive interactions between the patients, not in a condescending or parental manner, but in a collegial, admiring, and matter-of-fact way.

Properly managed, the group dynamics on the unit can be an important part, both of behavioral control and of new learning, in the recognition and expression of feelings through words rather than actions. The interpersonal skills of support and understanding can be greatly increased with this new opportunity for honest interaction.

The general therapeutic community and psychotherapy groups need to be augmented by speciality groups for those patients who require them. Chemical dependency treatment and education is almost always necessary, given that more than half of these youngsters are likely to have a complicating chemical dependency problem (Abel and Zeidenberg 1985; Buydens-Branchey et al. 1989). Treatment groups designed specifically for working through sexual and physical abuse issues should also be provided because a very high proportion of this population have been victimized in this way (Finkelhor 1984; Lewis et al. 1979; Marohn 1974).

Psychopharmacology

Medications alone are rarely sufficient to effectively treat CD. Early in the treatment process, when there is no alliance with the youngster, medications are often viewed as "chemical warfare" that the child psychiatrist appears to be using in an effort to force compliance with rules or to avoid behavioral difficulties with the adolescent patient.

However, many youngsters with CD do have underlying psychiatric or neurological illnesses that will respond to medication, with benefit to the overall treatment plan. The patient with attention-deficit hyperactivity disorder, major affective disorder, or seizure-like hyperdischarge in the temporal lobe may well benefit from appropriate medication. The medications used for children with CD who have these problems are the same as those used with other patients of this kind without CD (Stewart et al. 1990). These medications alleviate some of the problems underlying the CD, but alone will not reverse the maladaptive behavior unless they are combined with treatment programs that address skill deficiencies, family dysfunction, and maladaptive defenses. Psychopharmacotherapy with CD is described more fully in Chapter 14 of this book.

Family Intervention in Acute Hospital Treatment

The parents of hospitalized adolescents with CD are often completely dispirited and discouraged. They have lost any confidence in their ability to be helpful to their youngster and often feel extremely rejecting of the child because of the unacceptable behavior that has persisted over time and has grown so severe as to require inpatient treatment. The involvement of these parents in the treatment program needs to begin with an orientation and with education regarding the nature of CD. Since the patients themselves tend to portray themselves as actively choosing this life-style, it is not surprising that the parents often also believe that their youngsters are deliberately and maliciously choosing to be noncompliant. Recognizing the underlying disability and the purpose of the child's action defenses allows parents to be more sympathetic while also reinforcing their responsibility to maintain adequate limits and provide sufficient structure for their child. It is likewise important to evaluate the parents during this period to assess their own functioning and need for treatment, which may go beyond simple family therapy and counseling around their parenting duties. Many of these parents have impulse disorders and other difficulties that may also benefit from more direct treatment (Linnoila et al. 1989; Weissman et al. 1987).

It is useful to involve the parents in some experimental activity with their youngsters during the inpatient treatment program, since this method reaches beyond simple words to actively demonstrate both the kind of help that their child requires and the child's ability to respond positively to such help. This active involvement could go beyond family therapy to shared recreational activities or family involvement in the challenge program.

Of course, not every patient and family responds optimally, even if the treatment program is well designed. Some youngsters, for example, are successful in alienating other patients and even staff members, and maintain their "dependency shield" undented. They may even manage to disrupt the treatment program through provocation of other patients or directly dangerous acting out.

In these cases, an active reevaluation of the treatment effort should begin the moment the treatment effort appears to be failing. This mobilization should include emergency family meetings, staff evaluation of countertransference attitudes, active intervention in the patient group to support pro-therapy attitudes in patients, and a reassessment of the treatment plan to determine whether changes are necessary. In some cases these efforts are ineffective, and transfer to a different or more secure program may be in order. If discharge is done with clear recognition of the patient's inability to use the treatment and with honest regret, the experience can sometimes be a constructive reminder to the youngster that some effort at cooperation is essential for any treatment program to be effective. Some youngsters with CD become available for help only when it dawns upon them that they have come dangerously close to burning all their bridges.

> Mitch, a 16-year-old youth, had been expelled from three high schools before being hospitalized. From the beginning of his hospitalization, he was strongly motivated to understand and control his explosive temper. "I've got to learn to stop going off on people. There's only one more school that will take me," he explained.

In other cases, the parents may disrupt or interrupt the hospital treatment prematurely. Of course, every effort should be made to forge a therapeutic alliance with the parents—at least to the extent of gaining their trust that the program is generally on the right track. This objective requires individual evaluation of the reasons for parental dissatisfaction and an active response effort to gain or regain collaboration.

First of all, members of the treatment team need to evaluate their own roles in precipitating the crisis. Were the parents really understood and supported or was there overt or covert rejection, blaming, or neglect of them? Has communication been adequate for the needs of this particular family, especially early in the hospital course? Did the treatment team foresee potentially severe reactions to family separation—that is, evidence of enmeshment or symbiosis?

If the usual care was taken, there is the possibility that some family secrets are being threatened by the hospitalization. Unacknowledged child abuse, parental drug use, severe marital problems, and the like may be the hidden reason for the premature effort to remove the youngster from the hospital.

Often one never knows exactly why the treatment failed, but there is much to be gained for long-term treatment in the energetic effort to understand why the parents removed the youngster from treatment. Honest interest in the family, even in the face of anger, may build a base for more effective treatment efforts later.

Aftercare and Discharge

Youngsters with CD are ready for discharge from the hospital when they and their families achieve some recognition of the true nature of their illness and at least sporadic willingness to take positive steps to improve their situations.

It is obvious that brief, acute hospital care cannot completely reverse this chronic illness, and that aftercare with appropriate psychotherapy, educational remediation, and skills training will need to be provided. Arrangements for programming of this kind should occur in the last phase of hospital treatment. The youngster's progress and the family's strengths will offer clues as to whether aftercare should include a residential component or can occur on an outpatient basis, perhaps with a structured day program or special-education school that offers acceptance and skill for dealing with this patient population.

Outcome and Process Research

Outcome studies of treatment approaches to youngsters with CD are unavailable. One problem is the lack of criteria for defining equivalent patient populations, especially in view of the multiple etiological factors involved in creating conduct problems.

Follow-up data on hospitalized youngsters are even more sparse. Presumably, youngsters with CD who are hospitalized may be among the more complex or difficult cases. It is of interest that the Timberlawn Study (Gossett et al. 1983) revealed that about 20% of the youngsters diagnosed with CD at hospitalization were clearly suffering from a major psychiatric disorder at follow-up some years later.

Conclusion and Future Direction

Hospitalization will never be provided simply because treatment of one type or another is deemed best in the ivory towers of academia. Rather, hospitalization occurs in response to emergency situations, which take place with some frequency in youth with CD. Well-designed hospital care can provide safety, orientation, and a situation in which family, cognitive, and other therapies become possible.

References

Abel EL, Zeidenberg P: Age, alcohol and violent death: a postmortem study. J Stud Alcohol 46:228–231, 1985

Aichhorn A: Wayward Youth. New York, Viking, 1935

Aichhorn A: Delinquency and Child Guidance—Selected Papers. New York, International Universities Press, 1964

Alessi NE, McManus M, Grapentine WL: The characterization of depressive disorders in serious offenders. J Affect Disord 6:9–17, 1984

Biederman J, Newcorn J, Sprich S: Comorbidity of attention deficit hyperactivity disorder with conduct, depressive, anxiety and other disorders. Am J Psychiatry 148:564–577, 1991

Birmaher B, Stanley M, Greenhill L, et al: Platelet imipramine binding in children and adolescents with impulsive behavior. J Am Acad Child Adolesc Psychiatry 29:914–918, 1990

Brown GL, Ballenger JC, Minichiello MD, et al: Human aggression and its relationship to CSF 5-HIAA, MHPG and HVA, in Psychopharmacology of Aggression. Edited by Sandler M. New York, Raven, 1981, pp 131–147

Buydens-Branchey L, Branchey JH, Noumair D: Age of alcoholism onset, I: relationship to psychopathology. Arch Gen Psychiatry 46:225–230, 1989

Cloninger CR: A systematic method for clinical description and classification of personality variants: a proposal. Arch Gen Psychiatry 44:573–588, 1987

Coccaro EF, Siever LJ, Klar HM, et al: Serotonergic studies in patients with affective and personality disorders: correlates with suicidal and impulsive aggressive behavior. Arch Gen Psychiatry 46:587–599, 1989

Finkelhor D: Child Sexual Abuse: New Theory and Research. New York, Free Press, 1984

Gerstley L, McLellan AT, Alterman AI, et al: Ability to form an alliance with the therapist: a possible marker of prognosis for patients with antisocial personality disorder. Am J Psychiatry 146:508–512, 1989

Gossett JT, Lewis JM, Barnhart FA: To Find a Way. New York, Brunner/Mazel, 1983

Harrington R, Rutter M, Pickles A, et al: Adult outcomes of childhood and adolescent depression. Arch Gen Psychiatry 47:465–473, 1990

Hoffer W: Deceiving the deceiver, in Searchlights on Delinquency. Edited by Eissler KR. New York, International Universities Press, 1949, pp 150–155

Kazdin AE: Conduct disorder. The Psychiatric Hospital 20:153–158, 1990

Lewis DO, Shanok SS, Pincus JH, et al: Violent juvenile delinquents: psychiatric, neurological, psychological, and abuse factors. Journal of the American Academy of Child Psychiatry 18:307–319, 1979

Linnoila M, Virkkunen M, Scheinin M, et al: Low cerebrospinal fluid 5-HIAA concentration differentiates impulsive from nonimpulsive violent behavior. Life Sci 33:2609–2614, 1983

Linnoila M, DeJong J, Virkkunen M: Family history of alcoholism in violent offenders and impulsive fire setters. Arch Gen Psychiatry 46:613–616, 1989

Loeber R: Antisocial behavior: more enduring than changeable? J Am Acad Child Adolesc Psychiatry 30:393–397, 1991

Marohn RC: Trauma and the delinquent. Adolescent Psychiatry 3:354–361, 1974

Marohn RC: The negative transference in the treatment of juvenile delinquents. Annals of Psychoanalysis 9:21–42, 1981

Marohn RC, Dalle-Molle D, Offer D, et al: A hospital riot: its determinants and implications for treatment. Am J Psychiatry 130:631–636, 1973

Maziade M, Caron C, Cote R, et al: Extreme temperament and diagnosis. Arch Gen Psychiatry 22:286–295, 1983

Patterson GR: Coercive Family Processes. Eugene, OR, Castalia, 1982

Raine A, Venables PH, Williams M: Autonomic orienting responses in 15-year-old male subjects and criminal behavior at age 24. Am J Psychiatry 147:933–937, 1990

Robins LN: Deviant Children Grown Up: A Sociological and Psychiatric Study of Sociopathic Personality. Baltimore, MD, Williams & Wilkins, 1966

Ryan ND, Puig-Antich J, Ambrosini P, et al: The clinical picture of major depression in children and adolescents. Arch Gen Psychiatry 44:854–861, 1987

Ryback RS, Gardner EA: Limbic system dysrhythmia: a diagnostic electroencephalogram procedure utilizing procaine activation. J Neuropsychiatry Clin Neurosci 3:1–9, 1991

Shaffer D: Depression, mania and suicidal acts, in Child and Adolescent Psychiatry: Modern Approaches, 2nd Edition. Edited by Rutter M, Hersou L. Boston, MA, Blackwell Scientific, 1985, pp 698–719

Shaffer D: The epidemiology of teen suicide: an examination of risk factors. J Clin Psychiatry 49 (No 9, suppl):36–41, 1988

Stanton AH, Schwartz MS: The Mental Hospital. New York, Basic Books, 1954

Stewart JT, Myers WC, Burket RC, et al: A review of the pharmacotherapy of aggression in children and adolescents. J Am Acad Child Adolesc Psychiatry 29:269–277, 1990

Thomas A, Chess S, Birch HG: Temperament and Behavior Disorders in Children. New York, New York University Press, 1968

Turecki S: The Difficult Child, New York, Bantam, 1989

Weissman MM, Gammon GD, John K, et al: Children of depressed parents: increased psychopathology and early onset of major depression. Arch Gen Psychiatry 44:847–853, 1987

Chapter 16

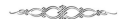

Residential Treatment

G. Pirooz Sholevar, M.D.

Residential treatment centers (RTCs) are psychiatric organizations that provide children with individually planned mental health treatment in conjunction with residential care. Their clinical programs are directed by either a psychiatrist or another mental health professional. They serve children and youths primarily under the age of 18. Fifty percent or more of these children and youths are mentally ill according to DSM-III-R diagnostic categories (American Psychiatric Association 1987; Lewis 1991; Stroup et al. 1988). There are continua of RTCs that are administered through social welfare, juvenile justice, and mental health systems.

Youth with conduct disorder (CD) are commonly admitted to RTCs, a phenomenon deriving from both the high prevalence of CD and the frequent failure of such children to respond to outpatient treatment. It is generally the more chronic and severely disturbed children and adolescents with CD who find their way to RTCs following failure to respond to psychiatric interventions in outpatient or short-term inpatient units. Furthermore, such children have frequently been reared in multiple foster homes or group homes and their maladaptive behavior has necessitated transfers in foster care. It is not unusual to encounter children with CD who have been subjected to multiple changes in their caregivers, from their natural parents to foster parents. The high incidence of physical and sexual abuse and of parental mental illness or alcoholism have also contributed to frequent changes in childcare arrangements.

History

RTCs emerged primarily from the custodial care model. The field of residential treatment for children subsequently developed on an empirical basis to provide multiple models of treatment to suit different needs. The centers were generally guided by different theoretical models of child development combining multiple viewpoints on a practical basis. In addition to the residential experience of having children live as a group in on-grounds schools or residential centers, children were provided with psychotherapy. The frequent communication among staff members assisted them in arriving at an understanding of the child in order to enhance therapeutic staff-child interactions. This knowledge was expected to be enhanced by individual treatment of the child and, later, by inclusion of the whole family in treatment. The combination of various treatment modalities with residential care, therefore, came to characterize milieu therapy. See the appendix to this chapter for guidance in matching symptomatology with specific therapeutic and milieu interventions.

Lewis (1991, p. 895) cites statistics (drawn from 1986 National Institute of Mental Health unpublished data) indicating that between 1972 and 1986, the number of RTCs increased from 340 to 437 and the number of resident children from 19,384 to 24,547. Therefore, RTCs would seem to be an expanding component of mental health care. RTCs account for roughly 6% of the total psychiatric beds in the United States (Lewis 1991). The majority of RTCs have 50 or fewer beds. Two-thirds of the residents in such centers are white, 22% black, and 9% Hispanic. Most children are between 5 and 15 years of age, and boys are referred more frequently than girls. RTCs tend to be somewhat selective: they reject three children for each child accepted for admission.

Indications for Residential Treatment

The lack of age-appropriate internal controls in children is the major reason for admission to RTCs, where they can receive consistent external controls (Lewis 1991). Children may present with moderate to severe symptoms of antisocial and aggressive behavior, psychotic symptoms, or severely infantile and regressive behavior. Serious learning problems are commonly observed in almost all of the children. A history of parental neglect, physical or sexual abuse, parental psychopathology, and multiple foster home placements is frequently reported. CD and attention-deficit hyperactivity disorder (ADHD) are the most common diagnoses in children admitted to RTCs.

It is difficult to estimate the exact number of children and adolescents with CD who are admitted to RTCs. Frequently, a clear majority of the children in RTCs exhibit some degree of conduct problem, regardless of their primary diagnosis. It is safe to estimate that more than one-half of the children and adolescents in RTCs are primarily conduct disordered. The number of children and adolescents with CD who are admitted to RTCs may be on the rise.

Staffing

RTC staff include both professional and childcare staff. The professional staff consist of child and adolescent psychiatrists, psychologists, social workers, and psychiatric nurses. The clinical or medical director has the crucial task of providing the conceptual framework for understanding the totality of the children's behavior to enable the staff to deal with the children in a therapeutic and corrective—rather than reactive—manner.

Childcare Staff

By far, the largest proportion of the child's life in a residential treatment setting is spent in group living. The childcare staff provide 24-hour care for the children and are the final agents of observation and intervention in the facility. In a well-run RTC, the observations of the childcare staff are systematically reported to the professional staff, who use these observations in shaping different aspects of the treatment plan—which in turn is implemented to a large degree through the efforts of the childcare staff. Members of the childcare staff may be called by different titles, such as childcare worker, residential counselor, psychiatric technician, or nurse's assistant.

The childcare staff provides a structured environment that constitutes a therapeutic milieu. The milieu defines tasks within the limits of the children's ability, provides incentives such as increased privileges for adaptive behavior, and encourages the children toward progressive adaptation rather than infantile and regressive behavior. Childcare staff members' high level of knowledge about the children enables them to make the necessary clarifications and interpretations to the children at appropriate times—a process defined as "life-space interview" (Redl 1959). The subjective feelings and experiences of staff members toward the children and their "countertransference" feelings are used therapeutically within this frame of reference. Frequently, these children have not previously encountered the degree of adequacy, sensitivity, and consistency of care provided by residential care staff, and they may rebel against it by frequent testing of the limits. The children quite often attempt to "split" the staff by causing staff members to fight each other on their behalf. This tactic is generally a repetition of these children's mode of operation with their parents at home. Splitting can result in staff members' blaming and counterblaming one another around the children's disruptive behavior and can force the staff to act punitively toward the children rather than relying on positive reinforcement (Lewis 1991).

The structured residential setting offers children a "corrective" emotional experience by helping them learn the value of positive interactions with peers and between children and the staff, striving toward the achievement of preset goals, mastery of the environment, and the satisfaction of having effect and impact on one's surroundings (White 1963). Such corrective experiences enable the child to recognize problems and conflict, to develop communication skills and self-control, and to learn problem-solving skills and behavior.

Staff Collaboration

The function of the staff is to provide the children with support, concern, guidance, and empathy. It is essential that the staff members be capable of exhibiting the same qualities toward each other. In general, the effectiveness of the program is either enhanced or reduced based on the level of cooperation or friction among the staff. Group cohesiveness among staff members improves performance. Such cohesiveness is promoted by holding regular meetings to discuss issues confronting the team as well as by establishing clear lines of authority, leadership, and role expectation (Lewis 1991).

Interstaff communication is necessary to help the total staff work as a cohesive group in providing children with integrated interventions. The participation of multiple staff members can make up for the blind spots of one or more of them but can also create role conflict. Therefore, clear policies in regard to expectations, limit setting, interpersonal contacts, and outside visits should be established. Treatment is most effective when there is clear staff cohesion and collaboration. In addition to psychoanalytic and learning theory, there has been a greater recent reliance on general systems theory to provide a framework for communication among staff members and between the staff and the family.

The staff members as a group participate in evaluating and establishing a diagnosis, which is usually consistently reevaluated. The diagnostic information should be considered from four developmental dimensions: biological, emotional, sociobehavioral, and cognitive-academic (Colligan et al. 1981).

Severely disturbed children have a significant impact on the individual and group functioning of the staff members. The supervisory process is designed to maintain the therapeutic quality of the staff-patient interaction in spite of persistent provocation from severely disturbed youths. In addition to intradepartmental supervisory and collaborative practices, staff members need to undertake interdisciplinary collaboration and conflict management activities. Brown (1983) provides a theoretical and systematic approach to managing conflict at departmental interfaces from a management perspective, focusing on six major opportunities for the following changes: 1) alter perceptions, 2) alter communications, 3) alter behavior, 4) alter interface, 5) alter one or both departments, and 6) alter organizational context.

Case Management

In many RTCs, a clinician—usually a social worker—is assigned to the child as a case manager responsible for coordination and integration of the work of the school, the childcare department, and the clinical department as well as that of the parent/guardian and accountable funding sources.

Treatment Process

The central therapeutic process in an RTC is milieu therapy that occurs within the context of a therapeutic milieu. The goal of the therapeutic milieu is to enhance not only self-control, self-observation, self-knowledge, and insight, but also the multiple ego functions that are the vehicles for achieving those goals. The ego capacities central to adequate adaptation are an adequately defined self-concept endowed primarily with positive emotions and a relatively well-defined and nonthreatening view of others. The process of enhancing these ego capacities can be delineated as achievement of clear self and object definitions. The failure of this process results in rapidly fluctuating self-esteem, or narcissistic vulnerability, and becoming mistrustful of others at the time of conflict. Other significant ego functions include the ability to control impulses, to tolerate frustration, and to sustain a "sense of reality" (Frosh 1983). Although reality testing is generally intact in most of the children in RTCs, their *sense of reality* is frequently impaired—that is, they function as though they were different people responding to different people in different situations. An example would be a child in a school who responds to a teacher as though the teacher were a stranger with no right to ask him or her to do a task, and as though the interaction were occurring in an undefined place, such as on the street, instead of in the classroom, where the context defines the nature of the task and the relationship. An important aspect of an adequate sense of reality is the feeling of "agency," whereby children feel that they can achieve their goals and have an effect on their circumstances through their own actions or through the use of routine processes. The feeling of agency protects a child from feeling helpless. Knowing the role of reinforcement and learning how to use it to achieve their goals helps children counter feelings of "learned helplessness" and pessimism about the future.

The primary instrument and vehicle for milieu therapy is the human interactions that occur within the residential program. These include guided interactions between the staff and the children, spontaneous interactions among the children, and staff-guided interactions among the children. Such interactions provide the child with the collective support of the staff who as a group will help him or her achieve the goals of self-control and self-observation. These, in turn, will evolve into an adaptive and realistic construction of self, object, and reality definitions.

Therapeutic milieu refers to an environment in which the child's symptomatic behavior is understood as an ego-dystonic element based on psychodynamic or familial contingencies. As such, the behavior is handled with insight, tolerance, and support for its correction rather than in a reactive fashion. This definition of the therapeutic milieu has much in common with the concept of the "holding environment" (Winnicott 1965): the therapeutic environment receives the pathogenic and pathological behavior of the child, examines and defines it within the context of the child's past and present experiences, and gives back to the child the redefined entity in a "detoxified" form.

The therapeutic milieu requires a physical setting that provides safety and containment for dangerous behavior, and that is conducive to interaction, feelings of community, relaxation, and pleasure. Another necessary foundation for creating a therapeutic environment is the presence of a "basic care" or "comprehensive care" climate in which the basic needs of the child for safety, acceptance, nurturance, guidance, and education are met on a continuous basis. Against these general and nonspecific functional backgrounds, the therapeutic environment provides for specific interventions with the child— both by the staff and by other children—based on understanding, feedback, and support for remediation of maladaptive behavior. This type of intervention furnishes the child with knowledge about the origin of his or her behavior (insight), a view of himself or herself as seen by the staff and other children (outsight) (Adams 1986), and an understanding of the nature of the interaction between people and reality.

Behavior modification principles are applied in all RTCs to promote socially adaptive and prosocial behavior and to reward children—by means of awarding points—for displaying such behavior. The points determine the level of privileges afforded the child. The requirements for moving from a less-privileged to a more-privileged level are clearly explained to the children.

The stresses of dealing with severely disturbed children may result in job dissatisfaction on the part of both the childcare and the professional staff. The "burnout" phenomenon can become even more severe for childcare staff members if they feel that they do not have the opportunity to cross interprofessional boundaries in their everyday jobs or in their future careers.

Treatment Modalities

In addition to milieu therapy within a therapeutic environment, all traditional modes of psychotherapy have an appropriate place in residential treatment. These modes include intensive individual psychotherapy, group therapy, treatment for parents, family therapy, and pharmacotherapy. Selected information from therapy sessions is generally shared with the entire staff to enhance their knowledge about the child's behavior and its psychodynamic underpinnings. Sharing such information among staff members allows them to continue the psychotherapeutic encounters with the children outside the therapist's office. The therapist is kept fully informed about the nature of the child's daily interactions with peers and staff in the residence.

However, maintaining the confidentiality of the child's communications with regard to other family members and other children in the RTC is necessary.

Intervention With Family and Parents

Concurrent psychotherapeutic work with the child's parents is essential. Major goals of working with parents are to help them assume a realistic posture toward the child (particularly regarding the possibility of his or her return home) and achieve a realistic view of the child's psychopathology and ego deficits, and to enhance their parental skills. It is very helpful to have the therapist who works with the child also undertake the work with the parents and family.

Wide swings between strong ambivalence and reaction formation toward the child are common in parents and need to be addressed therapeutically. Home visits are important tools for helping the parents to achieve a realistic view of the child's needs and behavior and to enhance their knowledge of their parenting skills and limitations.

Chapter 10 of this volume proposes the following classifications for families of children in RTCs:

— Available families
— Potentially available families
— Partially available families
— Totally unavailable families

Therapeutic guidelines for each of these family types are also presented in that chapter.

Medication

Medication in RTCs is used when there is a clear indication for or a target symptom responsive to a particular drug. Controlling the symptom can enhance the therapeutic relationship as well as the child's learning behavior. Well-established and clearly understood medication procedures are needed. The full staff generally participate in discussing the need for medication and in clarifying the anticipated goals of pharmacotherapy for the child. Impulsive proposals for the use of medication are sometimes made by staff members who feel frustrated and desperate in their efforts to manage especially difficult behavior. The child should be helped to understand the expected effect of the medication.

Recently, there has been an increased morbidity in the disorders of children entering RTCs. Many children may be admitted while on multiple psychopharmacological agents, such as antipsychotic, antidepressant, stimulant, and antiseizure medications. The RTC should be capable of administering medications in an appropriate and judicious fashion through child psychiatric and nursing supervision. However, the use of many psychopharmacological agents, particularly in a nontraditional and experimental fashion, may endanger the child, leave the facility vulnerable from a medicolegal point of view, and encourage the staff members to use medications inappropriately or punitively instead of attempting to develop a more comprehensive treatment strategy.

Learning Problems and the School Program

Learning disabilities are quite common in the backgrounds of children admitted to RTCs. A thorough diagnostic assessment of the child's learning behavior is necessary to arrive at a rational approach for the application of specific remedial measures. A special on-grounds school setting is usually required to enhance both supervision of the children and communication between educational and therapeutic staff. Unfortunately, a functional split between educational and therapeutic staff in RTCs can occur all too easily, with each group of staff members feeling demeaned or unappreciated by the other. The school staff should include teachers who are skilled in special educational assessment, special learning techniques, and some of the newer educational equipment, including computers. A low student-to-teacher ratio is necessary.

The teacher's relationship with the child assumes somewhat of a therapeutic quality similar to that of the childcare and mental health staff. Ideally, the teacher should be equipped with sufficient knowledge about the child's current behavior and background to judiciously provide clarifying commentaries (or interpretations) about the child's dysfunctional behavior. A major goal of the school is to motivate children to learn and to help them achieve multiple successful experiences at the appropriate level. In addition to educational goals, the teacher should use the learning and interpersonal opportunities to improve the children's self-esteem and motivation to learn as well as to provide opportunities for them to acquire adaptive skills.

Course of Treatment

Masterson (1956, 1967) has used psychoanalytic theory and the recent elaborations on separation-individuation theory to conceptualize the therapeutic process in an RTC. According to this model, children enter the RTC in a self-centered and isolated condition. In the next stage, they develop a symbiotic relationship with the facility and the staff. Toward the end of treatment, separation-individuation is established that allows the child to leave the center.

Upon entering an RTC, children may temporarily exhibit good behavior to please the staff. This honeymoon period usually is replaced by the reemergence of the children's symptomatic behavior, often modeled after their dysfunctional relationship with adults and peers prior to their admission to the RTC. Through milieu therapy supported by the administration of multiple treatment modalities by staff members, the child's self-observation toward his or her behavior (outsight) is enhanced, followed by the understanding of the internal and contextual triggers and reinforcers of that behavior (insight). Recognition of these factors on a repeated basis allows the child to work through his or her maladaptive behavior. Traditionally, 2 or more years have been required to complete this course. With pressure from funding sources, there has been a tendency to shorten this process, which frequently compromises the treatment outcome. Premature discharge can result in regression and reemergence of the old symptoms.

Because a full resolution of the symptoms is rarely attainable in an RTC, discharge planning for children in RTCs should emphasize the importance of follow-up care in both therapeutic and educational areas. Improved relationships with others, social adaptation, the ability to function in a community school, and the working through of certain kinds of traumas are realistic and necessary goals for the child.

The range of disposition plans include return to the family with or without outpatient or day treatment intervention, placement in a group or foster home, or boarding school.

Residential treatment is generally considered a phase of treatment rather than a comprehensive and complete regimen in itself. Children may remain vulnerable for a long period following discharge, and thus may still require treatment.

Favorable and Unfavorable Treatment Outcome

The high level of stability of antisocial behavior in spite of treatment requires a differentiation between the factors associated with poor therapeutic outcomes and those associated with favorable ones. Kazdin et al. (1987) have emphasized the need to identify those children likely to be most amenable to treatment. The idea would be to provide treatment to those youths with CD who are considered most likely to have a successful outcome and then to apply the successful intervention methods to increasingly more difficult youngsters. One can consider employing intensive, short-term treatment with those for whom a favorable outcome is likely, and using long-term, support-ive treatment with children who are unlikely to respond favorably to the former type of treatment. A variety of risk factors can help identify children who respond poorly to treatment. Such children tend to exhibit persistent delinquency and early antisocial and dysfunctional behaviors and may be at risk for parental abuse and neglect. They are typically from a troubled, discordant, low-income family in which one or both parents have a criminal record. The long-term prognosis for such children is poor and they are likely to pass their aggressive and delinquent behavior on to their offspring. In young adulthood, they spend time in jail and their lifespan may be cut short by violence (O'Malley et al. 1990).

Attempting to differentiate treatment responders from nonresponders, Fischer and Bersari (1979) and Force and Sebree (1985) have suggested that previous life experiences are more important than treatment program in the prediction of success. School performance and behavior, older age at admis-sion, and referral during crisis favor a successful treatment experience. In contrast, failure in a previous placement, commission of certain offenses, educational difficulties, nonsupportive parents (particularly in a high state of denial), and lower IQ correlate with an unsuccessful outcome (O'Malley et al. 1990).

Gilliland-Mallo and Judd (1986) found the following demographic data correlated with negative therapeutic outcome. Whites had a 70% success rate compared with 47% for nonwhites, and not being on probation was corre-lated with successful outcome 80% of the time compared with a rate of 54% for those on probation. Youngsters who were not using drugs, who had no prior runaway history, and who had home visits while in treatment all fared better than those with the opposite of these characteristics. "Success" in this study was defined as completing the residential program (O'Malley et al. 1990).

Neilson et al. (1982) examined the specific life events that led to more violent and delinquent behavior. They found a powerful relationship between frequency and age of parental separation and outcome. Physical aggression was related to separation at age 36–72 months, and sexual aggression dated back to age 0–12 months. The degree of parental abuse correlated with a number of aggressive and acting-out behaviors exhibited by the child (O'Malley et al. 1990).

The general factors correlated with posttherapeutic outcome relate to residential treatment as well. Among comorbid states coexisting with CD, ADHD is associated with more antisocial behaviors, a more adverse family environment, significantly lower intellectual/verbal scores, increased reading difficulties, poor motor ability, and persistent adult criminal behavior. Moffitt (1990) has proposed that family adversity and poor verbal ability may increase the risk of antisocial behavior later in life among those with ADHD (O'Malley et al. 1990).

A study to determine treatment efficacy undertaken at Devereux (an RTC in Devon, Pennsylvania) in 1988 (O'Malley et al. 1990) attempted to differentiate between children with CD who were discharged "negatively" (with an average length of stay of 11 months) and those who were discharged "positively" or "neutrally" (with an average length of stay of 12–26 months). The results showed that 70% of the youngsters had been negatively discharged, and that 78% of this group had been admitted on a "provisional" basis (i.e., they did not meet initial admission criteria). A subsequent study at Devereux in 1989 examined the concerns at the time of intake and found that there were no factors on admission that could reliably predict outcome; rather, the child's behavior in the institution was the best indicator for the success of treatment.

In 1990 a third study was conducted to determine the risk factors in residential treatment of CD. A group of children with successful treatment response was compared with an equal number of children with unsuccessful treatment response. The following factors were common to both groups: a disturbed home environment, an absent or relatively absent father, poor school behavior, academic deficits, peer difficulties, a history of substance abuse, a history of ADHD (60%), a history of depression, a history of previous treatment failure (70%), depressed affect (90%), impaired self-esteem, developmental disabilities, a history of multiple physical illnesses, and neurological impairment. Against this background, the group who did not respond to treatment could be differentiated from treatment responders by the following criteria:

— A larger number of caregivers
— Limited maternal contact (very significant)
— More parental psychopathology, including psychosis and alcoholism
— Court guardianship
— Little extended family involvement
— A history of abuse
— Serious sibling difficulties
— A limited capacity to relate to others
— Medications prescribed
— More severe DSM-III-R symptoms and less improvement in those symptoms at discharge
— Shorter length of stay (19.6 months compared with 30.6 months)
— Transfer from a hospital, an RTC, or a group home

The limited data in this study suggest that those children who came from home just prior to being admitted to an RTC had a much better chance of a successful outcome than those who had come from a hospital, a group home, or a foster home, particularly following frequent moves among multiple caregiving arrangements (O'Malley et al. 1990).

The data also suggest that children who were placed on probation were more likely to succeed in treatment—as if that action somehow caused the problem to be "nipped in the bud." This phenomenon, of course, should be differentiated from the poor outcomes of the children who have been involved in long-standing legal difficulty—a circumstance that is correlated with prolonged maladjustment and negative outcome (O'Malley et al. 1990).

Case Example

Shawn was almost 16 years old when admitted to an RTC. This admission was prompted by his stealing a few household items from the foster home in which he had lived between the ages of 10 and 16. The foster parents pressed charges, partly to enable the court and the Department of Human Services (DHS) to find an appropriate placement for him. Shawn had a history of multiple episodes of burglary and running away and a single incident of fire setting at the age of 7. At the time of the stealing from his foster parents, he was living with some friends for a few weeks. He denied that he had stolen the items and claimed that his foster brothers had let him into the house and given him the items.

Shawn was the middle of three children of a black mother and a white father. His father had been absent from the home since he was very young. At the age of 8 and following a period of neglect, Shawn was removed from his mother, who was alcoholic. Between the ages of 8 and 10, he was placed in a succession of shelters and detention homes before he went to live with his foster parents. His older brother had been placed earlier; his younger brother was placed with another foster family.

Shawn was admitted to the RTC with a diagnosis of CD–aggressive type, although there were very few historical incidents of confrontation. He was considered to be at risk for running away. His IQ was in the dull normal range and his reading ability and comprehension were age appropriate, but he was 3 years below grade level in math skills. Shawn's ability in the artistic area was quite remarkable, however. He seemed somewhat depressed at the time of admission and remained so for many months, although the diagnosis of depression as a comorbid state was never established. He exhibited the associated behavioral feature of blaming other people and taking no responsibility for his own actions.

Shawn was admitted to one of the larger cottages in the program. He readily achieved the highest behavioral level, did not get involved in fighting, and went AWOL only once to meet some girls. After 6 months in the center, it was felt that Shawn's involvement with the staff members and other children was superficial and that he needed a smaller program in which his interactions could be better monitored. Because he had developed an interest in sign language to communicate with some of the deaf children at the center, he was placed in a smaller cottage where hearing-impaired children were mixed with children with normal hearing. Shawn learned sign language readily and could relate well to hearing-impaired children. It was noticed that he watched the staff carefully and then tried to find ways of sneaking through and breaking the rules. He also seemed to provoke fights between other children in a subtle and sneaky fashion when staff members were not watching and he would not be caught. There were incidents of stealing on the unit and Shawn was suspected as the responsible person, although it could never be proven.

Whenever Shawn's role in different incidents were examined, he predictably blamed the incident on other people and claimed that he was being treated with prejudice because he was black—referring to his biracial origin. His tendency to blame others and to refuse responsibility for his own actions became the focus of therapeutic intervention in the milieu. In individual sessions, Shawn's negative view toward women and black women, who were "bitches," and who abandoned their children, became the focus of intervention. Shawn's defensive reaction of blaming DHS for removing him from his mother, denying his mother's neglectful behavior, and idealizing her image were other foci of intervention. The program also helped Shawn to recognize his interest and ability in the areas of art and music and to use them toward some type of future career.

The involvement of DHS in the treatment program occurred somewhat belatedly. DHS personnel were able to locate Shawn's mother, who lived about 300 miles from the RTC, and communication was established with her. However, it was seen as unlikely that she could be a resource to Shawn. The hope was that the mother would be able to make a trip to the program to help Shawn to sort out some issues. This never happened. Therefore, it was planned that Shawn would return to a closer neighborhood where his paternal uncle and father lived.

Shawn's residential treatment, which took $1\frac{1}{2}$ years, was considered to be a successful one. He exhibited many difficulties inherent in the treatment of "stealers" in comparison with "aggressors." Upon discharge, the clinical research team felt that the length of Shawn's treatment could have been shortened and treatment results enhanced by the following:

1. Locate the mother immediately following the admission and establish ties between Shawn and her.
2. Bring in the foster parents for a few family sessions to help Shawn understand that they are filing charges to ensure an appropriate placement for him.
3. Recognize that Shawn belonged to the group of "stealers" rather than "aggressors," and concentrate on the indirect and covert signs of aggression rather than the overt ones.

4. Place Shawn in a small program in which his "sneakiness" could be recognized early. Furthermore, his tendency to bypass the staff and to take events into his own hands should have been seen as a by-product of his neglectful background, in which parental authorities had not been present or could not be relied on for help.
5. Recognize Shawn's pattern of blaming others as a significant sign of his limited ability for self-observation and self-direction, and address this behavior early in individual, group, and milieu therapy.
6. Make a connection between Shawn's complaints about being treated with racial prejudice and his own negative feelings toward his mother for having abandoned him.

Evaluation of the Effectiveness of Residential Treatment Centers

Most of the outcome studies of RTCs are methodologically flawed and based on the global impressions of clinical staff. Such clinical impressions indicate that RTCs provide a beneficial experience for children during the residential phase and help them resume a satisfactory developmental course (Quay 1986). Lewis and Summerville (1986) found that the majority of children who had received about 2 years of residential treatment in one particular setting did poorly at follow-up according to the objective measures for outcome. They concluded that therapeutic gains in residential treatment did not correlate with sustained behavioral improvement on returning to the home and community. The authors emphasized the importance of the crucial attachments that form between the children and the staff members and recommended that these attachments be protected following discharge.

In summarizing the impact of the RTCs on children with CD, Quay (1986) emphasized that the progress in the conceptualization, the implementation, and especially the evaluation of residential treatment has not kept pace with advances in the understanding of other aspects of child and adolescent psychopathology. This situation is partially related to current thinking—on the part of both the mental health and the legal-correctional communities—deemphasizing the importance of residential treatment for children and favoring instead "the least restrictive environment." A shift has also occurred toward more punitive approaches in the face of both budgetary strictures and the influence of a "nothing works" philosophy. Therapeutic centers have contributed to this problem by failing to operationalize and to rigorously evaluate the effectiveness of their programs.

Quay (1986) concluded that, despite ample evidence for the effectiveness of residential treatment to bring about in-program behavior change, there is very little, if any, evidence for lasting change deriving from any of the different intervention modalities that have been studied. Progress, if any, in the last 6–8 years is almost nonexistent. Yet residential placement—if not treatment—is clearly here to stay, if only for the limited number of children and adolescents who are clearly dangerous to themselves or, more likely, to others. That certain types of residential intervention may work better with some disorders than with others is clear from extant research as well as from more recent reports by a number of investigators (Palmer 1984; Rutter 1982; Tramontana 1980); however, current studies of differential treatment are seriously lacking. As was the case in a number of earlier studies reviewed by Quay (1986), more recent follow-up studies of treated children have suggested that (undersocialized) CD symptoms—especially when pervasive and severe—are less amenable to change than are symptoms of anxiety, withdrawal, and dysphoria (Blotcky et al. 1984; Gossett et al. 1977; Nielson et al. 1982).

Evaluations of treatment in hospital and mental health settings (Craft et al. 1964) have suggested that individuals who manifest extreme CD are unresponsive to verbally oriented methods of behavior change. A study by Monkman (1972) examined the dimensions of progressive improvement, particularly in self-care behaviors and social functioning. The results showed a 53% improvement in problem behavior at home and a 7% relative improvement in school behavior.

The evaluation of treatment in a group-home setting is exemplified by Project Re-Ed (Bower et al. 1969; Hobbs 1966; Weinstein 1969, 1974). At the time of discharge from this program, 88% of the children were moderately or much improved, 12% were slightly improved, and none were the same or worse. The improved status of the children discharged from the RTC, in contrast to the control group, was particularly evident at 18 months after discharge.

The study of institutionalized delinquents has been exemplified by the Preston Typology Study (Jesness 1971), which was disappointing in terms of its effects on the postprogram rates of law violations.

Future Directions

The place of residential treatment in the continuum of child services is being significantly challenged by funding sources for economic reasons. Many state and federal policymakers emphasize "family preservation" or "alternative family placement" for children currently using RTCs. These recommendations represent attempts to cut costs and are not based on any research or clinical data. Staff burnout at RTCs is also a serious problem that needs to be addressed in a systematic way.

The traditional long-term residential treatment facilities are adapting their programs by shortening the length of treatment. New facilities may offer

90-day intensive assessment units or specialized units for children with histories of emotional and substance abuse.

The heightened emphasis on accountability has resulted in the intensification of the standards of the Joint Commission on Accreditation of Healthcare Organizations (JCAHO) and the stricter monitoring of such standards. There are now established standard requirements in the areas of administrative and clinical management, patient management, special treatment services, environmental management, and patient rights.

References

Adams PL: Individual psychotherapy, in Emotional Disorders in Children and Adolescents. Edited by Sholevar GP, Benson B, Blinder BJ. New York, Spectrum Publications Medical & Scientific, 1986

American Psychiatric Association: Diagnostic and Statistical Manual of Mental Disorders, 3rd Edition, Revised. Washington, DC, American Psychiatric Association, 1987

Blotcky MJ, Dimpiero TC, Gossett JT: Follow-up of children treated in psychiatric hospitals: a review of studies. Am J Psychiatry 141:1499–1507, 1984

Bower EM, Lourie RS, Strother CR, et al: Project Re-Ed: Evaluation by a Panel of Visitors. Nashville, TN, George Peabody College for Teachers, 1969

Brown D: Managing Conflict at Organizational Interfaces. Reading, PA, Addison-Wesley, 1983

Colligan RC, Roberts MD, Miner RA: An organizational grid for residential staff conference. Milieu Therapy 1:41, 1981

Craft M, Stephenson G, Granger C: A controlled trial of authoritarian and self-governing regimen with adolescent psychopaths. Am J Orthopsychiatry 34:543–554, 1964

Fischer BJ, Bersari CA: Self-esteem and institutionalized delinquent offenders: the role of background characteristics. Adolescence 53:197–214, 1979

Force RC, Sebree J: The validation of outcome predictors used in the admission decision at the St. Francis Boys' Home. Quality Review Bulletin 11:266–270, 1985

Frosh J: The Psychotic Process. New York, International Universities Press, 1983

Gilliland-Mallo D, Judd P: The effectiveness of residential care facilities for adolescent boys. Adolescence 21:311–321, 1986

Gossett JT, Barnhart D, Lewis JM, et al: Follow-up of adolescents treated in a psychiatric hospital: predictors of outcome. Arch Gen Psychiatry 34:1037–1042, 1977

Hobbs N: Helping disturbed children: ecological and psychological strategies. Am Psychol 21:1105–1115, 1966

Kazdin AE, Rodger A, Colbus D, et al: Children's Hostility Inventory: measurement of aggression and hostility in psychiatric inpatient children. J Clin Child Psychol 16:320–328, 1987

Lewis M (ed): Child and Adolescent Psychiatry: A Comprehensive Textbook. Baltimore, MD, Williams & Wilkins, 1991

Lewis M, Summerville J: Residential treatment, in Child and Adolescent Psychiatry: A Comprehensive Textbook. Edited by Lewis M. Baltimore, MD, Williams & Wilkins, 1986, pp 895–909

Jesness CF: The Preston Typology Study: an experiment with differential treatment in an institution. Journal of Research in Crime and Delinquency 8:38–52, 1971

Masterson J: Prognosis in adolescent disorders and schizophrenia. J Nerv Ment Dis 124:219–232, 1956

Masterson J: Psychiatric Dilemmas of Adolescence. Boston, MA, Little, Brown, 1967

Moffitt TE: Juvenile delinquency and attention deficit disorder: boys' developmental trajectories from age 3 to age 15. Child Dev 61:893–910, 1990

Monkman MM: A Milieu Therapy Program for Behaviorally Disturbed Children. Springfield, IL, Charles C Thomas, 1972

Nielson G, Young D, Latham S: Multiply acting out adolescents: developmental correlates and response to secure treatment. International Journal of Offender Therapy and Comparative Criminology 25:195–207, 1982

O'Malley J, Sholevar GP, Norton J, et al: Risk factors in residential treatment of conduct disorders: a pilot project. Paper presented at the annual meeting of the American Academy of Child and Adolescent Psychiatry, Chicago, IL, October 1990

Palmer T: Treatment and the role of classification: a review of basics. Crime and Delinquency 30:245–267, 1984

Quay HC: Residential treatment, in Psychopathological Disorders of Childhood, 3rd Edition. Edited by Quay HC, Werry JS. New York, Wiley, 1986, pp 558–582

Redl F: A strategy and technique of the life space interview. Am J Orthopsychiatry 29:1–18, 1959

Rutter MP: Psychological therapies in child psychiatry: issues and prospects. Psychol Med 12:723–740, 1982

Stroup A, Witkin M, Atay J, et al: Residential Treatment Centers for Emotionally Disturbed Children—1983 (Mental Health Statistical Note No. 188). Rockville, MD, National Institute of Mental Health, 1988

Tramontana MG: Critical review of research on psychotherapy outcome with adolescents: 1967–1977. Psychol Bull 88:429–450, 1980

Weinstein L: Project Re-Ed schools for emotionally disturbed children: effective as viewed by referring agencies, parents and teachers. Exceptional Children 35:703–711, 1969

Weinstein L: Evaluation of a program for re-educating disturbed children: a follow-up comparison with untreated children. Final report to the Bureau for the Education of the Handicapped, Office of Education, U.S. DHEW. Project Nos. 6-2974 and 552023, December 1974

Winnicott D: Psychiatric disorders in terms of infantile maturational processes, in The Maturational Process and the Facilitating Environment. New York, International Universities Press, 1965, pp 230–241

White P: Competence and the psychosexual stages of development, in Jones E: Ego and Reality in Psychoanalytic Therapy: A Proposal Regarding Independent Ego Energies. Psychological Issues, Monograph 11, 1963

Appendix: Matching Symptomatology and Classification With Specific Therapeutic and Milieu Therapeutic Interventions in Conduct Disorder

The following outline can serve as a clinical protocol to provide specific interventions for different symptoms and risk factors in conduct disorder. It can enhance therapeutic effectiveness for the severe cases of conduct disorder by increasing therapeutic integration and reducing fragmented efforts by the treatment team.

Symptomatology

Overt and covert aggressive symptoms of conduct disorder represent different therapeutic challenges and require different techniques applied in the milieu and in multiple therapeutic modalities (the numbers in parentheses refer to each symptom's order within the DSM-III-R listing of diagnostic criteria for conduct disorder).

I. *Aggressive (Overt)*

   A. Has deliberately engaged in fire setting (4)
   B. Has broken into someone else's house, building, or car (6)
   C. Has deliberately destroyed others' property (other than by fire setting) (7)
   D. Has been physically cruel to animals (8)
   E. Has forced someone into sexual activity with him or her (9)
   F. Has used a weapon in more than one fight (10)
   G. Often initiates physical fights (11)
   H. Has stolen with confrontation of a victim (e.g., mugging, purse snatching, extortion, armed robbery) (12)
   I. Has been physically cruel to people (13)

II. *Nonaggressive (Covert)*

   A. Has stolen without confrontation of a victim on more than one occasion (1)
   B. Has run away from home overnight at least twice while living in parental or parental surrogate home (or once without returning) (2)
   C. Often lies (other than to avoid physical or sexual abuse) (3)
   D. Is often truant from school (for older person, absent from work) (5)

III. *Symptoms of Comorbid States*

   A. Attention-deficit hyperactivity disorder
   B. Learning disability

C. Depression
D. Suicidality
E. Substance abuse

IV. *Associated Features (Symptoms)*

   A. Blames others
   B. Has poor interpersonal relations with peers and adults
   C. Engages in boisterous and show-off behavior
   D. Exhibits cognitive and attributional deficits (problem solving)
   E. Displays cognitive-perceptual characteristics (suspiciousness, instability, and resentment)
   F. Shows academic disinterest

V. *Residual Symptoms or Risk Factors*

   A. Attention-deficit hyperactivity disorder
   B. Parental neglect and rejection
   C. Physical abuse
   D. Sexual abuse
   E. Multiple caretakers
   F. No consistent mother figure
   G. Absence of father
   H. Parental substance abuse
   I. Large family size
   J. Association with delinquent peer group
   K. Early living in institutions
   L. Ineffective and inconsistent parenting
   M. Marital problems in parents
   N. Low IQ
   O. Socioemotionally disturbed (SED) educational classes
   P. Learning disabled (LD) educational classes
   Q. Legal problems
   R. Low socioeconomic status
   S. History of oppositional defiant disorder

VI. *Assets*

   A. High IQ
   B. Consistent mothering
   C. Two involved parents
   D. Adequate educational achievement
   E. Middle socioeconomic status
   F. Special abilities and talents (sports, art, etc.)

Classification

Clinical classification according to DSM-III-R or DSM-IV (American Psychiatric Association 1994) subtypes and comorbid states allows additional assessment of the interpersonal, psychological, familial, educational, and vocational levels of the child. Other diagnostic conclusions include the assessment of risk factors and assets of the child.

I. *Classification*
    A. Clinical classification (DSM-III-R; DSM-IV)
    B. Subtyping (according to DSM system)
    C. Social level of behavior
        1. Socially compliant
        2. Dyssocial
        3. Antisocial
    D. Interpersonal levels
        1. Egocentric, self-directed, isolated
        2. Needs-satisfying, sadomasochistic relationships
        3. Narcissistic relationships
        4. Other-directed
        5. Reciprocal, cooperative, collaborative
        6. Other types
    E. Psychological levels
        1. Self-regulation
        2. Self-definition
        3. Identity formation
    F. Family types
        1. Family available
        2. Potentially available family
        3. Unavailable family (structural deficiency, defensiveness)
        4. Disengaged, disintegrated family
        5. Disintegrated natural and foster families (serial and network disintegrations)
    G. Educational level
        1. Achievement levels according to grades in
            a. Reading
            b. Math
            c. Other subjects
    H. Prevocational level
        1. Vocational readiness
        2. Vocational level

II. *Subtypes*

    A. Solitary aggressive behavior
    B. Group delinquent behavior
    C. Undifferentiated

III. *Comorbid States*

    A. Attention-deficit hyperactivity disorder
    B. Learning disabilities
    C. Depression
    D. Suicidality
    E. Substance abuse

Specific Therapeutic Modalities

Specific interventions can be applied in the course of multiple treatment modalities. Different treatment approaches can address the child's disabilities and risk factors while capitalizing on the child's assets. The best results can be obtained through judicious integration of multiple treatment modalities.

I. *Clinical Interventions*

    A. Individual psychotherapy
    B. Behavior therapy
    C. Group psychotherapy
    D. Family therapy
    E. Medication
    F. Recreational and occupational therapy
    G. Art therapy
    H. Music therapy
    I. Pair therapy
    J. Pet-assisted therapy

II. *Educational Interventions*

III. *Prevocational and Vocational Interventions*

IV. *Cognitive Interventions*

Milieu Therapeutic Interventions

Preplanned interventions in the milieu are specifically designed to address the child's disabilities. They make use of the child's assets to promote therapeutic relationships with the staff and to enhance development and rehabilitation.

I.   *Community Meetings*

II.   *Staff-Patient Interactions*

III. *Peer Interactions*

VI.   *Planned Interventions by Peer Group*

Chapter 17

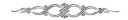

Prevention

Ronald J. Prinz, Ph.D.

The prevention of conduct disorder (CD) is an area of research just beginning to come into its own (Muehrer and Koretz 1992; Offord 1989). Communities, public policymakers, juvenile corrections departments, the juvenile justice system, and mental health services agencies are recognizing that it is often futile to wait until youths commit serious crimes to begin the intervention process in earnest (Seidman 1987). Prevention programming is being increasingly touted as the strategy of choice in addressing the burgeoning adolescent crime rate. However, research on prevention and data in support of successful prevention efforts have not yet caught up with the ambitious goals associated with the proposed public policy changes.

Levels of Prevention

In the area of child and adolescent CD, prevention can take many different forms, depending on 1) what the implementers are trying to prevent, 2) the point(s) of intervention in the developmental timeline, 3) who is targeted, and 4) the theoretical and conceptual assumptions driving the preventive intervention. The notions of primary, secondary, and tertiary prevention are both helpful and confusing when applied to CD. *Primary prevention* is invoked when the intervention is implemented prior to the onset of CD. *Secondary prevention* refers to intervention in the early stages of CD to prevent its continuation. *Tertiary prevention* targets the reduction or elimination of adverse consequences associated with CD. Under this scheme, the distinction between treatment and—particularly—tertiary (but also secondary) prevention is somewhat obscured, perhaps because prevention and treatment can be viewed as a continuum rather than as two distinct entities. On the front end of that continuum, what appears to be primary prevention might also be construed as secondary prevention when diagnostic criteria are not rigidly invoked. For example, 7-year-old children who exhibit markedly aggressive behavior at home and school technically may not qualify for a diagnosis of CD according to the current diagnostic system, but their behavior is nonetheless characteristic of the prodromal phase of the disorder. Strictly speaking, intervention at this point could be called primary prevention because the children do not yet "have" the disorder. However, such a definition would not allow us to distinguish this type of preventive endeavor from another preventive intervention targeting young children who are at high risk for CD because of other factors besides marked aggressive behavior but who have not yet exhibited a prodromal form of the disorder.

The level of prevention is affected by the choice of outcome target as well. Traditionally, mental health services have focused on the prevention of disorders. However, the prevention of CD is part of a larger context in which the targets are the prevention of serious crime in adolescence and of adult criminality, neither of which qualify explicitly as disorders. If serious juvenile crime is the focal point, then treatment of CD in the early stages prior to the commission of serious crimes would be considered a preventive measure. Similarly, if adult criminality is the focus, then programs for juvenile offenders could also be construed as preventive interventions. Even when the goal is the prevention of adult criminality, however, it is widely believed that preventive efforts begun after the onset of puberty are often too late to be effective.

Universal Versus Targeted Interventions

Although a number of variations for preventive interventions are available, two general strategies are universal intervention and targeted intervention. A *universal preventive intervention,* as the name suggests, is applied to all individuals in a population, regardless of risk status. The administration of the polio vaccine to the entire child population is an example of a universal intervention. In the CD area, a program that is applied to all of the children in a school or to all children at a certain age would be considered universal. For example, Prothrow-Stith (1987) and colleagues have developed a violence prevention curriculum that is implemented broadly in high schools.

The contrasting method of prevention involves specific targets of application. Instead of directing the intervention at everyone, a *targeted preventive intervention* focuses on individuals at increased risk for developing the adverse outcome to be prevented. Acquired immunodeficiency syndrome (AIDS) prevention programs that focus on users of intravenous needles or on sexually active adolescents are examples of targeted interventions. In the CD area, programs that select children on the basis of one or more risk factors would be considered targeted preventive interventions. For example, a home-based family intervention such as the Homebuilders Program (Kinney et al. 1991) works with families who are experiencing problems of child abuse, other family violence, or adverse parental mental health. Even apart from the exorbitant cost, such a targeted program would not be appropriate for all families in a community.

Universal programs have some advantages. Because children are not singled out, the potential adverse consequences of labeling or stigmatization are avoided (Lorion 1987; McCord 1978). A universal program does not put pressure on the interventionists to guess who is likely to develop the outcome selected for prevention and thus minimizes the problem of missed cases or false negatives. However, the universal approach also has some disadvantages. For outcomes such as CD, which has a relatively low base rate of occurrence, universal interventions are inefficient and potentially cost ineffective. Intervening with 1,000 children to help the 100 who were destined to develop the disorder is a costly and cumbersome strategy. The issue is compounded if an intensive—and therefore expensive—intervention is required to successfully prevent the disorder. CD is an unquestionably difficult problem to treat or prevent, requiring comprehensive and intensive interventions (Miller and Prinz 1990; Patterson et al. 1992). Coie and his colleagues (Conduct Problems Prevention Research Group 1992) recently concluded that "no known study to date has been successful in the long-term prevention of conduct disorder" (p. 510). Given this state of affairs, interventions that are restricted in comprehensiveness, intensity, or duration due to the cost of universal administration are unlikely to successfully prevent CD.

Targeted preventive interventions also have advantages and disadvantages. Concentrating on the individuals who are at greatest risk is a more cost-effective use of services and in addition might be a better matching arrangement. The type of program necessary for addressing serious difficulties would probably be of limited interest or applicability to the general population. By targeting the individuals at greatest risk, more comprehensive programs of longer duration can be considered. With respect to disadvantages, the targeted approach might miss some of the children who need the programming, either because of incorrect selection (false negatives) or because of refusal to participate. Targeted interventions also have a greater likelihood of stigmatizing the children and families who use such services and so must be implemented with extreme caution.

Risk Factors and Points of Intervention

Many risk factors are associated with the ontogeny of CD (Loeber 1990; Offord 1989). Some risk factors predate a child's birth, such as parental criminality or psychopathology (Offord 1982; Robins 1981), parental substance abuse (M. O. West and Prinz 1987), parental social insularity (Dumas 1986; Wahler and Dumas 1987), and sometimes marital discord (Offord and Boyle 1986; Rutter and Giller 1983). Other risk factors pertain more to the family environment in infancy, toddlerhood, and childhood, such as inadequate parental supervision (Farrington 1978; Patterson 1982, 1986; Snyder et al. 1986), poor parental discipline (Farrington and D. J. West 1981; McCord 1988; Patterson 1982), and parental uninvolvement or rejection (Loeber and Stouthamer-Loeber 1986; Patterson and Bank 1989; Wadsworth 1980). After school entry, a number of additional risk factors come into play, including academic difficulties (Dishion et al. 1991; Offord and Waters 1983; Rutter and Giller 1983; Wolfgang et al. 1972), poor "bonding" with school (Hawkins and Lishner 1987; Hawkins and Weis 1985; Hirschi 1969), rejection by peers and inadequate development of social skills (Bierman 1986; Dishion et at. 1991; Parker and Asher 1987; Snyder et at. 1986), and association with deviant peers (Elliot et al. 1985; D. J. West and Farrington 1977). Community factors associated with the combination of poverty and social disorganization also contribute to risk (Dumas and Wahler 1983; Offord et al. 1986; Rutter et al. 1975), although risk for CD is lower in poor but socially cohesive communities (Sampson and Groves 1989).

Risk for the development of serious and chronic forms of CD is also associated with particular dimensions of child behavior. For example, "early starters," or children between the ages of 4 and 8 who have an early onset of behavior problems (Dumas 1992; Loeber 1988, 1990; Patterson et al. 1989), are at greatest risk. The early onset of covert antisocial activities such as stealing, lying, and fire setting (Loeber and Stouthamer-Loeber 1987) is problematic, as is also the persistence of a difficult and impulsive temperament (Campbell et al. 1986; Moffitt 1990).

These constellations of risk factors suggest several points for initiation of preventive interventions. For the factors that predate childbirth, intervention with prospective parents who qualify for one or more of the identified risk factors is an obvious early starting point. However, the base rate in this population for subsequent development of CD in the offspring may not be very high. To address family child-rearing practices, intervention could be initiated between birth and 6 years of age, although the younger the child, the more the low-base-rate problem comes into play. School entry seems to be an important nexus for a number of reasons. At this point (age 5 or 6 years), parenting practices are still amenable to change, school-related risk factors have not yet taken their toll, and prediction of CD based on early onset of behavior problems is more reliable. Another logical point of intervention is during the early years of elementary school (e.g., second or third grade) after the onset of behavior problems but before deviant peers exert their strongest influence.

Selected Examples of Prevention Efforts

Although no intervention study has yet achieved unconditional success in preventing serious forms of CD, several prevention efforts have made laudable attempts. To illustrate different points and targets of intervention, some of these prevention studies are briefly presented here.

The Prenatal/Early Infancy Project (Olds 1988) focused on maternal factors during pregnancy and infancy through the child's second birthday. The proximal goals were improved maternal and infant health—including a reduction of premature and low-weight births—through improved health practices. The broader goals included a reduction in subsequent child behavior problems and abusive parenting. The targeted risk group was young single mothers of low socioeconomic status. The intervention program consisted of home visits by nurses throughout pregnancy to help the mothers improve their diets, maintain hygiene, and refrain from drug/alcohol and cigarette use, and throughout infancy to improve maternal childcare skills. Although not explicitly focused on prevention of child conduct problems, the intervention did address a number of risk factors for CD. Compared with minimal intervention (limited services without frequent home visits), the preventive intervention produced a lower incidence of child abuse and neglect, fewer emergency room visits, higher birthweights, reduced maternal smoking, and higher levels of maternal employment. It is an open question whether these kinds of gains can be linked to later prevention of CD in the children.

The Houston Parent-Child Development Center (H-PCDC) focused on primary prevention of behavior problems in young children (Johnson 1975, 1988; Johnson and Breckenridge 1982; Johnson and Walker 1987). This 2-year program targeted Hispanic children at age 1 year who were at risk because of socioeconomic disadvantage. Services delivered in the home and in the program center included workshops on child behavior management, preacademic enrichment, and personal management; coaching in child care; individual counseling; and social support. The children were assessed at follow-up in second and third grades. Compared with control children, intervention children showed less aggressive or disruptive behavior in the classroom, performed at a higher level intellectually, and were less likely to be referred for special services. This program represents a promising approach that warrants replication. The investigators were able to demonstrate that by addressing an important set of risk factors during early childhood, later risk factors such as early onset of classroom behavior problems and academic difficulties could be reduced. The linkage to prevention of subsequent CD is again an unanswered question.

A school-based intervention program was tested by Bry and her colleagues (Bien and Bry 1980; Bry 1982; Bry and George 1979, 1980). Youths who presented discipline problems and had low academic performance were selected in the sixth and seventh grades and randomly assigned to an intervention condition or a no-intervention control condition. Three different intervention conditions were tested: 1) teacher conferences to focus on programs that would help individual children with problems, 2) teacher conferences plus group meetings with children to help them with classroom behavior and academic performance, and 3) teacher conferences, group meetings with children, and parent conferences to expand the programming. At follow-up (up to 5 years after the intervention), the one and two-component interventions had produced no significant improvement over the no-intervention condition. However, youths who received all three components showed less criminal behavior, fewer school problems, less drug abuse, and better employment records than youths in the control condition. This approach to prevention, which included components for teachers, children, and parents, demonstrated that a viable preventive intervention must focus on multiple contexts. The investigators were also able to demonstrate some preventive effects with respect to antisocial outcomes.

McCord (1978) described the 30-year follow-up of the Cambridge-Somerville Youth Study, in which, beginning in 1939, 506 boys between 5 and 13 years of age who exhibited "delinquency-prone histories" were randomly assigned to a treatment program or a control group. The treatment program, which lasted an average of 5 years, consisted of a collection of various services, including counselor visits to the home twice a month, academic tutoring, medical or psychiatric treatment, summer camps, and community programs such as the Boy Scouts and the YMCA. The 30-year follow-up revealed that although the men who had received the treatment reflected subjectively that the program had benefited them, they actually fared worse than the control subjects with respect to criminal behavior, health, age at death, and employment variables. Because the fidelity and uniformity of treatment (or lack thereof) might not have met current standards, the mechanism of these effects is not clear. Nonetheless, the McCord (1978) study underscores the importance of considering adverse or iatrogenic effects when implementing targeted interventions.

Davidson and his colleagues (Davidson and Redner 1988; Davidson et al. 1990) developed an intervention program to divert delinquent adolescents from the juvenile justice system. Their program was designed to intervene early in the sequence of events in the juvenile justice system (i.e., after apprehension but before adjudication) to reduce recidivism. The intervention was implemented by paraprofessionals (college students) who were trained to provide behavioral contracting, child advocacy, and linkage to community resources and to promote greater youth involvement in positive community activities. The intervention, which was tested in a series of controlled studies, significantly reduced recidivism (police contacts) compared with the results of either the traditional justice system approach or an attention-placebo control condition. Although late in the developmental course, such interventions with adolescents who have already gotten into trouble hold some promise and are needed to reduce growing demands on the juvenile justice system.

Conclusion

Epidemics require extraordinary countermeasures. The proliferation of violence, delinquency, and adult criminality in society must be met with a concerted response from the entire public health sector. Although prevention or early intervention with high-risk children seems to be the most promising (albeit underutilized) mode of attack, the field has yet to document long-term preventive effects. As we move closer to tackling the urgent challenge of preventing serious and chronic CD in childhood and adolescence, a clear need exists for systematic evaluation of comprehensive interventions that combine targeted and universal strategies.

References

Bien NZ, Bry BH: An experimentally designed comparison of four intensities of school-based prevention programs for adolescents with adjustment problems. Am J Community Psychol 8:110–116, 1980

Bierman KL: The relationship between social aggression and peer rejection in middle childhood, in Advances in Behavioral Assessment of Children and Families, Vol 2. Edited by Prinz RJ. Greenwich, CT, JAI Press, 1986, pp 151–178

Bry BH: Reducing the incidence of adolescent problems through preventive intervention: one- and five-year follow-up. Am J Community Psychol 10:265–276, 1982

Bry BH, George FE: Evaluating and improving prevention programs: a strategy from drug abuse. Evaluation and Program Planning 2:127–136, 1979

Bry BH, George FE: The preventive effects of early intervention on the attendance and grades of urban adolescents. Professional Psychology 11:252–260, 1980

Campbell SB, Breaux AM, Ewing LJ, et al: Correlates and predictors of hyperactivity and aggression: a longitudinal study of parent-referred problem preschoolers. J Abnorm Child Psychol 14:217–234, 1986

Conduct Problems Prevention Research Group (CPPRG): A developmental and clinical model for the prevention of conduct disorder: the FAST Track program. Development and Psychopathology 4:509–527, 1992

Davidson WS II, Redner R: The prevention of juvenile delinquency: diversion from the juvenile justice system, in Fourteen Ounces of Prevention: A Casebook for Practitioners. Edited by Price RH, Cowen EL, Lorion RP, et al. Washington, DC, American Psychological Association, 1988, pp 123–137

Davidson WS II, Redner R, Amdur RL, et al: Alternative Treatments for Troubled Youth: The Case of Diversion From the Justice System. New York, Plenum, 1990

Dishion TJ, Patterson GR, Stoolmiller M, et al: Family, school, and behavioral antecedents to early adolescent involvement with antisocial peers. Dev Psychol 27:172–180, 1991

Dumas JE: Indirect influence of maternal social contacts on mother-child interactions: a setting event analysis. J Abnorm Child Psychol 14:203–216, 1986

Dumas JE: Conduct disorder, in Handbook of Clinical Behavior Therapy, 2nd Edition. Edited by Turner SM, Calhoun KS, Adams HE. New York, Wiley, 1992, pp 285–316

Dumas JE, Wahler RG: Predictors of treatment outcome in parent training: mother insularity and socioeconomic disadvantage. Behavioral Assessment 5:301–313, 1983

Elliott DS, Huizinga D, Ageton SS: Explaining Delinquency and Drug Use. Beverly Hills, CA, Sage, 1985

Farrington DP: The family background of aggressive youths, in Aggression and Antisocial Behavior in Childhood and Adolescence. Edited by Hersov LA, Berger M, Shaffer D. Oxford, UK, Pergamon, 1978, pp 73–93

Farrington DP, West DJ: The Cambridge study in delinquent development (United Kingdom), in Prospective Longitudinal Research: An Empirical Basis for the Primary Prevention of Psychosocial Disorders. Edited by Mednick SA, Baert AE. New York, Oxford University Press, 1981

Hawkins JD, Lishner D: Etiology and prevention of antisocial behavior in children and adolescents, in Childhood Aggression and Violence: Sources of Influence, Prevention, and Control. Edited by Crowell DH, Evans IM, O'Donnell CR. New York, Plenum, 1987, pp 263–282

Hawkins JD, Weis JG: The social development model: an integrated approach to delinquency prevention. Journal of Primary Prevention 6:73–97, 1985

Hirschi T: Causes of Delinquency. Berkeley, University of California Press, 1969

Johnson DL: The development of a program for parent-child education among Mexican-Americans in Texas, in The Exceptional Infant, Vol 3. Edited by Friedlander BZ, Sterritt GM, Kirk GE. New York, Brunner/Mazel, 1975, pp 374–398

Johnson DL: Primary prevention of behavior problems in young children: the Houston Parent-Child Development Center, in Fourteen Ounces of Prevention: A Casebook for Practitioners. Edited by Price RH, Cowen EL, Lorion RP, et al. Washington DC, American Psychological Association, 1988, pp 44–52

Johnson DL, Breckenridge JN: The Houston Parent-Child Development Center and the primary prevention of behavior problems in young children. Am J Community Psychol 10:305–316, 1982

Johnson DL, Walker T: The primary prevention of behavior problems in Mexican-American children. Am J Community Psychol 15:375–385, 1987

Kinney J, Haapala D, Booth C: Keeping Families Together: The Homebuilders Model. New York, Aldine De Gruyter, 1991

Loeber R: The natural history of juvenile conduct problems, delinquency, and associated substance use: evidence for developmental progressions, in Advances in Clinical Child Psychology, Vol 11. Edited by Lahey BB, Kazdin AE. New York, Plenum, 1988, pp 73–124

Loeber R: Development and risk factors of juvenile antisocial behavior and delinquency. Clinical Psychology Review 10:1–41, 1990

Loeber R, Stouthamer-Loeber M: Family factors as correlates and predictors of juvenile conduct problems and delinquency, in Crime and Justice: An Annual Review of Research, Vol 7. Edited by Morris N, Tonry M. Chicago, IL, University of Chicago Press, 1986, pp 29–149

Loeber R, Stouthamer-Loeber M: Prediction, in Handbook of Juvenile Delinquency. Edited by Quay HC. New York, Wiley, 1987, pp 325–382

Lorion RP: The other side of the coin: the potential for negative consequences of preventive interventions, in Preventing Mental Disorders: A Research Perspective. Edited by Steinberg JA, Silverman MM. Rockville, MD: Alcohol, Drug Abuse, and Mental Health Administration, 1987, pp 243–250

McCord J: A thirty-year follow-up of treatment effects. Am Psychol 33:284–289, 1978

McCord J: Parental behavior in the cycle of aggression. Psychiatry 51:14–23, 1988

Miller GE, Prinz RJ: Enhancement of social learning family interventions for childhood conduct disorder. Psychol Bull 108:291–307, 1990

Moffitt TE: Juvenile delinquency and attention deficit disorder: boys' developmental trajectories from age 3 to age 15. Child Dev 61:893–910, 1990

Muehrer P, Koretz DS: Issues in preventive intervention research. Current Directions in Psychological Science 1:109–112, 1992

Offord DR: Family backgrounds of male and female delinquents, in Delinquency and the Criminal Justice System. Edited by Gunn J, Farrington DP. New York, Wiley, 1982, pp 203–220

Offord DR: Conduct disorder: risk factors and prevention, in Prevention of Mental Disorders, Alcohol and Other Drug Use in Children and Adolescents. Edited by Shaffer D, Philips I, Enzer NB. Rockville, MD, Office for Substance Abuse Prevention, 1989, pp 273–308

Offord DR, Boyle MH: Problems in setting up and executing large-scale psychiatric epidemiological studies. Psychiatr Dev 3:257–272, 1986

Offord DR, Waters BG: Socialization and its failure, in Developmental-Behavioral Pediatrics. Edited by Levine MD, Carey WB, Crocker AC, et al. Philadelphia, PA, WB Saunders, 1983, pp 229–257

Offord DR, Alder RJ, Boyle MH: Prevalence and sociodemographic correlates of conduct disorder. American Journal of Social Psychiatry 6:272–278, 1986

Olds DL: The prenatal/early infancy project, in Fourteen Ounces of Prevention: A Casebook for Practitioners. Edited by Price RH, Cowen EL, Lorion RP, et al. Washington, DC, American Psychological Association, 1988, pp 9–23

Parker JG, Asher SR: Peer relations and later personal adjustment: are low accepted children at risk? Psychol Bull 102:357–389, 1987

Patterson GR: Coercive Family Processes. Eugene, OR, Castalia, 1982

Patterson GR: The contribution of siblings to training for fighting: a microsocial analysis, in Development of Antisocial and Prosocial Behavior: Research, Theories and Issues. Edited by Olweus D, Block J, Radke-Yarrow M. New York, Academic Press, 1986, pp 90–112

Patterson GR, Bank CL: Some amplifying mechanisms for pathologic processes in families, in Systems and Development: Symposia on Child Psychology. Edited by Gunnar M, Thelen E. Hillsdale, NJ, Lawrence Erlbaum, 1989, pp 167–210

Patterson GR, DeBaryshe ED, Ramsey E: A developmental perspective on antisocial behavior. Am Psychol 44:329–335, 1989

Patterson GR, Reid JR, Dishion TJ: A Social Interactional Approach, Vol 4: Antisocial Boys. Eugene, OR, Castalia, 1992

Prothrow-Stith D: Violence Prevention Curriculum for Adolescents. Boston, MA, Education Development Center, 1987

Robins LN: Epidemiological approaches to natural history research: children's antisocial disorders. Journal of the American Academy of Child Psychiatry 20:566–580, 1981

Rutter M, Giller H: Juvenile Delinquency: Trends and Perspectives. New York, Penguin, 1983

Rutter M, Cox A, Tupling C, et al: Attainment and adjustment in two geographical areas, I: the prevalence of psychiatric disorder. Br J Psychiatry 126:493–509, 1975

Sampson RJ, Groves WB: Community structure and crime: testing social-disorganization theory. American Journal of Sociology 94:774–802, 1989

Seidman E: Toward a framework for primary prevention research, in Preventing Mental Disorders: A Research Perspective. Edited by Steinberg JA, Silverman MM. Rockville, MD, Alcohol, Drug Abuse, and Mental Health Administration, 1987, pp 2–19

Snyder J, Dishion TJ, Patterson GR: Determinants and consequences of associating with deviant peers. Journal of Early Adolescence 6:29–43, 1986

Wadsworth MEJ: Early life events and later behavioral outcomes in a British longitudinal study, in Human Functioning in Longitudinal Perspective. Edited by Sells SB, Crandell K, Roff M, et al. Baltimore, MD, Williams & Wilkins, 1980, pp 168–180

Wahler RG, Dumas JE: Stimulus class determinants of mother-child coercive interchanges in multidistressed families: assessment and intervention, in Prevention of Delinquent Behavior. Edited by Burchard JD, Burchard SN. Beverly Hills, CA, Sage, 1987, pp 190–219

West DJ, Farrington DP: The Delinquent Way of Life. London, Heinemann, 1977

West MO, Prinz RJ: Parental alcoholism and childhood psychopathology. Psychol Bull 102:204–218, 1987

Wolfgang ME, Figlio RM, Sellin T: Delinquency in a Birth Cohort. Chicago, IL, University of Chicago Press, 1972

Chapter 18

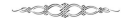

New Directions for Research

Steven I. Pfeiffer, Ph.D.

Conduct disorder (CD), one of the most common psychiatric disorders among children and adolescents, is distinguished by a persistent pattern of behavior in which the basic rights of others and societal norms are violated (DSM-IV [American Psychiatric Association 1994]). For a number of reasons, this disorder is a priority concern in the mental health field:

— Its high referral rate—between one-third and one-half of all child and adolescent clinic referrals involve aggressive, antisocial behavior and conduct problems (Kazdin 1987b)
— Its high prevalence—it accounts for 4%–10% of all child psychiatric disorders (Kazdin 1987a)
— Its stability and poor prognosis (Loeber 1982, 1991)
— The wide range of deficits associated with the disorder (Kazdin 1988)
— Evidence that antisocial behaviors are transmitted across generations, at tremendous ongoing cost to society

Along with these factors, which make CD one of the more difficult disorders to treat, many unanswered questions add to the need for continuing research on CD. For example, some argue that the central problem in CD is

The author wishes to express his appreciation to Rosalie Greim and Fran Mues for their assistance in preparing this chapter.

the child's alienation from conventional values (e.g., Jessor and Jessor 1984), whereas others suggest a number of possible biological, familial, and environmental reasons for the child's failure to learn, accept, or incorporate societal norms. In addition to uncertainty about the essence of the disorder, researchers still have not reached a consensus about how many distinct subtypes or dimensions constitute CD (Loeber and Lahey 1989; Martin and Hoffman 1990), the reasons for CD's substantial overlap with other psychiatric disorders (Lewis 1986; Lewis et al. 1984), or even whether CD actually meets the strict medical criteria for being considered a valid syndrome or disorder (Hinshaw 1987). The seriousness of the problem is further exacerbated by the absence of interventions that clearly demonstrate long-range efficacy.

Thus, it is painfully obvious that there is still much that we don't know about CD. Our circumscribed knowledge, however, offers challenging opportunities for researchers who seek to better understand CD's etiology, developmental course, and risk factors as well as the various pathways leading to antisocial behavior in order to design more effective interventions to prevent, treat, or decelerate the development of CD.

This chapter does not offer a comprehensive review of the extant research literature on CD—such a review would require a volume at least equal to the length of this entire book. Rather, in this chapter I focus on some recent promising research findings. The findings are grouped within three models of developmental psychopathology: *parent/family models, cognitive/information-processing models,* and *biological vulnerability models.* I then briefly review unanswered research questions about *risk factors, syndromal validity,* and *subtypes,* and conclude with suggestions on how best to design research studies on *treatment outcome.*

Parent/Family Models

Perhaps the largest number of research studies have explored the relationship between parental and family factors and the development of CD. The seminal work of Patterson (1980, 1982, 1986) has provided strong support for a relationship between CD and a pattern of dysfunctional parental disciplinary practices, such as hostility, permissiveness, lack of monitoring, and erratic limit setting. These poor parental disciplinary practices help to create a home environment in which a vicious cycle of hostile exchanges is reinforced, ultimately fueling the child's aggressive behavior.

Following Patterson's model, a number of investigators have explored the relationship of CD to parental psychopathology, marital discord, child-management techniques, and family child-rearing climate (e.g., Brody and Forehand 1986; Farrington et al. 1988; Hops et al. 1987; Jouriles et al. 1988; Panaccione and Wahler 1986). One possible causal pathway to CD that has recently received attention is the combined effect of maternal depression and marital discord. Researchers have found that depressed mothers are more critical, disapproving, and aversive in their interactions with other family members than nondepressed mothers (Dumas 1986; Hops et al. 1987; Webster-Stratton 1988). Marital discord has been found to adversely affect the parents' ability to provide a stable, secure, and supportive home environment (Barkley 1990; Bond and McMahon 1984; Christensen et al. 1983; Dodds et al. 1987; Emery 1982; Jouriles et al. 1987). The combination of maternal depression and marital discord contributes to higher rates of child deviance, parent-child conflict, and child aggressive behavior (McCord 1990).

A set of related studies has found, not surprisingly, that children of criminal and alcoholic parents are at greater risk for CD (Quinton et al. 1990; Robins 1991; Rutter 1985a). Furthermore, teenage motherhood—because of its common associations with lower socioeconomic status and parental antisocial personality—has been found to correlate with CD problems (Christ et al. 1990).

In a particularly well-designed study that evaluated the combined effects of parent management training and cognitive-behavioral problem-solving skills training, inpatient children 7–12 years of age showed significant improvement in antisocial behavior and overall adjustment compared with children randomly assigned to a contact-control experimental condition. Reduction in the children's aggressive symptoms at home and in school and enhanced prosocial behavior were evident both immediately after treatment and at a 1-year follow-up assessment (Kazdin et al. 1987). This study is noteworthy for a number of reasons: the investigators 1) adopted a rigorous research design, including random assignment of subjects; 2) relied on multiple sources of information and multiple methods of assessment; and 3) incorporated a follow-up assessment 1 year after treatment to permit testing of generalization and transfer of treatment gains to the child's home and school environments. Too few treatment outcome investigations adhere to carefully designed research protocols (Pfeiffer 1989), a point that will be discussed in greater detail later in this chapter.

Research has also documented that parent and family interventions based on social learning theory can be effective, particularly if the training programs are used with younger children from less-dysfunctional families (Kazdin 1985; Patterson 1986, 1992). However, a substantial number of families exhibit high levels of resistance, poor engagement, and inadequate maintenance of treatment gains with social learning family interventions (Miller and Prinz 1990). In addition, parents who are more dysfunctional predictably respond less favorably (Strain et al. 1981), because the social learning approach places several demands on the parents—most notably, in requiring their active participation and their learning of the educational materials.

Exploration of the role of parental and family influences has generated rich dividends. As the preceding examples suggest, a host of parental and marital factors, child management techniques, and family climate characteristics help explain the etiology, developmental course, and eventual outcome of CD in children and adolescents. However, fertile territory remains for future research on parent and/or family interventions. More investigations comparing parent management training with alternate treatments are needed. Researchers need to examine how to broaden the focus of parent training interventions to mitigate the negative impact of marital discord and parental psychopathology on treatment outcome. Future studies are needed on which innovative therapeutic procedures enhance the positive effects of parent training (Dodds et al. 1987; Robins 1991). Researchers may also want to classify dysfunctional families within some agreed-upon diagnostic system, detail the severity of youngsters' clinical dysfunction, and then correlate these data with amenability and response to the parent training intervention. This line of inquiry will provide a valuable opportunity to demonstrate which types of families and children are most likely to benefit from treatment that focuses on parent and/or family interactions.

Cognitive/Information-Processing Models

A second model of developmental psychopathology with significant heuristic value for furthering our understanding of CD is based on the theory that overly aggressive youngsters are prone to overperceive hostile intentions in others and, as a result of their defensive attitudes, elicit aggressive responses that serve to reinforce their biased perceptions. Such aggressive responses have been regarded as illustrative of insufficient cognitive activity (cognitive deficiencies) (Goldstein and Glick 1987), dysfunctional thinking processes (cognitive distortions) (Dodge and Newman 1981), and the defense mechanisms of projection and denial (Burlingame 1973). A number of investigators have explored the relationship of cognitive and perceptual processes and aggression (e.g., Dodge and Frame 1982). A particularly productive and exciting line of research is based on Dodge's (1986, 1993) social information-processing model. Dodge proposes that a tendency to make hostile attributions about others' behavior becomes a self-fulfilling prophecy—that is, biased attributions elicit aggressive responses, which then contribute to peer rejection and adult condemnation. Such reactions, in turn, leave the child affectively primed to respond with further retaliatory behaviors and attuned to process social information in ways that insulate the child from any threat to his or her biased view of the world as a hostile environment (Dodge 1985).

Most recently, Dodge (1986) has expanded his model and delineated five sequential cognitive steps (encoding, interpretation, response search, response decision, and enactment) necessary for an individual to respond appropriately to social situations. The implication for the CD youngster is that such a child may evidence a deficiency in one or more of these steps:

1. **Encoding deficits**: The child conducts an incomplete search of social cues before evaluating another person's intentions.
2. **Interpretation deficits**: Presumably based on a history of actual victimization, parental psychopathology (e.g., Webster-Stratton 1988), or neuropsychiatric vulnerabilities (Lewis et al. 1989), the youngster is biased toward perceiving hostile intent in others.
3. **Response search deficits**: The child generates too few—and often less-appropriate—alternative solutions.
4. **Response decision deficits**: The child awards more value to aggressive responses and evaluates them more favorably.
5. **Enactment deficits**: The child lacks prosocial negotiation skills.

To date, too few clinical research studies have directly investigated these five cognitive steps, particularly as antecedents of aggression in CD. Dodge and Frame (1982) provided evidence for a tendency by aggressive boys to over-attribute hostile intentions to peers, and Dodge and Newman (1981) offered the provocative finding that attentional deficits may play a role in the over-attribution of hostile intent. Finally, Richard and Dodge (1982) reported that aggressive boys verbalize fewer potential solutions to interpersonal situations. These three research studies only begin to provide empirical validation for Dodge's theoretical model of CD.

Future researchers may want to investigate more carefully each of the five cognitive steps in the social information-processing model and also to examine how these biased attributions first develop. Other unanswered questions include whether the substantial overlap between CD and attentional deficits (Hinshaw 1987; Hinshaw et al. 1993; Kazdin 1985; Naglieri et al. 1994) explains, in part, why aggressive youngsters pay less attention to available social cues and respond more impulsively in selecting less-appropriate solutions in social situations. We may also want to explore the extent to which neuropsychiatric (Lewis et al. 1989) and neuropsychological factors (Tramontana and Hooper 1987, 1989) influence the alleged dysfunctional information processing of the CD youngster. As recommended earlier, research will further our understanding of CD only when dysfunctional clinical populations are included as subjects. Presently, much of the research investigating the efficacy of problem-solving skills training and related cognitive/information-processing interventions has relied on nonclinical students rated as "overly aggressive."

Biological Vulnerability Models

A small but persuasive body of literature implicates hormonal, physiological, and biochemical factors in CD. Hare (1978) found that psychophysiological abnormalities underlie impulsivity and the failure to inhibit aggressive behavior, and Lewis (1986) demonstrated an association between minor neurological anomalies and aggressive behaviors. Mednick and Gabrielli (1983) provided evidence to support the hypothesis that antisocial youngsters have an autonomic system inherently hyporesponsive to intense and punishing stimuli, and Alpert et al. (1981) identified a relationship between levels of certain neurotransmitters—such as serotonin and norepinephrine and their metabolites—and aggression. However, although these findings supporting a biological predisposition to the disorder are highly promising, there still is too little unequivocal empirical support. For example, only one genetic study exists that specifically addressed CD (Jary and Stewart 1985), no investigation has found a significant relationship between adolescent testosterone levels and aggression, and no chromosomal abnormalities have been documented in antisocial persons.

Early research investigating the neurological basis for many violent and aggressive behaviors did not receive widespread or general acceptance. "Episodic dyscontrol" was viewed as the result of drives overwhelming compromised control mechanisms, presumed to be deficient because of subcortical dysfunction, most likely within the limbic system (Balis and McDonald 1978). A small number of studies have implicated abnormal electrophysiological, neurological, and neuropsychological findings in the aggressive behavior of CD youngsters (Coble et al. 1984; Elliott 1982; Korhonen and Sillanpaa 1976; Krynicki 1978; Luchins 1983; Tramontana and Hooper 1987; Woods and Eby 1982).

One particularly promising biological theory that has gained recent attention proposes that CD is the result of both excessive activity in an energizing behavioral activation system (BAS) and deficits in a complementary behavioral inhibition system (BIS) (Gray 1987). This two-factor biobehavioral theory recently received support in a carefully designed clinical investigation (Walker et al. 1991), and in the near future we can expect considerable research activity testing the hypothesis of an underactive BIS (lower adrenaline and serotonin) and concomitantly overactive BAS. The neural systems hypothesized to govern both the BIS and the BAS are interconnected with the hypothalamic-pituitary-adrenal (HPA) axis (Gray 1982), and advances in neurodiagnostic technology may permit more direct testing of Gray's theory.

Although Gray's biobehavioral theory implicates a specific area of the brain in CD, at present there is little evidence of specificity in type or pattern of brain dysfunction (Boll and Barth 1981; Tramontana and Hooper 1989). More carefully designed research using sophisticated diagnostic procedures will be needed to test localization hypotheses and to examine the various pathways in which brain dysfunction contributes to increasing the risk of CD. Very likely a number of possible combinations of largely nonspecific and indirect biological vulnerabilities lower the youngster's adaptive capacity, increase his or her exposure to deleterious environmental circumstances, and contribute to his or her alienation from and rejection by the nondisturbed peer group. (See Lytton 1990 for a discussion of the relative strength of child effects versus environmental effects.)

Risk Factors

Risk factors increase the likelihood of a child's developing a psychiatric disorder (Garmezy 1983). In a series of epidemiological studies, Offord and his associates (Offord 1989; Offord et al. 1979; Rae-Grant et al. 1989) identified a number of factors that increase the probability of a child's developing CD:

— Paternal criminality and maternal psychiatric history
— Belonging to a dysfunctional family
— Large sibship (4 or more siblings)
— Being male and the eldest child
— Early-onset CD associated with lower socioeconomic status
— Severe perinatal complications
— Developmental delays

Future research will want to analyze the relative contributions of the various risk factors and their interrelationships and to investigate whether they serve as causal or moderating variables. Prospective longitudinal studies of the early developmental predictors of CD are scarce (Robins 1991), and investigators need to explore a wider range of risk factors. Potentially relevant and yet infrequently investigated factors include the child's difficult temperament, the father's presence and involvement within the family, the child's academic status and psychoeducational learning profile, and the impact of single-parent and two-parent working families.

In addition to focusing on risk factors that increase a child's vulnerability to developing CD, investigators may also want to examine those prophylactic factors that serve to reduce the risk of the child's acquiring CD (Rutter 1985b). Offord (1989) identified six risk-compensatory factors that offer opportunities for designing and testing more effective interventions to prevent and treat CD:

1. Voluntary change to a less-deviant peer group
2. Employment
3. Improved social circumstances
4. Positive, warm, close relationship with a parent or other adult
5. Compensatory positive experiences
6. Effective coping mechanisms

A comprehensive exploration of biopsychosocial factors (Pfeiffer 1985; Whittaker and Pfeiffer, in press) that incorporates examination of the continual interplay between the inner life of the child and his or her family and environment will help to identify ameliorative, protective, neutral, and malignant factors. (See Sameroff and Chandler 1975 for a discussion on the transactional view of causality.)

Syndromal Validity

CD represents heterogeneous clinical phenomena with a number of different etiologies, several known developmental markers, more than one single pathway, and a multiplicity of signs and symptoms shared with other psychiatric disorders (Lewis et al 1984; Loeber 1991; Quay 1986). Based on strict medical criteria, CD does not yet constitute a valid syndrome—studies have not documented a specific pattern of biological/etiological precursors or evidence of a specific response to known interventions (Hinshaw 1987).

In an article entitled "Conduct Disorder: Diagnosis of Dubious Validity and Usefulness" (1984), Lewis and her colleagues reported that CD overlaps with many other diagnoses. They maintained that CD is often an interim diagnosis that lacks clear exclusionary criteria and that obfuscates other potentially treatable neuropsychiatric disorders (Lewis et al. 1984). Similarly, Kazdin (1985) emphasized that antisocial behaviors emerge from a variety of clinical syndromes.

CD's co-occurrence with other psychiatric syndromes or disorders' is substantial, although researchers have identified important distinctions between CD and attention-deficit disorder (Hinshaw 1987; Kazdin 1985; Offord et al. 1979), academic underachievement (Frick et al. 1991), depression (Puig-Antich 1982), oppositional disorder (Loeber and Schmaling 1985; Robins 1991), and learning disability (Cannon and Compton 1980; Funk and Ruppert 1984; Lahey et al. 1978; Robbins et al. 1983; Wardell and Yeudall 1980; Zinkus and Gottlieb 1978). Multivariate statistical analyses have not consistently confirmed independent factors that reflect the defining characteristics of the disorder, and this circumstance has led some to suggest that a dimensional rather than a categorical conception of CD might be more useful (Martin and Hoffman 1990).

Although we know that CD is often accompanied by other psychiatric disorders, we know very little about why, or about how the co-occurrence with other disorders—such as anxiety, depression, attention deficits, and learning disability—alters the expression and chronicity of CD. Prospective longitudinal work will help identify which markers differentiate those youngsters whose CD is likely to desist from those whose CD is likely to persist; which child and family causal factors affect stability; and the orderly developmental sequences in the unfolding of the disorder over time (Loeber 1991). Future research will benefit from employing multiple informants and multiple sources of information; greater specification of the various sources of clinical information; and agreed-upon, reliable diagnostic criteria (Kazdin 1985; Naglieri et al. 1994; Pfeiffer 1989; Routh 1990).

Subtypes

A number of factor analytic studies have provided evidence for at least two distinct factors or dimensions of CD (Martin and Hoffman 1990; Quay 1986). Researchers are optimistic that more carefully designed investigations will eventually distinguish several subtypes (Kazdin 1987a; Loeber and Lahey 1989).

Quay (1986) reviewed 61 studies published in the last 40 years and concluded that an *undersocialized aggressive subtype* of CD (*solitary aggressive type* in DSM-III-R [American Psychiatric Association 1987]) appears in almost all of the studies. Quay's review also indicated strong support for a *socialized aggressive subtype* of CD that was restricted primarily to the adolescent age group. However, a number of the youngsters in the studies evidenced characteristics of both dimensions.

Loeber and Schmaling (1985) conducted a meta-analysis of 28 studies of various child behavior rating scales. They concluded, using multidimensional scaling, that CD falls along a single bipolar dimension with confrontative/overt behaviors at one extreme and clandestine/covert behaviors at the other. They also identified a third group of CD children—labeled "versatiles"— who present with both types of symptoms.

Rey et al. (1988) compared youngsters diagnosed with CD and oppositional defiant disorder (ODD) and found that the two groups differed only in magnitude of social impairment and severity of antisocial behavior. This finding raised a provocative issue that future research will need to resolve regarding whether CD and ODD are separate disorders or simply two points along a single continuum or different phases of one chronic psychiatric disorder.

Three research studies independently found that the combination of aggression and shyness was most predictive of later drug abuse or criminality (Kellam et al. 1983; McCord 1987; Moskowitz and Schwartzman 1989). The presence of shyness with aggression challenges the putative two dimensions of "externalizing" and "internalizing," since shyness is not a symptom of any of the three subclasses of disruptive behavior disorders (i.e., attention-deficit hyperactivity disorder [ADHD], CD, and ODD) (Robins 1991).

Time of onset has also been suggested as a dimension that may distinguish two subtypes of CD. Early onset of symptoms suggests a less benign course, at least based on the delinquency literature (Loeber 1982; Robins 1991).

As the preceding discussion suggests, much work remains to be done to increase our understanding of the distinct subtypes of CD and of their implications for etiology, pathogenesis, and prognosis. Investigators will need to reach a consensus on objective classificatory criteria and measurement strategies to help us answer the following questions:

— Will epidemiological studies help validate different subtypes?
— Are CD and ODD distinct syndromes?
— Do different statistical procedures (e.g., factor analysis versus cluster analysis) identify the same dimensions?
— Do particular subtypes respond differently to specific treatment regimens?

Treatment Outcome Studies

Although CD is one of the more difficult psychiatric disorders to treat, no large-scale efforts have been undertaken to systematically study its treatment or prevention (Robins 1991). Controlled studies of treatment outcome are rare, and few studies have investigated the impact of treatment with clinically identified populations; in addition, studies typically fail to measure or report the severity of the subjects' dysfunction (Kazdin 1985; Pfeiffer and Strzelecki 1990).

Recent reviews of treatment research highlight the need for more carefully designed and rigorously implemented studies of outcome (e.g., Kazdin et al. 1990; Pfeiffer 1989). Treatment outcome studies frequently evidence the following methodological problems:

— Failure to carefully describe the characteristics of the sample group and its degree of clinical dysfunction
— Absence of suitable comparison groups
— Lack of comprehensive assessment of multiple areas of functioning
— Failure to delineate the critical aspects of the treatment regimen, and no assurance of treatment integrity
— Small sample sizes
— Little follow-up data on the long-term effects of treatment
— Use of global outcome measures to the exclusion of more specific criteria

As mentioned in an earlier section, parent management training (Patterson 1986) and cognitive problem-solving skills training (Glick and Goldstein 1987) are particularly promising approaches that warrant more investigation.

Behavior therapy is a third promising therapeutic strategy. Future treatment outcome research will need to demonstrate that change in highly specific social behaviors is associated with decreases in concurrent and future antisocial behaviors, and that improvements in clinically relevant areas are maintained after treatment is terminated (Kazdin 1985; Kazdin et al. 1990). Too often, outcome studies fail to demonstrate *generalization, maintenance,* and *durability* of gains.

Very few outcome studies have documented the efficacy of individual, group, or family therapy with youngsters who have CD (Kazdin 1985). It is reasonable to hypothesize that children with CD are not amenable to talking therapies because their distrust, defensiveness, narcissism, and lack of insight impede their developing a trusting relationship and working alliance with a therapist. We know that young people with CD are hedonistic and risk takers. Nonstandard therapeutic interventions like Outward Bound might provide legitimate expressions for these risk-taking tendencies by easing boredom and teaching prosocial skills that require physical daring (Robins and Earls 1986).

The following suggestions are offered to guide future studies on treatment outcome. They are not necessarily specific to CD, but can be applied to all outcome research investigations.

Ensure treatment integrity. Monitoring quality assurance throughout the study will ensure that the treatment is consistently carried out as intended and is satisfactorily received by the patient. Developing treatment manuals and reliability checks on adherence to specific therapeutic regimens are but two of many ways to reduce threats to the internal validity of the outcome project (Elkin et al. 1988; Kazdin 1985; Yeaton and Sechrest 1981).

Collect unquestionably successful treatment cases. One useful outcome research strategy is to collect a bank of unquestionably successful cases. This approach can guide future intervention research by generating clusters of correlated risk-compensatory factors. Researchers can also compare the clearly successful cases with the treatment-resistant and poor-response cases (Gendlin 1986).

Obtain consensus on defining success or improvement. A review of the extant treatment outcome literature clearly indicates an absence of consensus in how investigators define improvement. Treatment outcome should be viewed and measured as multidimensional and multidirectional, allowing for both positive and negative effects across a variety of dimensions. "Symptoms among children and adolescents often wax and wane, suggesting that simply looking at the diminution in symptoms may be too narrow a perspective. Enhanced coping capacity and adjustment in the community seem like two of many possible ways for researchers to define success" (Pfeiffer and Strzelecki 1990, p. 852). Additional outcomes might include long-term impact, consumer satisfaction, potential side effects in nontargeted areas, drug and alcohol use, educational attainment, and social competence (Miller and Prinz 1990; Mirin and Namerow 1991; Pfeiffer and Strzelecki 1990).

Use multiple outcome perspectives.   Strupp and Hadley (1977) have eloquently described the use of multiple perspectives as a means of obtaining a comprehensive measure of outcome. Their tripartite model views outcome from three vantage points: the child, the child's significant others (e.g., parents and teachers), and the clinician. Self-reports and peer ratings (Robins 1991), as well as greater specification of the various sources of information (Routh 1990), enhance the validity of this measurement strategy.

Examine amenability to treatment.   It is likely that children with CD who vary in their responsiveness to therapeutic intervention can be identified. Clinical trials can test which subtypes are most responsive to which specific treatment (Kazdin 1987b). Likely candidates to help define amenability are severity, frequency, and diversity of the antisocial behavior; number of family risk factors; academic functioning; presence of attention-deficit hyperactivity; intelligence; motivation to change; level of insight; social circumstances; and availability of a close relationship with a parent or other adult.

Increase the strength of treatment.   Our inability to demonstrate treatment efficacy may reflect, in part, the fact that we have not yet attacked CD with sufficiently potent treatment dosages. Kazdin (1985) persuasively states that "current clinical trials have not shown that CD can be ameliorated and that the poor prognosis can be controverted" (p. 280). Increasing the comprehensiveness of treatment and intensifying the treatment are two exciting new directions for outcome research. In designing clinical trials, we may need to provide treatment with the strongest possible dosage to see if we can create an intervention package that truly interrupts the deleterious processes (Coleman et al. 1992; Kazdin 1987a; Loeber 1991). Asked in another way, is CD a chronic, intractable disorder, or have we not yet devised sufficiently powerful interventions?

Conclusion

CD is one of the more difficult psychiatric disorders to treat—based, in part, on a number of unanswered questions that provide the impetus for continued research on this disorder. Future research will most quickly advance our understanding of CD by incorporating what we already know about biological vulnerabilities, attributional bias, and familial and environmental risk factors.

Innovative treatments will require carefully designed outcome studies. Our clinical efforts will be most productive when we can demonstrate generalization, maintenance, and durability of treatment gains. We face exciting opportunities to better understand CD and to design more effective interventions to prevent and treat CD.

References

Alpert JE, Cohen DJ, Shaywitz BA, et al: Neurochemical and behavioral organization: disorders of attention, activity, and aggression, in Vulnerabilities to Delinquency. Edited by Lewis DO. New York, Spectrum, 1981, pp 109–171

American Psychiatric Association: Diagnostic and Statistical Manual of Mental Disorders, 3rd Edition, Revised. Washington, DC, American Psychiatric Association, 1987

American Psychiatric Association: Diagnostic and Statistical Manual of Mental Disorders, 4th Edition. Washington, DC, American Psychiatric Association, 1994

Balis GU, McDonald M: Episodic dyscontrol: definitions, descriptions, and measurement, in Brain Dysfunction in Aggressive Criminals. Edited by Monroe R. Lexington, MA, DC Heath, 1978, pp 1–14

Barkley RA: Attention Deficit Hyperactivity Disorder: A Handbook for Diagnosis and Treatment. New York, Guilford, 1990

Boll T, Barth J: Neuropsychology of brain damage in children, in Handbook of Clinical Neuropsychology. Edited by Filskov SB, Boll TJ. New York, Wiley, 1981, pp 418–452

Bond CR, McMahon RJ: Relationships between maternal distress and child behavior problems, maternal personal adjustment, maternal personality, and maternal parenting behavior. J Abnorm Psychol 93:348–351, 1984

Brody GH, Forehand R: Maternal perceptions of child maladjustment as a function of the combined influence of child behavior and maternal depression. J Consult Clin Psychol 54:237–240, 1986

Burlingame WV: Jerry—a case of behavior disorder, in Disturbed and Troubled Children. Edited by Freehill MF. New York, Spectrum, 1973, pp 177–199

Cannon I, Compton C: School dysfunction in the adolescent. Pediatr Clin North Am 27:79–96, 1980

Christ MAG, Lahey BB, Frick PJ, et al: Serious conduct problems in the children of adolescent mothers: disentangling confounded correlations. J Consult Clin Psychol 58:840–844, 1990

Christensen A, Phillips S, Glasgow RE, et al: Parental characteristics and interactional dysfunction in families with child behavior problems: a preliminary investigation. J Abnorm Child Psychol 11:153–166, 1983

Coble P, Taska L, Kupfer D, et al: EEG sleep "abnormalities" in preadolescent boys with a diagnosis of conduct disorder. Journal of the American Academy of Child Psychiatry 23:438–447, 1984

Coleman M, Pfeiffer SI, Oakland T: Aggression replacement training with behavior disordered adolescents. Behavioral Disorders 18:54–66, 1992

Dodds MR, Schwartz S, Sanders MR: Marital discord and treatment outcome in behavioral treatment of child conduct disorders. J Consult Clin Psychol 55:396–403, 1987

Dodge KA: The future of research on the treatment of conduct disorder. Development and Psychopathology 5:311–319, 1993

Dodge KA: Attributional bias in aggressive children, in Advances in Cognitive-Behavioral Research and Therapy, Vol 4. Edited by Kendall PC. New York, Academic Press, 1985, pp 73–110

Dodge KA: A social information processing model of social competence in children, in Minnesota Symposium on Child Psychology, Vol 18. Edited by Perlmutter M. Hillsdale, NJ, Lawrence Erlbaum, 1986, pp 77–125

Dodge KA, Frame CL: Social cognitive biases and deficits in aggressive boys. Child Dev 53:620–635, 1982

Dodge KA, Newman JP: Biased decision-making processes in aggressive boys. J Abnorm Psychol 90:375–450, 1981

Dumas JE: Indirect influence of maternal social contacts on mother-child interactions: a setting event analysis. J Abnorm Child Psychol 14:203–216, 1986

Elkin I, Pilkonis PA, Docherty JP, et al: Conceptual and methodological issues in comparative studies of psychotherapy and pharmacotherapy, I: active ingredients and mechanisms of change. Am J Psychiatry 145:909–917, 1988

Elliot FA: Neurological findings in adult minimal brain dysfunction and the dyscontrol syndrome. J Nerv Ment Dis 170:680–687, 1982

Emery RE: Interparental conflict and the children of discord and divorce. Psychol Bull 92:310–330, 1982

Farrington DP, Gallegher B, Morley L, et al: Are there any successful men from criminogenic backgrounds? Psychiatry 50:116–130, 1988

Frick PJ, Kamphaus RW, Lahey BB, et al: Academic underachievement and the disruptive behavior disorders. J Consult Clin Psychol 59:289–294, 1991

Funk JB, Ruppert E: Language disorders and behavioral problems in preschool children. J Dev Behav Pediatr 5:357–360, 1984

Garmezy N: Stressors of childhood, in Stress, Coping and Development in Children. Edited by Garmezy N, Rutter MP. New York, McGraw-Hill, 1983, pp 43–84

Gendlin ET: What comes after traditional psychotherapy research? Am Psychol 41:131–136, 1986

Glick B, Goldstein AP: Aggression replacement training, special issue: counseling and violence. Journal of Counseling and Development 65:356–362, 1987

Goldstein AP, Glick B: Aggression Replacement Training: A Comprehensive Intervention for Aggressive Youth. Champaign, IL, Research Press, 1987

Gray JA: The Neuropsychology of Anxiety: An Enquiry Into the Functions of the Septo-Hippocampal System. Oxford, UK, Oxford University Press, 1982

Gray JA: The Psychology of Fear and Stress, 2nd Edition. Cambridge, UK, Cambridge University Press, 1987

Hare RD: Electrodermal and cardiovascular correlates of psychopathy, in Psychopathic Behaviour: Approaches to Research. Edited by Hare RD, Schalling D. Chichester, UK, Wiley, 1978

Hinshaw SP: On the distinction between attentional deficits/hyperactivity and conduct problems/aggression in child psychopathology. Psychol Bull 101:443–463, 1987

Hinshaw SP, Lahey BB, Hart EL: Issues of taxonomy and comorbidity in the development of conduct disorder. Development and Psychopathology 5:31–49, 1993

Hops H, Biglan A, Sherman L, et al: Home observations of family interactions of depressed women. J Consult Clin Psychol 55:341–346, 1987

Jary ML, Stewart MA: Psychiatric disorder in the parents of adopted children with aggressive conduct disorder. Neuropsychobiology 13:7–11, 1985

Jessor R, Jessor SL: Adolescence to young adulthood: a twelve-year prospective study of problem behavior and psychosocial development, in Handbook of Longitudinal Research, Vol 2. Edited by Mednick SA, Harway M, Finello KM. New York, Praeger, 1984

Jouriles EN, Barling J, O'Leary KD: Predicting child behavior problem in maritally violent families. J Abnorm Child Psychol 15:165–173, 1987

Jouriles EN, Pfiffner LJ, O'Leary SG: Marital conflict, parenting, and toddler conduct problems. J Abnorm Child Psychol 16:197–206, 1988

Kazdin AE: Treatment of Antisocial Behavior in Children and Adolescents. Homewood, IL, Dorsey Press, 1985

Kazdin AE: Conduct Disorders in Childhood and Adolescence. Newbury Park, CA, Sage, 1987a

Kazdin AE: Treatment of antisocial behavior in children: current status and future directions. Psychol Bull 102:187–203, 1987b

Kazdin AE: Social learning family therapy with aggressive children: a commentary. Journal of Family Psychology 1:286–291, 1988

Kazdin AE, Esveldt-Dawson K, French NH, et al: Effects of parent management training and problem-solving skills training combined in the treatment of antisocial child behavior. J Am Acad Child Adolesc Psychiatry 26:416–424, 1987

Kazdin AE, Bass D, Ayers WA, et al: Empirical and clinical focus of child and adolescent psychotherapy research. J Consult Clin Psychol 58:729–740, 1990

Kellam SG, Simon MB, Ensminger ME: Antecedents in first grade of teenage substance use and psychological well-being: a ten-year community-wide prospective study, in Origins of Psychopathology. Edited by Ricks DF, Dohrenwend BS. Cambridge, UK, Cambridge University Press, 1983, pp 17–42

Korhonen T, Sillanpaa M: MBD-like behavior and neuropsychological performances. Acta Paedopsychiatrica 42:75–87, 1976

Krynicki VE: Cerebral dysfunction in repetitively assaultive adolescents. J Nerv Ment Dis 166:59–67, 1978

Lahey BB, Stempniak M, Robinson EJ, et al: Hyperactivity and learning disabilities as independent dimensions of child behavior problems. J Abnorm Psychol 87:333–340, 1978

Lewis DO: Conduct disorder, in Psychiatry. Edited by Michels R, Cavenar JO Jr, Brodie HKH. Philadelphia, PA, JB Lippincott, 1986, pp 275–284

Lewis DO, Lewis M, Unger L, et al: Conduct disorder and its synonyms: diagnoses of dubious validity and usefulness. Am J Psychiatry 141:514–519, 1984

Lewis DO, Lovely R, Yeager C, et al: Toward a theory of the genesis of violence: a follow-up study of delinquents. J Am Acad Child Adolesc Psychiatry 28:431–436, 1989

Loeber R: The stability of antisocial and delinquent child behavior: a review. Child Dev 53:1431–1446, 1982

Loeber R: Antisocial behavior: more enduring than changeable? J Am Acad Child Adolesc Psychiatry 30:393–397, 1991

Loeber R, Lahey BB: Recommendations for research on disruptive behavior disorders of childhood and adolescence, in Advances in Clinical Child Psychology, Vol 12. Edited by Lahey BB, Kazdin AE. New York, Plenum, 1989, pp 221–245

Loeber R, Schmaling KB: Empirical evidence for overt and covert patterns of antisocial conduct problems: a meta-analysis. J Abnorm Child Psychol 13:337–352, 1985

Luchins D: Carbamazepine for the violent psychiatric patient. Lancet 1:766, 1983

Lytton H: Child and parent effects in boys' conduct disorder: a reinterpretation. Dev Psychol 26:683–697, 1990

Martin B, Hoffman JA: Conduct disorders, in Developmental Psychopathology. Edited by Lewis M, Miller SM. New York, Plenum, 1990, pp 109–118

McCord J: Another perspective on aggression and shyness as predictors of problems. Paper presented at the biannual meeting of the Society for Research and Child Development, Baltimore, MD, April 23–26, 1987

McCord J: Long-term perspectives on parental absence, in Straight and Devious Pathways from Childhood to Adulthood. Edited by Robins LN, Rutter MP. Cambridge, UK, Cambridge University Press, 1990

Mednick SA, Gabrielli WF: Biological, psychological, and sociofamilial factors in crime (part II), in Longitudinal Study of Social and Biological Factors in Crime. Edited by Mednick B, Mednick SA, Baker R, et al. Washington, DC, Department of Justice, 1983

Miller GE, Prinz RJ: Enhancement of social learning family interventions for childhood conduct disorder. Psychol Bull 108:291–307, 1990

Mirin SM, Namerow MJ: Why study treatment outcome, in Psychiatric Treatment: Advances in Outcome Research. Edited by Mirin SM, Gossett JT, Grob MC. Washington, DC, American Psychiatric Press, 1991, pp 1–14

Moskowitz DS, Schwartzman AE: Painting group portraits: studying life outcomes for aggressive and withdrawn children. J Pers 57:723–746, 1989

Naglieri JA, LeBuffe PA, Pfeiffer SI: The Devereaux Scales of Mental Disorders Manual. San Antonio, TX, Psychological Corporation, 1994

Offord DR: Conduct disorder: risk factors and prevention, in Prevention of Mental Disorders, Alcohol and Other Drug Use in Children and Adolescents. Edited by Shaffer D, Philips I, Enzer NB. Rockville, MD, U.S. Department of Health and Human Services, 1989, pp 273–307

Offord DR, Sullivan K, Allen N, et al: Delinquency and hyperactivity. J Nerv Ment Dis 167:734–741, 1979

Panaccione VF, Wahler RG: Child behavior, maternal depression, and social coercion as factors in the quality of child care. J Abnorm Child Psychol 14:263–278, 1986

Patterson GR: Mothers: the unacknowledged victims. Monogr Soc Res Child Dev 45:1–64, 1980

Patterson GR: Coercive Family Processes. Eugene, OR, Castalia, 1982

Patterson GR: Performance models for antisocial boys. Am Psychol 41:432–444, 1986

Patterson GR: Age effects in parent training outcome. Behavior Therapy 23:719–729, 1992

Pfeiffer SI: Clinical Child Psychology: An Introduction to Theory, Research and Practice. Orlando, FL, Grune & Stratton, 1985

Pfeiffer SI: Follow-up of children and adolescents treated in psychiatric facilities: a methodology review. The Psychiatric Hospital 20:15–20, 1989

Pfeiffer SI, Strzelecki S: Inpatient psychiatric treatment of children and adolescents: a review of outcome studies. J Am Acad Child Adolesc Psychiatry 29:847–853, 1990

Puig-Antich J: Major depression and conduct disorder in prepuberty. Journal of the American Academy of Child Psychiatry 21:118–128, 1982

Quay HC: Conduct disorders, in Psychopathological Disorders of Childhood, 3rd Edition. Edited by Quay HC, Werry JS. New York, Wiley, 1986, pp 35–72

Quinton D, Rutter MP, Gulliver L: Continuities in psychiatric disorders from childhood to adulthood in the children of psychiatric patients, in Straight and Devious Pathways From Childhood to Adulthood. Edited by Robins LN, Rutter MP. Cambridge, UK, Cambridge University Press, 1990

Rae-Grant N, Thomas BH, Offord DR, et al: Risk, protective factors, and the prevalence of behavioral and emotional disorders in children and adolescents. J Am Acad Child Adolesc Psychol 28:262–268, 1989

Rey JM, Bashir MR, Schwartz M, et al: Oppositional disorder: fact or fiction? J Am Acad Child Adolesc Psychiatry 27:157–162, 1988

Richard BA, Dodge KA: Social maladjustment and problem solving in school-aged children. J Consult Clin Psychol 50:226–223, 1982

Robbins DM, Beck JC, Pries R, et al: Learning disability and neuropsychological impairment in adjudicated, unincarcerated male delinquents. Journal of the American Academy of Child Psychiatry 22:40–46, 1983

Robins LN: Conduct disorder. J Child Psychol Psychiatry 32:193–212, 1991

Robins LN, Earls F: A program for preventing antisocial behavior for high-risk infants and preschoolers: a research prospectus, in Psychiatric Epidemiology and Prevention: The Possibilities: Papers Resulting From a Research Planning Workshop Held Through The Neuropsychiatric Institute, The University of Carolina, February 14–16, 1982. Edited by Hough R, Brown VP, Goldston S. Los Angeles, CA, Neuropsychiatric Institute, University of California at Los Angeles, 1986, pp 73–83

Routh DK: Taxonomy in developmental psychopathology, in Handbook of Developmental Psychopathology. Edited by Lewis M, Miller S. New York, Plenum, 1990, pp 53–62

Rutter MP: Family and school influence on behavioral development. J Child Psychol Psychiatry 26:349–368, 1985a

Rutter MP: Resilience in the face of adversity: protective factors and resistance in psychiatric disorder. Br J Psychiatry 147:598–611, 1985b

Sameroff A, Chandler M: Reproductive risk and the continuum of caretaking causality, in Review of Child Development Research, Vol 1. Edited by Horowitz F. Chicago, IL, University of Chicago Press, 1975, pp 197–244

Strain PS, Young CC, Horowitz J: Generalized behavior change during oppositional child training: an examination of child and family demographic variables. Behav Modif 5:15–26, 1981

Strupp HH, Hadley SW: A tripartite model of mental health and therapeutic outcomes. Am Psychol 32:187–196, 1977

Tramontana MG, Hooper SR: Discriminating the presence and pattern of neuropsychological impairment in child psychiatric disorders. International Journal of Clinical Neuropsychology 9:111–119, 1987

Tramontana MG, Hooper SR: Neuropsychology of child psychopathology, in Handbook of Child Neuropsychology. Edited by Reynolds C, Fletcher-Janden E. New York, Plenum, 1989

Walker JL, Lahey BB, Russo MF, et al: Anxiety, inhibition, and conduct disorder in children, I: relations to social impairment. J Am Acad Child Adolesc Psychiatry 30:187–191, 1991

Wardell D, Yeudall L: A multidimensional approach to criminal disorders: the assessment of impulsive and its relation to crime. Advances in Behavioral Research and Therapy 2:159–177, 1980

Webster-Stratton C: Mothers' and fathers' perceptions of child deviance: roles of parent and child behaviors and parent adjustment. J Consult Clin Psychol 56:909–915, 1988

Whittaker J, Pfeiffer SI: Research priorities for residential group child care. Child Welfare 73 (in press)

Woods BT, Eby MD: Excessive mirror movements and aggression. Biol Psychiatry 17:23–32, 1982

Yeaton WH, Sechrest L: Critical dimensions in the choice and maintenance of successful treatments: strength, integrity, and effectiveness. J Consult Clin Psychol 49:156–167, 1981

Zinkus PW, Gottlieb MI: Learning disabilities and juvenile delinquency. Clin Pediatr 17:775–780, 1978

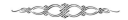

Afterword

Conduct disorders, as a group of pervasive, chronic, and disabling emotional disorders, are the most common reason for a child's referral to mental health services. A much larger number of adolescents and children frequently engage in antisocial behavior; however, because their actions are not detected or reported, they often evade psychiatric evaluation and treatment. The etiology of conduct disorder is complex and poorly understood. Parental psychopathology and skill deficits, children's narcissistic vulnerabilities and developmental lags in socialization, and high-risk environmental and school conditions are common contributors to the genesis and maintenance of the disorder. Disturbances in psychobiological functioning—particularly in the reward-inhibition system—are suspected to play a role in some types of conduct disorder. A child's temperament may also play a significant role in the development of conduct disorder, although this role is poorly defined.

Conduct disorders as a group have proven quite resistant to various treatment modalities. Parent management training, which focuses on enhancing parental skills, may be one of the more promising interventions in comparison with individual, family based, or residential treatment and medication. A comprehensive approach combining many of these intervention techniques may be necessary, particularly with the most treatment-resistant groups.

Considering the large number of children at risk for or suffering from conduct disorder, early prevention programs may ultimately prove to be the most realistic approach to early intervention. However, the development of highly effective intervention programs will require a fuller understanding of the role of biological, developmental, psychological, familial, and sociological factors in the genesis of conduct disorder.

G. Pirooz Sholevar, M.D.

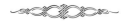

Index

*Page numbers printed in **boldface** type refer to tables or figures.*